NORTH
STAR
WAY

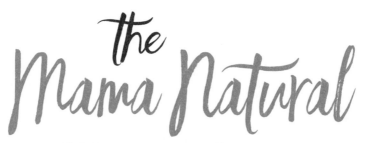

the Mama Natural

WEEK-BY-WEEK GUIDE TO

PREGNANCY & CHILDBIRTH

GENEVIEVE HOWLAND

NORTH STAR WAY

New York   London   Toronto   Sydney   New Delhi

The author is donating 10 percent of her net income from this book (excluding agency commissions, taxes, and illustrator and marketing expenses) to charities that support maternal and children's health, including Mercy in Action, Mother Health International, and Samaritan's Purse.

North Star Way
An Imprint of Simon & Schuster, Inc.
1230 Avenue of the Americas
New York, NY 10020

First North Star Way trade paperback edition April 2017

NORTH STAR WAY and colophon are trademarks of Simon & Schuster, Inc.

For information about special discounts for bulk purchases, please contact Simon & Schuster Special Sales at 1-866-506-1949 or business@simonandschuster.com.

The North Star Way Speakers Bureau can bring authors to your live event. For more information or to book an event, contact the North Star Way Speakers Bureau at 1-212-698-8888 or visit our website at www.thenorthstarway.com.

DESIGN BY Karla Baker
ILLUSTRATIONS BY Alice Rutherford

Manufactured in the United States of America

10 9 8 7 6 5 4

Library of Congress Cataloging-in-Publication Data

Names: Howland, Genevieve, author.
Title: The mama natural week-by-week guide to pregnancy and childbirth / by
    Genevieve Howland.
Description: First North Star Way trade paperback edition. | New York : North
    Star Way, 2017.
Identifiers: LCCN 2016059018 (print) | LCCN 2017002183 (ebook)
    Subjects: LCSH: Pregnancy—Popular works. | Childbirth—Popular works. | Obstetrics—
Popular works. | BISAC: HEALTH & FITNESS / Pregnancy & Childbirth. | FAMILY &
RELATIONSHIPS / Parenting / General. | FAMILY & RELATIONSHIPS / Parenting /
Motherhood.
Classification: LCC RG551 .H69 2017 (print) | LCC RG551 (ebook) | DDC
    618.2—dc23
LC record available at https://lccn.loc.gov/2016059018

ISBN 978-1-5011-4667-1
ISBN 978-1-5011-4668-8 (ebook)

This book is dedicated
to my mom, Alyce, who
taught me the depth
of the mama heart.
I love you.

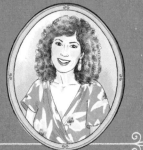

A NOTE TO READERS

This publication contains the opinions and ideas of its author and contributors. It is intended to provide helpful and informative material on the subjects addressed in the publication. It is sold with the understanding that the author and publisher are not engaged in rendering medical, health, or any other kind of personal professional services in the book.

Any statements or claims about the possible health benefits conferred by any foods or supplements have not been evaluated by the Food and Drug Administration and are not intended to diagnose, treat, cure or prevent any disease.

Information found in the book is meant to motivate the reader to make healthy choices based on the reader's own research in partnership with her or his healthcare provider. It should not be relied upon to determine dietary changes, a medical diagnosis, or courses of treatment. The content of this book is not intended to be a substitute for professional medical advice, diagnosis, or treatment. Always seek the advice of your midwife, physician, or other qualified health provider with any questions you may have regarding a medical condition. Never disregard professional medical advice or delay in seeking it because of something you have read in this book. Reliance on any information provided by Mama Natural, whether in the book or on the website or elsewhere, is solely at your own risk.

The author and publisher specifically disclaim all responsibility for any liability, loss, or risk, personal or otherwise, that is incurred as a consequence, directly or indirectly, of the use and application of any of the contents of this book.

Finally, the author wishes to affirm that you are a beautiful and intelligent individual, and she looks forward to walking through this wondrous pregnancy journey with you!

contents

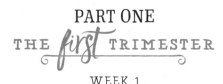

PART THREE
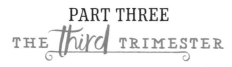
THE *Third* TRIMESTER

INTRODUCTION

THE BIRTH OF *"Mama Natural"*

So, there I was, stark naked and crouched on all fours in the birthing tub, grunting and straining, overcome with a primal urge—a desperate need—to bear down and *push*. In the background, I could just barely make out the hypnosis track I'd insisted on playing during labor and delivery in hopes that it would take the pain away. (Um, not so much.) Behind me, perched on the edge of the tub, my husband was working hard to apply pressure to my lower back. (I had the dreaded "back labor," meaning baby was positioned face-up and the hardest part of his head pressed against my spine during each and every contraction.) Surrounding us were my midwife, a video camera resting atop a tripod, and not one but *two* doulas.

I was 8.5 centimeters dilated. I'd been in labor for more than twenty-four hours. I'd been actively pushing for what felt like a year. Once more, I tucked my chin to my chest, tightened my abs, and let out a guttural groan. Then I looked into the encouraging face of my midwife and thought: *What in the heck am I doing here?*

Me: a former junk food junkie. Me: who used to be sixty-plus pounds overweight. Me: who once couldn't make it past ten in the morning without a cigarette and a gallon or two of diet soda.

Me: a woman who was ready to throw everything she had planned and prayed for out the window and request—no, *demand*—an epidural. Or a C-section! Or maybe some kind of miraculous body swap, so someone *else* could deal with birthing this baby.

You see, I wasn't always "Mama Natural."

⚬✳⚬

Though I ate mostly balanced, healthy meals growing up, food always had a kind of magnetic hold over me. When I was two years old, for example, I scarfed down a bottle of Flintstones vitamins (and promptly had to have my stomach pumped). At summer camp, I volunteered for kitchen duty just so I could wolf down multiple plates of food. Once I'd reached high school, I swung the other way, living off rice cakes, Diet Coke, and carrot sticks. During that phase, I climbed aboard a Stairmaster and flipped through a women's magazine when an attention-grabbing headline caught my eye: "Are You a Compulsive Overeater?" I figured the answer would be a big fat no—how could I be a compulsive eater if I was thin and wasn't eating all that much?

I answered yes to almost every single question.

By college, I'd graduated from excessive working out and dieting to the (increasingly common) late-night binge. The weight started to pile on, but I wasn't ready to give up my comfort crutch. Food may have been making me fat and depressed, but to feel better about myself—irony of ironies—I just ate more food. Fast-forward another few years, and I'd packed on more than 65 pounds. I knew, deep down, that I was slowly killing myself. I was only twenty-three, but I felt dead already—emotionally, mentally, and spiritually.

That New Year's Eve, I ate a super-sized McDonald's Value Meal—my "last supper," as I called it—and though I wasn't a particularly religious person at the time, I started writing a letter: to God, to the angels, to anyone out there who would listen and help me. The pain of overeating had finally become bigger than the fleeting pleasure it provided. The fear of facing the world without my emotional crutch now seemed small compared to the misery of waking each day with a puffy face, cramping bowel, and bloated waistline. I had hit my rock bottom, and I made a "soul decision" to get well. The next morning, I woke up and changed my life. I joined a support group for overeaters, where I learned that I had a sugar *addiction*. (Whereas some people can eat a cookie or two and call it quits, my brain was telling me to eat the entire box.) I sought out a nutritionist, got myself on a food plan, and decided to cut refined sugar from my diet completely. *Not* bingeing became my new normal. I watched, awestruck, as month after month went by with no sugar. Soon, I was ready to give up other crutches, like nicotine, caffeine, and NutraSweet. The weight fell off, of course. But something much more incredible happened: No longer smoking and eating my anxieties away, the fog lifted. I began to experience fuller emotions and a greater sense of clarity.

I started to choose organic, nutrient-filled foods. I flipped my house upside down, tossing out harsh cleaning supplies and chemical-laden beauty products. I went all-in on a natural lifestyle.

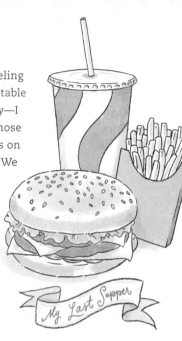

My Last Supper

Six years later—feeling confident and comfortable in my own skin, *finally*—I "winked" at a man whose profile I'd come across on a popular dating site. We agreed to meet for dinner, and by the time our waiter brought the menus over, I was intrigued. He was cuter than his photo, not to mention witty and whip-smart. He had an exciting job, too, as a creative director at a large advertising agency. (I may have been living a healthier life, but I was listless and uninspired by my corporate career.)

Michael, however, was not exactly smitten with me.

He asked if I wanted a cocktail. I told him I didn't drink.

He asked if I wanted an appetizer. I told him I wouldn't have room for my entrée.

He asked if I wanted to split a dessert. I told him I didn't eat sugar.

He asked for the check, and the date was over before it had really started.

I went home and actually cried. It's a cliché, but Michael had stirred something in me. I emailed him a thank-you note as a courtesy, and though he'd written me off as aloof, something in that note struck a chord. Our second date went much better than the first, and that stirring I'd felt eventually grew into a deep love, mutual respect, and a committed partnership. It's why I say our relationship was love at *second* sight.

We were married in a beautiful church wedding in 2007. Less than three years later, I was

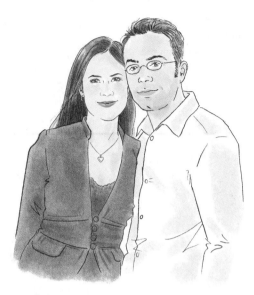

pregnant with our first child. Given my clean lifestyle, it's probably not surprising that I was interested in a natural pregnancy and childbirth.

Don't get me wrong. Like many—if not most—women, I was scared of a vaginal delivery. (Has any woman ever been truly *excited* about the prospect?) But I wasn't particularly thrilled about the alternative, either.

I'd grown up ogling the long, raised scar running from my mother's pelvis practically up to her sternum (the result of a Cesarean performed using an older surgical technique). So I decided to approach natural birth like a reporter: reading everything I could get my hands on and grilling friends who had already been through it. I was amazed at what I discovered, and the more I read, the more I *knew* that going natural was the right choice for me. I upped my natural living game: more veggies, more exercise, more sleep. I interviewed midwives and doulas and chose my birth team. And because our apartment in the Chicago area was a bit cramped, I made plans to have

the baby at a birthing center—midway on the natural scale between an at-home birth and a more conventional feet-in-the-stirrups sort of delivery.

Of course, I read all the baby books, too. But I couldn't find anything that addressed pregnancy—an actual week-by-week or month-by-month guide—from a natural perspective.

Most of the advice out there, I realized, was written from a medicalized and fear-based point of view.

When I *did* find a natural treatment or tip, it was usually referred to as a "grandmother's remedy." And that's when my husband and I came up with a crazy idea: why not be a voice for a different kind of approach to pregnancy, birth, and beyond? By the end of my first trimester, we'd started documenting our pregnancy via weekly videos uploaded to YouTube. A short time later, we began blogging as Mama Natural.

Gradually, our audience grew. We began to realize that making videos and writing blog posts could become more than just a creative outlet. I never would have predicted that the birth of our online careers would coincide with the birth of our actual baby!

As it turned out, birthing the website was a heck of a lot easier.

༺✳༻

After more than an hour of hard-core pushing—and still no baby—I wanted out of the tub.

I may have committed to a natural pregnancy, but I hadn't done consistent exercises to keep my hips open and aligned—something I was regretting now, since my midwife explained that my son was sort of stuck underneath my pelvis. I'd tried drinking red raspberry leaf tea—commonly thought of as a "uterine tonic," helping to tone and strengthen the muscles of the pelvic floor in preparation for labor—but given up way back in the first trimester. I was regretting that decision now, too, since my uterus felt *exhausted*. I no longer had strong or effective contractions, nor the strength to bear down and push. I realized I hadn't done very much mental prep for childbirth, either. Sure, I'd brought the hypnosis soundtrack with me to the hospital, but I'd listened to it only a handful of times during the pregnancy. Now—after *four* hours of pushing—I was adrift: tired, cranky, and a little bit delirious. At one point, I actually thought I could just go to sleep for the night and resume pushing the baby out in the morning.

That's when my midwife started talking about possible interventions: the labor-inducing drug Pitocin, forceps assistance, even vacuum extraction—all things I'd read about and *didn't* want.

But I'd entered my second day of labor and was quickly running out of steam, so I chose the most natural option to accelerate delivery: using a breast pump. (It encourages the production of oxytocin, the hormone that stimulates contractions.)

Great idea: the contractions intensified, but still no baby. Eventually, I consented to a Pitocin drip, mostly because we settled on the lowest dose possible.

The "hit of Pit" kicked in quickly. Within 10 minutes, the urge to push was surging. I waddled over to the birthing stool, grabbed my husband's arms for support, and before long the baby was crowning. In the video (yes, you can watch all this on my YouTube channel), there's a moment where I literally go wide-eyed in disbelief before reaching for my son, instinctively bringing him to my breast, and at the sound of his strong, healthy cry, bursting into tears of gratitude.

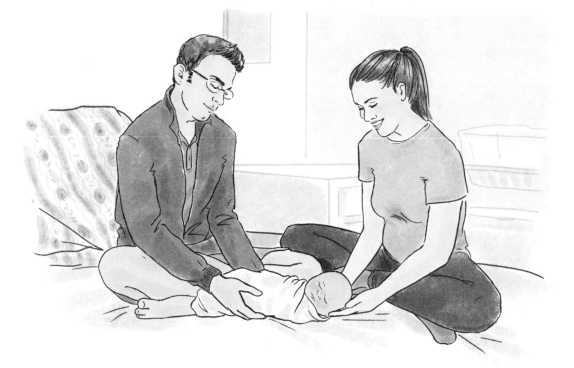

Griffin was born at 11:03 p.m. after a
twenty-seven-hour marathon of labor. The pain
was gone—it had been since the instant he
made his debut—because my body was flooded
with endorphins, a perk of going (mostly)
natural. Though I'd been exhausted and out of
it only moments earlier, I was suddenly energized, chatting and laughing with my husband
and birth team. Baby Griffin was very alert, too.
In fact, that's what everyone kept saying about
him—how alert he was, those beautiful steel-
gray eyes taking it all in, processing the new
world around him.

Later that night, as our baby slept for the
very first time, Michael and I ordered a huge
batch of Mexican takeout and chowed down in
the birth center, marveling at each other—and
at Griffin—the entire time. Neither of us could
quite believe what we'd just been through.

This violent, beautiful, scary, joyous
experience had easily been the most
transformational moment of our lives.

I already knew that I wanted to do it all over
again. I knew I wanted to have more children. I
believed in the natural process.

But I also knew that—next time around—
things were going to be different.

WHY GO NATURAL?

Making babies is still pretty standard stuff.
Sperm meets egg. Sperm fertilizes egg.
Mama gets pregnant. Mama feels nauseated,
exhausted, and increasingly huge for nine long
months. The question of how best to nurture
the developing child in the womb, though,
and—especially—how best to bring that baby
into the world, is where the debate rages. There
are a lot of competing voices out there. There's
a lot of righteousness and finger pointing. It's
an extremely personal debate, as well as a
highly politicized one, and it's been going on for
hundreds and hundreds and *hundreds* of years.

So, what's everybody yelling about?

Until the advent of modern medicine, babies
were typically born at home, and mamas-to-
be were attended to almost exclusively by
women—either female relatives or, in most
cases (even as far back as antiquity), hired
midwives. By the mid- to late 1800s, however,
a kind of turf war broke out. Midwifery became
associated with old-world folk medicine,
whereas newly licensed physicians—exclusively men, many of whom had never even
seen a live birth—began to advertise their more
"modern" and "sophisticated" techniques. A

few decades later, an American obstetrician by the name of Joseph DeLee called for a ban on the use of midwives altogether—he referred to them as "evil" and "barbaric." He also put forth a bold new notion: that pregnancy, rather than being a natural process, was "pathogenic" in nature. In other words, pregnancy was like a sickness or a disease, and he thought it was best treated as such. By the 1930s, hospital birth had replaced home birth as the norm. And things continued that way, with midwife-attended birth declining year after year after year.

That is, until recently.

Before we get ahead of ourselves, it's important to point something out: in the old days, the practice of medicine—in all fields, not just obstetrics—was pretty brutal. There is plenty of evidence, for example, that the earliest doctor-attended births did not exactly go *well*. Back in the day, giving birth in a hospital was far more dangerous than giving birth at home, and the maternal death rate actually *increased* at the beginning of the twentieth century. (Infection rates in hospitals were sky-high, for one thing, in part because doctors didn't know to wash their hands between patients.) Those early, hard-won discoveries, however, paved the way for astonishing medical breakthroughs. Doctors learned about the transmission of infection and disease via bacteria. They developed smarter and safer surgical techniques. They helped make pregnancy and childbirth—once a pretty serious health risk—exceedingly safe for most women and babies.

But with all those lifesaving breakthroughs has come a steady rise in some other *not-so-great* trends.

Case in point: the ideal Cesarean rate is between 10 percent and 15 percent, according to the World Health Organization; yet 33 percent of American women—double the recommended rate—are currently giving birth via C-section. Why? There are plenty of theories, including the idea that some women

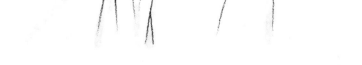

Don't worry — I got this!

are just "too posh to push." (Total myth, by the way. Only 1 percent to 2 percent of women just "decide" to have a completely elective, medically unnecessary C-section.) But the most likely culprit is the modern, medicalized approach to labor and delivery.

These days, a standard hospital birth may go a little something like this: Mama is induced on her due date. She spends the majority of labor flat on her back. She's likely strapped to a machine for continuous electronic fetal monitoring. If she doesn't progress rapidly enough, she may have her water broken or be put on a Pitocin drip, for anywhere from six to twenty-plus hours. And rather than being guided through natural pain-relief techniques, she may be encouraged to just go ahead and get that epidural.

Guess what? Every single one of those totally standard, commonplace procedures is associated with a higher likelihood of eventual C-section.

If you're wondering why that matters—who cares if the C-section rate is kinda high?—well, there are a whole host of reasons. For one thing, it's easy to forget that a Cesarean is serious, invasive abdominal surgery; the associated risks and side effects are considerably higher than in uncomplicated vaginal births. Babies born via C-section, meanwhile, have a higher chance of developing asthma, allergies, obesity, and diabetes later in life; they're also less likely to successfully breastfeed. While it's certainly true that not *every* woman can or should deliver vaginally (C-sections can be life-saving for mamas and babies who need them!), it seems to me that we should be doing what we can to *lower* the rates.

Unfortunately, other forms of medical intervention are on the rise, too. The use of Pitocin, for example, has doubled since 1990,

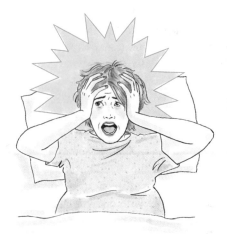

even though it may be less safe than we previously thought: a 2013 study at Beth Israel Medical Center in New York found that Pitocin was associated with lower APGAR scores (a test to evaluate a newborn's health), as well as unexpected admission to the neonatal intensive care unit (NICU). Epidurals—administered to roughly 60 percent of laboring women—can mess with mama's natural production of oxytocin, thereby *extending* labor and increasing the risk of perineal tear. (Who knew?)

Aside from all these potential medical complications, there are plenty of emotional side effects to this approach, too.

The further we get from the idea that women were *designed* to give birth—the more we treat mamas-to-be like sick people—the more likely they are to accept interventions they neither want nor actually need. We have so sanitized and anesthetized the birth experience that many women have no idea what their bodies are actually capable of doing and no awareness of the potential side effects of all those "modern" medical services. Perhaps, for example, you figured getting an epidural was just standard care, but no one told you that it would lower your body's natural production of oxytocin, the hormone that stimulates contractions. Without the urge to push, you may find that you need more drugs (Pitocin this time) to kick-start your labor. When the Pitocin-induced contractions become too intense, you may need more pain meds. The pain meds dull the urge to push again, so you need more Pitocin. You can see how quickly this becomes a vicious cycle. In fact, it's called the "Cascade of Intervention" for good reason. And once it starts, the birth experience you may have planned for can begin to slip through your fingers. Before you know it, the baby is in distress and you're being prepped for an emergency C-section. Rather than being something *you* did, it can feel as though childbirth was something that was done *to* you. When that happens, mamas might feel anything from overwhelmed and scared to violated and depressed.

It's no wonder the pendulum is swinging away from the medical management view and toward a more natural approach to delivering babies.

In 1989, midwives were the lead care providers at just 3 percent of American births. These days, the number is closer to 9 percent, and it's been rising steadily for the last twenty-five years. Consistent midwife care throughout pregnancy is associated with *better* birth outcomes for both baby and mama. While you can reap plenty of rewards by sticking with a natural-minded obstetrician in a hospital setting, there are benefits to getting out of the hospital, too: among women who choose to deliver at birth centers, only 6 percent do so by C-section.

The most compelling reason to go natural, however, might be the simplest to understand, as well as the easiest to overlook: **women were designed to give birth**. The hips that some of us loathe can turn out to be our very best friends during labor. The hormones that make us weep during those touching TV commercials work in a finely calibrated balance during birth—interfere with that balance, and you risk stalling labor, stressing the baby, increasing mama's anxiety, and complicating breastfeeding. Even the pain associated with childbirth is part of the grand plan: it signals mama to change positions so that baby can move toward the birth canal; it tells her when it's time to push (and when not to).

Childbirth is primal and instinctual—it's wild and unpredictable; but in most cases, it is *not* something that needs to be medically managed, treated, or tamed.

When mamas are encouraged to trust the ancient wisdom of their bodies, when they're allowed to focus on the process without distraction, they don't just have shorter labors and deliver healthier babies—they feel empowered.

CALLING ALL MAMAS

It's my belief that many more women would choose to go natural if they knew the benefits. But the arguments in favor of natural birth can sometimes feel just as agenda-driven and politically charged—not to mention *polarizing*—as the medical management view. In the push for alternative birthing solutions, for example,

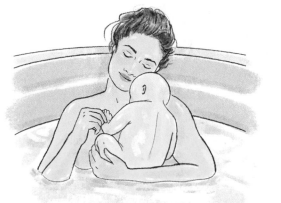

THE SURPRISING BENEFITS OF
natural childbirth

Natural birth is more than going drug-free for its own sake or delivering like you've got something to prove. Did you know that mamas who go natural can (*usually*) do the following?

Get Their Snack On

There's a long-held consensus in the medical world that women shouldn't be allowed to eat—at all—during labor. Why? Because back in the 1940s, when C-sections were typically performed under general anesthesia, concerns emerged about the dangers of aspiration. (That is, inhaling food or fluid into the lungs while unconscious.) These days, the threat of aspiration during delivery is almost nonexistent, and a number of organizations, including the American Society of Anesthesiologists, have since argued that restricting food is both unnecessary and unwarranted. But in the majority of hospitals, mamas-to-be are still expected to make do with ice chips, especially if they've had an epidural.

Here's the good news: Most midwives actually *support* eating a bit of (light, easily digestible) food during labor. (I remember the boost of energy I got from sipping apple juice between contractions.) Mamas who go natural can also eat immediately *after* the birth, whereas mamas who deliver via C-section will have to hang in there for a few more hours, until their bodies have recovered from surgery.

Move Around Freely

Sign up for an epidural, IV fluids, or continuous electronic fetal monitoring and you may be confined to a bed, unable to get up, walk around, or even go to the bathroom. (Mamas often don't realize that when they ask for an epidural, they may be asking for a catheter, too!) In fact, the standard laboring position in most hospitals is for mama to be flat on her back, which only compresses the pelvis, making the passage for baby tighter and smaller. Going natural, however, allows you to move freely, to listen to your body's cues, and to work with gravity. I delivered my second baby on all fours, simply because that's what felt most comfortable to me.

Inoculate Their Babies with Good Bacteria

True, the idea of pushing something the size of a watermelon out from between your legs can seem pretty, uh, *strange*, but there are benefits to delivering your child via the birth canal: Babies delivered vaginally pick up protective bacteria that help to build their brand-new immune systems. (When born via scheduled C-section, babies may pick up bacteria from the room they were born in, including potentially harmful bacteria like staph.) Passing through the birth canal also helps a baby to expel amniotic fluid from the lungs, which may lower his risk for developing respiratory problems.

$\longrightarrow$

Enjoy a Hormonal High

Mamas who go natural experience a hormonal "high" at the moment of birth—a rush of endorphins (for energy) and a wave of oxytocin, the "feel-good" hormone that stimulates bonding. Cuddling baby, making eye contact, skin-to-skin touching, and breastfeeding only enhance the hormonal cascade. Interventions, however, disrupt the body's delicate hormonal balance, which means mama likely won't receive the same emotional pay-off—the otherworldly elation—from all that pushing.

Experience Better Breastfeeding

We know that breastfeeding within an hour or so of birth ups your chances for a long and happy nursing relationship, in part because skin-to-skin contact is associated with better bonding, increased milk production, and—believe it or not—*less crying*. (Key!) Early breastfeeding also ensures that baby receives the colostrum, a thick, yellowish, milk-like substance that's high in protein, vitamin A, immune cells, and antibodies. Colostrum also has a digestive effect, helping baby to pass his or her first stools. Narcotic pain medications, however, tend to affect babies the same way they affect mamas: resulting in drowsiness and disorientation. Perhaps not surprisingly, sleepy babies have trouble nursing. Mamas who need to deliver via C-section also aren't always able to breastfeed right away, as they may still be recovering.

Go Home Sooner

Cesareans constitute major abdominal surgery, while epidurals increase the likelihood of perineal tear and instrument-assisted birth—all of which only elongate recovery time. Mamas who are able to go natural, however, are often up and walking shortly after baby makes his or her debut.

doctors and hospitals sometimes become demonized.

Too often, women who elected to have an epidural or who delivered via C-section feel excluded from the "natural club," as if their birth experience was somehow "less than" or inferior.

It pains me that women who wanted to give birth naturally but couldn't—perhaps due to a high-risk pregnancy or an unforeseen medical complication—might feel judged.

I certainly felt remorseful after my hit of Pit. Even though it was a minor dose—even though my labor had stalled and my body needed the help—I couldn't help but feel a little disappointed. Birth, however, is unpredictable. We can steer the ship as best we can, but ultimately the process is much bigger than us. It's neither possible nor safe for *every* woman to have a 100 percent intervention-free experience. There is no one "right" way to deliver, and as much as I believe in the power of going natural, no mama should ever be made to feel

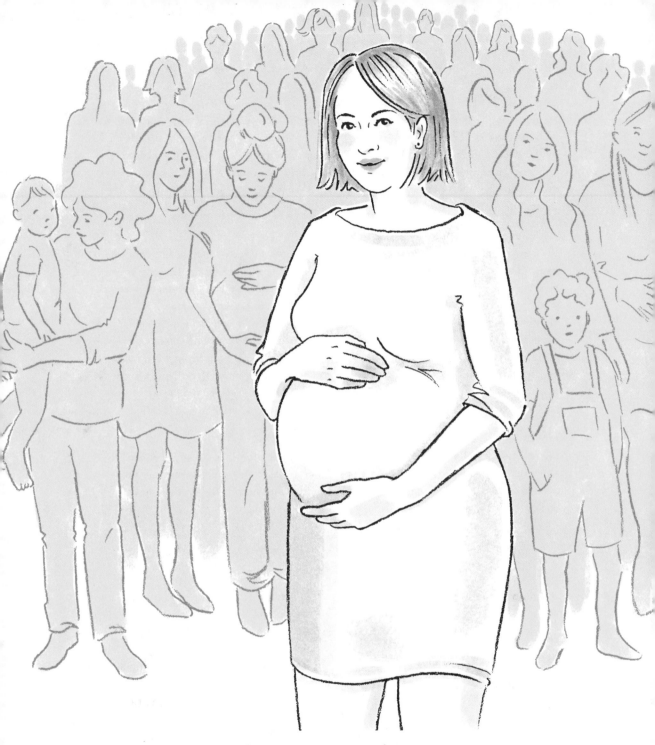

Welcome to a sacred path that billions
of women have walked before you

bad about her choices. That's why this book was written with *all* mamas in mind—from those who only want to cut back on processed foods or experiment with natural remedies for heartburn and morning sickness, to those who are all-in for an at-home water birth. No matter where you fall on the natural mama spectrum, this guide is for you.

Empowerment—rather than judgment—is what this book is about.

Together, we'll talk about everything from pregnancy nutrition to performing a toxic sweep of your home. We'll discuss routine tests and screenings (which ones you actually *need* versus which you might want to steer clear of), as well as determine who should be on your birth team—a midwife, a doula, an obstetrician, or all three. I'll provide loads of natural remedies for pregnancy ailments, from sore breasts to morning sickness and more, as well as tips on how best to set yourself up for an intervention-free labor and delivery. You'll get evidence-based medical insights from Cynthia Mason, a certified nurse-midwife—who happened to deliver both of my children!—and Maura Winkler, RN, certified doula, lactation consultant, and placenta encapsulator (as well as cohost of the Mama Natural online birth course). You'll read stories and receive feedback, too, from plenty of "crunchy" mamas who are part of the Mama Natural community. It's all the stuff I wished I'd known during my first pregnancy, organized in the simplest, least overwhelming format possible: week by week. But as you read, feel free to pick what resonates with you and leave the rest. No woman should have to keep up with any Mama Natural Joneses!

When I got pregnant again (two and a half years after birthing Griffin), I was armed with the knowledge I hadn't had the first time around, and I was much better prepared—emotionally, physically, and spiritually. True, second births are often easier, but I was absolutely *amazed* at the difference. No twenty-seven hours of labor. No climbing in and out of the birth tub. My daughter Paloma was born within 20 minutes of my arrival at the birth center. She practically shot out of me like a cannonball, which is why I call hers my "supernatural" birth.

I can't claim that going natural is always easy or entirely painless, but the benefits are profound. You can choose to be present for all of it—the blood, sweat, and tears, as well as the ecstasy, joy, and elation.

Welcome to pregnancy: a sacred path that billions of women have walked before you. Best wishes as you embark on this transformative journey. But most of all, congratulations!

Can you *believe* it?
You're having a baby.

MEET *cynthia mason*, CNM, APN, MSN

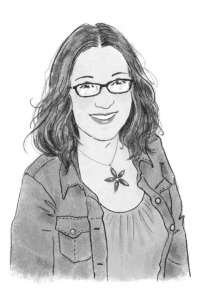

hello and congratulations on your pregnancy! As a midwife who's attended more than five hundred births—more than one thousand if you count my time working as a registered nurse at a county hospital in Cleveland—I've seen firsthand how sacred and life-altering having a baby can be.

When I started my career, I wanted to become a pediatrician—I loved children and I wanted to help people, so pediatrics seemed like a natural fit. Several internships and opportunities to shadow physicians later, however, I realized that I wasn't philosophically aligned with the standard model of medical care that exists in the United States. Most of the talented physicians I trailed were focused entirely on what was going *wrong* with the body, rather than figuring out how to make things go right. And there was *zero* emphasis on preventive medicine or holistic living.

It wasn't until my junior year in college that I understood how different things could be. I was working as a receptionist and patient educator at a family planning clinic, and I saw firsthand how certified nurse-midwives cared for their patients while encouraging a healthier, more holistic lifestyle. It was like a lightbulb went off; I knew this was what I was supposed to do. In the world of midwifery, we call this our *calling*.

A year later, I graduated with a degree in biology and went on to receive my master's-level training at the Frances Payne Bolton School of Nursing at Case Western Reserve University. And these days, I'm living my dreams: I'm married to an amazing husband, we have a pair of loving fur babies, and every morning (sometimes in the middle of the night, too!) I rush out of bed, full of adrenaline, ready to welcome a new life to the world.

MEET *Maura Winkler*, RN, CD, IBCLC

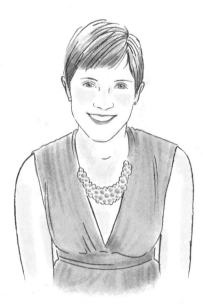

hey, there! I'm Maura Winkler, registered nurse, certified doula, student midwife, placenta encapsulator, and board-certified lactation consultant. I'm also a wife and mother of two.

I always knew that I wanted to help mamas-to-be deliver their babies, so I moved from my hometown of Buffalo, New York, to Chicago to attend medical school. But after more than a year of hands-on training, I realized the medical management view of labor and delivery just wasn't for me. What I found was an "intervention-first" approach to childbirth—the opposite of what I knew, intuitively, the experience of having a baby could be.

I remember one night at the hospital in particular: a young mother's labor was progressing more slowly than some of the residents would have liked. So they suggested "pitting and breaking" her—medical shorthand for putting her on a Pitocin drip and breaking her bag of waters. Luckily, cooler heads prevailed, and the woman was able to deliver drug-free, at her own pace. But the scary part came later: the "pit and break" resident told me that hers was the first low-intervention birth he had *ever* witnessed.

A few months later, I dropped out of med school to pursue my doula and midwife education and certification. To date, I've attended more than one hundred fifty births—including my own (I delivered both of my children in the comfort of my own home)—and have seen how awesome it can be to go natural.

PART ONE

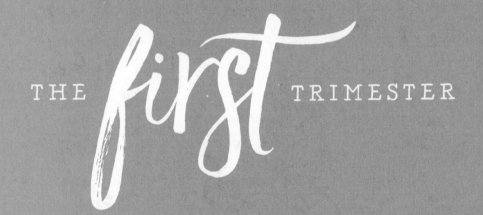

THE *first* TRIMESTER

A LITTLE BIT
pregnant

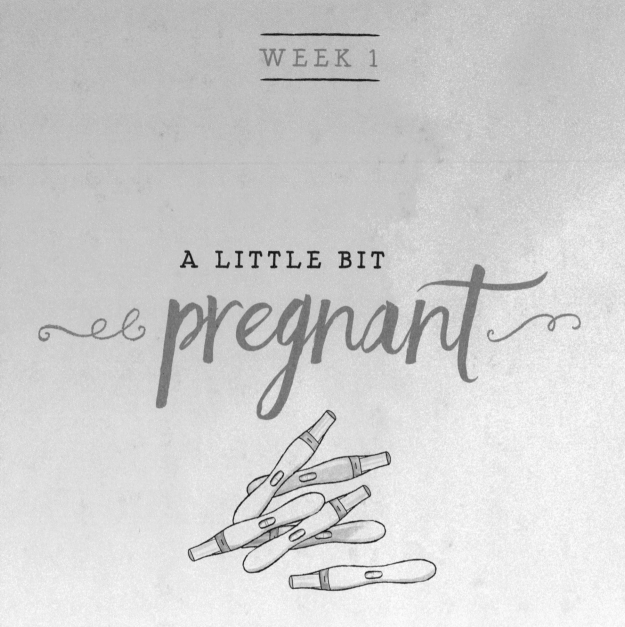

I was hovering near the pharmacy at Walgreens, scanning the vast array of home pregnancy tests lining the shelves. Michael and I had only recently started trying for baby #1. And though my period wasn't due for another five or six days, I—like most women who are actively trying to conceive—had spent the past week or so obsessing over every *possible* early sign and symptom. Were my boobs sore? Was I peeing more than usual? Was I feeling nauseous? I couldn't wait anymore. I *had* to know. I scanned the shelves, feeling both anxious and awestruck, and soon experienced the first of many wondrous discoveries on the journey to motherhood: Pregnancy tests are *expensive*.

Overwhelmed by choice and high on adrenaline, I went with a middle-of-the-road option: One line for no, two lines for yes, and a promise to give me an answer as soon as five days before my missed period. Bingo. I bought a three-pack of tests and headed home. Then I ripped open the box and pored over the directions, which is when I realized that I was supposed to use my "first morning urine."

Also, that 99 percent accuracy guarantee? Not so accurate, it turns out, if you take a home pregnancy test *too* early.

At five days out, my chances of getting a false negative were high, so I stuck the test back in the box and tried not to think about it for a few days. Easier said than done, I can tell you.

Two days later, I bounded out of bed, took care of business in the bathroom, and waited the two or three (excruciating) minutes for my results, pacing back and forth across the apartment like a caged cheetah. Finally, what felt like a year later, I stepped forward, took a deep breath, and picked up the test . . . only to find the *faintest possible hint* of a second pink line.

"Is this a second line?" I said aloud, though I was alone in the bathroom. "IS THIS A SECOND LINE?!" Next thing I knew I was running around the apartment like a crazy person, holding the test up to the skylight to view it in the most natural daylight possible, then I was shoving it in my (now bewildered) husband's face while simultaneously going online and texting all my girlfriends. "Does this count?" I wailed, typing frantically in the Google search box. In the middle of the madness, it dawned on me that perhaps something was wrong with the test. Perhaps this test had been defective? Immediately, I peed on sticks two and three, and laid them out on the bathroom counter in a neat little row. Unfortunately, each of them produced the exact same reading: one very dark pink line, one very faint, practically invisible one.

You have got to be kidding me, I thought to myself.

From the other room, I suddenly heard the *ping!* of an incoming text. I lunged for my phone, and saw that one of my dearest friends (a mother of two) was telling me to get one of the tests that actually spell out "pregnant" or "not pregnant." Why hadn't I thought of that? I pulled myself together and got in the car.

Trip to Walgreens: round 2.

It wasn't until I was back at the store, however, digital pregnancy test in hand, that I realized I had a problem. I had used up all my good "first morning urine." I was out of the quality pee. I hesitated briefly; should I chance it? Would I risk wasting an expensive test on a subpar urine sample? You bet I would!

But then I looked at my watch, which brought me to problem No. 2: I only had 20 minutes or so to get to a meeting. If I was going to do this, it would have to go down in a Walgreens bathroom. Not exactly what I'd pictured as the magical moment in which I would discover that I was bringing a new life into the world. Bravely, I forged ahead and locked myself in the stall, which is when I discovered problem No. 3: I wasn't just out of the good urine; I was out of urine entirely. I squeezed out every last drop I could muster, set the test on top of the toilet paper dispenser, and looked at it dubiously. I watched, wide-eyed, as the little hourglass in the indicator window began to flip and flip and flip . . . until the thing just timed out.

Nooooooooooooo!!

I scanned the directions, and discovered that "lack of urine" might result in an error message. Guilty as charged.

I'm not sure how I managed, but I made it through the business meeting and the rest of my workday, as well as my after-work plans—it was New Year's Eve, and Michael and I stayed out pretty late. But at six thirty the next morning, I flew out of bed. I had a bladder full of the good stuff and the digital test in hand. I did my thing in the bathroom. I waited. I paced around nervously. Finally, I checked my results.

Pregnant.

And it took me only five tests (and a near nervous breakdown) to get a positive reading that I actually believed.

MAMA FERTILITY TIP: DITCH FAT-FREE DAIRY!

Trying to conceive? Make sure you're eating a well-balanced, low-sugar, preferably organic diet and, if tolerated, a few servings per day of organic full-fat dairy. Think: organic whole milk from pastured cows, whole-milk Greek yogurt, and grass-fed cheese (the real stuff, not the bright orange imitation bricks or singles). Why? Recent research out of the Harvard School of Public Health suggests a strong link between women who ate two or more daily servings of low-fat or fat-free dairy products and "ovulatory infertility" (that is, when the ovary doesn't release an egg). Intake of *full*-fat dairy, on the other hand, may decrease that risk. Looking for more baby-makin' tips? Type "fertility" in the search box at mamanatural .com.

PAPA FERTILITY TIP: GO ORGANIC!

When it comes to conception, Mama's not the only one who should be making adjustments and preparations. Papa needs to step up his game, too! The Boston-based Environmental and Reproductive Health (EARTH) study, for example, found that men who ate fruits and vegetables with high levels of pesticide residue had lower sperm counts and fewer "normal" sperm than men who ate produce with low pesticide residue. The lesson here? Dad may need to clean up his diet before you get busy. You'll find more info on how to help him do that in the next few chapters.

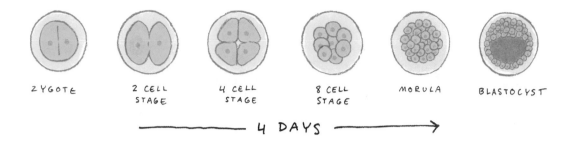

ZYGOTE   2 CELL STAGE   4 CELL STAGE   8 CELL STAGE   MORULA   BLASTOCYST

← 4 DAYS →

HOW ACCURATE ARE HOME PREGNANCY TESTS?

It's exciting to be in the throes of trying to conceive—chasing your partner around like a teenager, keeping track of your temperature with a basal body thermometer, pinpointing your ovulation. Every session could be *The One.*

Of course, having sex 'round the clock in the sole interest of procreation can be a little, well, *unsexy.* (I'll never forget holding my legs up in the air afterward, desperately trying to coax my husband's sperm to meet my egg.) But there may be no stranger phenomenon in the journey to motherhood than peeing on stick after stick to confirm a possible pregnancy.

When I posted a version of my story on Facebook, mamas from coast to coast chimed in to share their equally wacky and anxiety-ridden experiences. "I took five!" one mama wrote. "I took eight!" said another. These women, by the way, are not in the minority. In a recent survey by a popular baby-goods company, 62 percent of respondents said they took *at least* two tests to confirm the happy news. I wouldn't be surprised if the figures went much, much higher. Finding out that you're pregnant can be so shocking, so amazing, so utterly life-changing that one little pee-on-a-stick test doesn't seem monumental or scientific enough to be trustworthy. *Can this really be right?* you may think, staring suspiciously at the little strip of plastic in your still trembling hands.

What I hadn't known during my first pregnancy, however, is that one test would likely have been plenty. Home testing kits screen for the presence of something called human chorionic gonadotropin (hCG), a hormone produced by the cells of the placenta during a pregnancy. There are a few *very* rare medical conditions that can cause the body to produce hCG for other reasons (fertility treatments sometimes contain hCG, too).

But in the vast majority of cases, even the faintest double line or plus sign is a sure indication that you are with child.

While the chances of getting a false positive are relatively low, though, the chances of getting a false negative—a negative result when you really *are* pregnant—are quite high, especially if you take a test too early. A lot must happen before your body begins producing hCG.

First things first: Papa's sperm has to meet and fertilize Mama's egg. If you and your partner managed to time things right, the fertilized egg will begin transitioning into a single-celled zygote, a process that'll take 12 to 24 hours. Then the zygote will begin a leisurely three- to five-day journey through the fallopian tube on its way to your uterus (dividing and multiplying, growing from one cell to two and from two cells to four, etc., the entire time). Once inside, the zygote will transition again—this time into

claire: "I knew even before I took the test that I was pregnant. But then I took another one a few weeks later—just to make sure!"

ashton: "I have three sons, and with each pregnancy I took at least three tests. I even made my husband take one, just to make sure they weren't rigged!"

megan: "I was sure that I was pregnant, but the tests kept coming back negative. I ended up taking nine—and after all that, I still went in for a blood test."

something called a blastocyst, or a tiny mass of cells with a fluid-filled center. It will implant itself into the lining of your uterus, snuggling deep into the sponge-like tissue. And soon, it will split into two—half will become the embryo (a.k.a. your growing baby) and half will become the placenta (the organ that nourishes baby during pregnancy). It's now been any-where from six to twelve days since ovulation, and your body has only *just* begun to produce hCG. It may be several more days before there's enough of the hormone in your urine to be detectable via a home-based pregnancy test.

If you haven't taken that first test yet (oth-erwise known as the most nerve-wracking pee of your life), your best chance for an accurate reading is to wait until at least a day or two *after* your missed period. If you can manage to wait a whole week, the likelihood of getting an accurate result shoots up to nearly 100 percent. These days, many tests no longer require you to use your "first morning urine," but doing so will only further increase the accuracy: hCG levels are usually at their highest in the morn-ing, when your urine is the most concentrated. But if you can't wait (who can blame you?!) and you get a negative result, don't lose hope. You may not have had enough hCG in your urine, or the test you purchased might not be especially sensitive. Wait a week and then try again.

COULD IT BE TWINS?

Once I got my positive pregnancy test, the next thing I started obsessing about was whether I had two buns in the oven, instead of just one. I was kinda *hoping* for twins, in fact—a boy and a girl. But what were the chances?

Turns out, it depends on which *kind* of twins you're talking about.

Identical twins occur in only about 3.5 out of every 1,000 births, and the rate hasn't budged in the last few decades. That's because identical babies are a rare and random event: spontane-ously, a single fertilized egg must split into two.

Fraternal twins, on the other hand, are much more common—rates have jumped

I'M ALREADY PREGNANT.
WHEN SHOULD I CALL MY DOCTOR?

It's my opinion that hiring a midwife is one of the best decisions you can make on the way to a natural childbirth. As we've discussed, midwifery care is associated with lower rates of interventions, as well as better birth outcomes for mama and baby—in low-risk, uncomplicated pregnancies. In some cases, a midwife is *not* your best option. Women with chronic medical conditions (such as diabetes, high blood pressure, or epilepsy) or who have a history of complicated pregnancies or difficult births are almost always better off seeing an obstetrician, who may even refer them to a maternal-fetal medicine specialist, also known as a perinatologist.

Regardless of whom you choose, however, keep in mind that most practitioners won't schedule your first prenatal appointment until you're at least six to eight weeks along, if not later. In a low-risk pregnancy, there's just not a lot for *any* doctor to do during those first few weeks. Although that can strike a lot of women as mildly terrifying (I remember phoning my midwife when I found out I was pregnant with my second child and being shocked when she said, "Congratulations, see you in ten weeks"), remember that pregnancy is a natural biological process—*not* a medical emergency.

When Michael and I were trying for our first child, we got pregnant immediately, so I hadn't yet assembled my birth team. Some women choose to interview midwives, doulas, and obstetricians before they conceive; others just assume they'll stick with their regular ob-gyn from conception to delivery. But if you don't know whom you want to deliver with—or if you've chosen a healthcare provider but you are having second thoughts—don't worry. We'll go over all that in the next few chapters. We'll talk about managing "high-risk" pregnancies, too. (Because even "high-risk" mamas can be part of the natural journey. Keep reading!)

more than 75 percent in the last thirty years. The reason? Mostly, it's fertility treatments. In vitro fertilization, for example, ups your odds by about 20 percent to 40 percent, depending on how many embryos were implanted in the womb. Fertility drugs such as Clomid, meanwhile, stimulate the ovaries to release more eggs, increasing your chances by roughly 10 percent to 30 percent.

There are other reasons for the recent rise in multiples, though. We're taller and heavier than our parents and grandparents.

Women are waiting longer to get pregnant, and women over the age of 35 produce more follicle-stimulating hormone (FSH), which is associated with twin pregnancies. You're also more likely to have two babies if you're African American and this isn't your first birth.

Want a more personalized assessment of your risk, er, chances? Check out the quiz at mama natural.com.

THE FIRST STEP TO A NATURAL CHILDBIRTH

Whether you're still months away from trying or you're already pregnant, now's the time to start making some important lifestyle changes. From conception to delivery, your baby will be at the mercy of her environment. But you likely won't even realize you're carrying a child until Week 5 or 6 of your pregnancy. That's because—ready for some bizarro math?—the *instant* papa's sperm meets and fertilizes your egg, even though it'll be far too early to confirm the pregnancy with a home-based test, you'll already be *two weeks pregnant*.

Say what?

A normal, full-term pregnancy, as you probably know, lasts anywhere from 39 to 42 weeks, or 40 weeks on average. Your due date, however, isn't calculated from the precise moment of conception—which would be nearly impossible to determine with any accuracy—but rather from the first day of your last menstrual period. Since ovulation (and possible fertilization) doesn't occur until two weeks *after* menstruation, you're not actually pregnant at all during Weeks 1 and 2 of your pregnancy. You're what I like to call *a little bit pregnant*.

And at this early stage, the best thing you can do to increase your odds of having a natural childbirth isn't signing up for a prenatal yoga class or touring alternative birth centers; it's making the decision that you *want* one.

That might sound outrageously simple—or painfully obvious—but the truth is that very few mamas just stumble into a natural childbirth. The modern medical world, for all its positives, is frankly working against you. After all, the vast majority of mamas—we're talking 80 percent to 90 percent—have *at least* one intervention during labor (that might include electronic fetal monitoring, an IV drip for fluids or medication, an epidural, or Pitocin to kick-start contractions). Most women, in fact, have several. So while it may be tempting to think, "I'm just going to *try* for a natural birth" or "We'll just see how it goes," in the end, that attitude may not serve you. Better to make the commitment early on in your pregnancy if going natural is your end goal.

WHAT'S YOUR "WHY"?

Defining your "why," or motivation for going natural, is a crucial first step. Because when the going gets tough—and it will, in some way or another—your "why" will become your North Star, guiding you through the darker moments.

Pause and think about all the compelling reasons you might want to go natural, then use the following space to write down three, four—or more!

1 ....
....

2 ....
....

3 ....
....

4 ....
....

5 ....
....

WHAT OTHER *natural mamas* SAY

jennifer: Funny enough, at the beginning of my pregnancy I thought I wanted a C-section—it sounded easier! Then I began to read and research, and discovered that interventions often get in the way of birth and affect breastfeeding. Having those babies growing inside me motivated me to take my health to a whole other level.

carolyn: I knew that if my grandma could have eight kids at home—naturally—then I could definitely do it!

jessica: I wanted a natural birth, but my pregnancy ended with an unplanned, unwanted, possibly unnecessary C-section. Now I'm doing the opposite of what I did the first time around—a natural VBAC is my biggest motivator!

baby steps

PREPARING YOUR BODY AND HOME FOR YOUR LITTLE BAMBINO

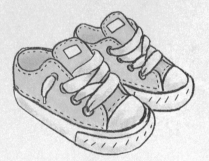

So you've made the decision to go natural—whatever "going natural" might mean to you. Next on the agenda, then, is to make baby's home for the next nine months as safe and welcoming as possible. That means taking a closer look inside the four walls of your home, as well as thinking about what's going on in your womb. Whether you're actively trying to conceive or you're already expecting, it's time to clean up your insides and outsides.

So long, triple-shot latte.
Au revoir, sushi.
Good-bye, bubbly Prosecco,
I hardly knew ye.

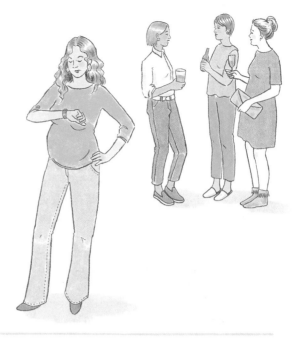

GIVE UP YOUR VICES

These days, most women—especially those who are *actively* trying to conceive—already know plenty about the dangers of taking illicit drugs and smoking during pregnancy. No need to go into too much detail here, except to say that illicit drug use (cocaine, heroin, methamphetamine, etc.) has been linked with an increased risk of miscarriage, preterm birth, birth defects, and stillbirth, not to mention serious dangers to your own health. Cigarette smoking while pregnant has been associated with those same complications, as well as low birth weight and an increased risk of sudden infant death syndrome (SIDS). If you're a smoker, you'll want to stop immediately. If you can't quit cold turkey, discuss with your doctor the benefits (and risks) of smoking cessation aids. Also look into natural tools that can help, like exercise, deep breathing, or meditation. If you share a home with a smoker, have a serious conversation with him or her about quitting—or at an absolute minimum, smoking outside the home—as secondhand smoke can be nearly as harmful. And while medical marijuana may help various health conditions, the American College of Obstetricians and Gynecologists urges mamas to avoid pot while pregnant. Some studies have shown links between

ACK! I GOT A LIL' TIPSY JUST LAST WEEK!!

It's not uncommon for women to discover they're pregnant, feel elated for a moment or two, then flip to panic mode when they remember a recent alcohol-infused night on the town. *What if I unknowingly harmed my baby?!*

Mama? Take a deep breath. Your baby almost certainly is—and will be—just fine. The important thing to focus on now is that you *are* pregnant, and therefore this *won't* happen again. Eat well, get some exercise, rest, and cut yourself some slack. If you're overcome with concern, talk to your midwife or doctor.

marijuana consumption and babies with low birth weight, an increased need for neonatal care, and learning and developmental issues.

When it comes to alcohol consumption, on the other hand, things get a little more controversial. In 2016, the Centers for Disease Control (CDC) released a report warning that American women—as many as 3.3 million of them—were at risk for having an "alcohol-exposed pregnancy" because they were (1) sexually active, (2) drinking alcohol, and (3) not taking birth control. Reporters labeled the press release both alarmist and sexist, and a media firestorm promptly erupted. "CDC says women shouldn't drink unless they're on birth control" became a headline at outlets ranging from *Forbes* and *USA Today* to CNN and the *Washington Post*. Just one problem: that's not actually what the CDC meant.

While there's no hard evidence that having an *occasional* drink—especially while trying to get pregnant—poses serious risks to a baby in utero, the dangers of drinking too much alcohol while pregnant are well known. Fetal alcohol syndrome, the most serious of several fetal alcohol spectrum disorders, causes severe neurological impairment, growth deficiencies, and birth defects. Alcohol crosses the placenta and enters baby's bloodstream, so it's fair to say that when you drink, baby drinks. And yet, 75 percent of women who report wanting to get pregnant "as soon as possible" don't stop

drinking. What's more, upwards of 50 percent of pregnancies in the United States are unplanned. That means that lots of women may continue drinking without realizing that they are carrying a child, which is exactly why the CDC issued such a dire (if poorly worded) report.

It's true that in some cultures, having an occasional glass of wine or half pint while pregnant is common. (For centuries, it was thought that beer could actually help with breastfeeding, though we now know it's likely the barley and hops present in beer—as opposed to the alcohol—that helps to encourage milk production and letdown.) There is no amount of alcohol, however, that's been proven safe to consume for an expectant mama. If you're trying to conceive, you'll want to quit altogether or have only an occasional drink. Once you're pregnant (keeping in mind that you may not know for sure for several more weeks), total abstinence is the way to go.

CLEAN UP YOUR MEDICINE CABINET

When it comes to figuring out which medications are safe for mamas-to-be, the short answer is to run everything past your midwife or doctor. If you take prescription drugs, for

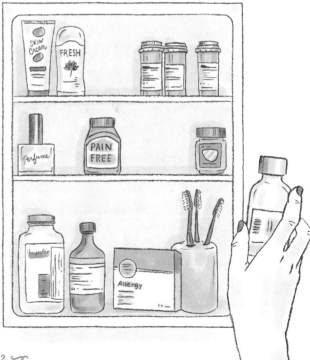

example—think blood pressure pills, antidepressants, or an asthma inhaler—you may need to switch to a different brand or stop taking them altogether *before* attempting to get pregnant. Unfortunately, loads of over-the-counter (OTC) meds aren't particularly safe to take, either. Some cold, cough, and allergy medications, as well as aspirin, naproxen, and ibuprofen are all generally not recommended for pregnant women.

For many years, Tylenol (acetaminophen) was considered the best choice if a pregnant mama needed to treat a headache or some other minor ailment. Two recent studies, however, have cast some doubt on that drug, too. One, published in *JAMA Pediatrics* in 2014, found that babies born to pregnant women who took acetaminophen for six weeks or longer had a higher risk of developing attention-deficit/hyperactivity disorder (ADHD). The other, published in the *International Journal of Epidemiology* in 2013, suggested that acetaminophen, when taken by pregnant women for 28 days or longer, contributed to behavioral problems, language delays, and slow motor development. Both studies are considered preliminary—there's not much evidence that taking Tylenol once or twice would have adverse effects on your growing baby. Certainly, a fever is one instance where acetaminophen may be quite helpful—sustained fever in the first trimester can lead to both miscarriage and birth defects. (Full disclosure: I took Tylenol for a few days during my first pregnancy after having a tooth pulled—more on that in Week 11.) But the point remains: even drugs that we once thought were safe might not be.

And certainly, long-term use of any OTC drug is almost definitely a no-go.

Always check with your midwife or doctor before using herbal remedies during pregnancy. However, gingerroot, nettles, dandelion root, cranberry, chamomile, and red raspberry leaf tea are generally considered safe for use in moderate doses. On the flip side, steer clear of Oregon grape, mugwort, goldenseal, red clover, pokeroot, pennyroyal oil, thuja, and tansy, as these can be dangerous for mamas-to-be.

The thing is, most OTC drugs are sort of frowned upon in the natural community, anyway. There's been evidence floating around for years that some pain relievers and fever reducers can be hard on the liver. Most OTC drugs contain a fair amount of inactive "filler" ingredients—dyes, stabilizers, and preservatives—that crunchy mamas like to steer clear of. However, you'll want to be careful with natural and herbal supplements, too. Echinacea, St. John's wort, and ginkgo biloba, for example, have been associated with fertility problems in women who are trying to conceive. Just because something is "natural" doesn't mean it's always safe to take during pregnancy. I'll provide loads of natural remedies that *are* safe, though—for everything from headaches to morning sickness and more—so don't worry. Help (if you find that you need it) is on the way!

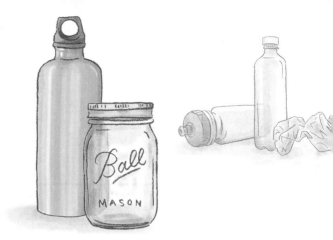

DO A CHEMICAL SWEEP OF YOUR HOME

If you're into natural and green living, you may have already started to reduce your exposure to noxious chemicals—perhaps by tossing out harsh cleaning supplies or opting for a gentler laundry detergent, free of irritating dyes and fragrances. But if you haven't yet, now is a great time to start. Certain chemicals (many of them found in common household items) have been linked to fertility issues, an increased risk of miscarriage, and health problems later in life. Yuck—let's clean it up! Here are some of the biggest offenders that may be lurking in your home:

BANISH BISPHENOL A (BPA)

Found in everything from plastic bottles and plastic food storage containers to the linings of certain canned foods (to prevent corrosion), BPA is ubiquitous—but it's also a "known endocrine disruptor," meaning it can mess with your hormones and interrupt normal fetal development. Though the FDA has not yet banned BPA, nor recommended that pregnant women avoid it, it has stated that there is "some concern about the potential effects of BPA on the brain, behavior, and prostate gland of fetuses, infants, and children." As of 2012, it is illegal to use BPA in the manufacture of baby bottles and sippy cups.

But it's somehow safe for us adults? No, thank you.

To lessen your exposure to BPA:

♡ Opt for stainless steel or glass water bottles, baby bottles, and drinking cups, not plastic. Even "BPA-free" plastics have been shown to potentially leach BPA-*like* chemicals that mimic the hormone estrogen.

♡ Never heat your food in plastic or put hot food or liquids into plastic containers. This can cause chemicals to leach into your food. Instead, choose glass storage containers, such as Pyrex or Mason jars.

♡ Avoid canned foods as much as possible, or choose brands that don't use BPA in the lining, like Eden Organics or Native Forest.

GO ORGANIC TO KNOCK OUT PESTICIDE RESIDUE

Well, now that you've tossed out about a mountain of those plastic food storage containers (you can recycle them, by the way), you'll want to make sure the produce you're bringing home isn't laced with chemicals, either. We already know that high levels of pesticide residue affect the health of men's sperm, so it shouldn't come as a particularly big shock that pesticides may affect the health of your growing baby, too. A study published in *PNAS Early Edition*, for example, found that high levels of exposure to the insecticide chlorpyrifos (which the EPA proposed banning in 2015) may lead to abnormalities in a child's cortex, the area of the brain responsible for memory, language, personality, and muscle movement. Research out of the University of California, Berkeley's School of Public Health, meanwhile, suggests that high pesticide exposure in utero leads to lower IQ scores. We also know that babies who are conceived during the late

DIRTY DOZEN	THE CLEAN 15
Apples	Avocados
Bell Peppers	Asparagus
Celery	Cabbage
Cherries	Cantaloupe
Cherry tomatoes	Cauliflower
Cucumbers	Eggplant
Grapes	Grapefruit
Nectarines	Honeydew
Peaches	Kiwi
Spinach	Mangoes
Strawberries	Onions
Tomatoes	*Papayas
	*Pineapple
	*Sweet corn
	Sweet peas

*May still be GMO (see page 18).

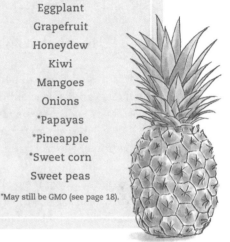

spring and early summer (April through July)—coincidentally, when the concentration of pesticides in groundwater is at its highest—have an increased risk of birth defects, according to a study published in *Acta Paediatrica*.

True, organic fruits and vegetables are almost always more expensive than conventionally grown produce, but it's likely worth the cost to bring home pesticide-free food. If your budget is tight, opt for organic produce whenever you're eating from among the "Dirty Dozen," the fruits and veggies with the highest residual pesticides. You can stick with conventional produce when you're eating from the "Clean 15" (crops that contain less chemical residue).

SURVIVE MOSQUITO SEASON

If you're pregnant during the summer months, you'll want to think about mosquito protection. Most bites are harmless, of course, but some of these little bloodsuckers carry infectious diseases like Zika and West Nile virus, both of which can be harmful to mama and baby. Luck-ily, there are some easy ways you can reduce your exposure:

♥ Remove all sources of standing water around your home—they're literal breeding grounds for mosquito larvae.

- To keep your skin covered, choose long, flowing maxi dresses or long-sleeved linen shirts—light fabrics will prevent you from melting in the summer heat.

- When the sun starts to set, head inside. Mosquitos are most active (and most likely to bite) at dusk.

- Explore natural mosquito spray. There's no doubt that DEET-based bug repellent is effective, and while not *ideal* (DEET is a known neurotoxin), a bit of bug spray may present a lower risk to you than a mosquito-borne illness. If you live in a low-risk area of the country, however, look into natural mosquito repellents that are safe for pregnant moms. Finally, beware of citronella candles, which often contain artificial fragrance rather than pure essential oil. If you have an outdoor outlet, you're better off diffusing citronella oil instead.

CHECK YOUR PERSONAL CARE PRODUCTS

Unfortunately, the vast majority of personal care products—shampoo, conditioner, body wash, cosmetics, toothpaste, shaving cream, and laundry detergent, to name but a *few*—contain loads of chemicals that may be harmful in ways we are only just beginning to fully understand. Phthalates, for example, are known endocrine disruptors (just like BPA); they've been linked to childhood obesity, infertility in men, and higher risks of attention-deficit/hyperactivity disorder (ADHD). Yet, they can show up in everything from deodorant, hairspray, and virtually anything fragranced to pesticides, carpeting, and shower curtains. Parabens and sodium lauryl/laureth sulfate (SLS/SLES) meanwhile are *suspected* endocrine disruptors, and there's some concern that both might be carcinogenic. Eek!

The thing is, it's just not possible to completely avoid exposure to these kinds of chemicals 100 percent of the time (unless you want to live in a bubble!). It is possible, however, to lessen your exposure, and to prioritize what's most important to you. (For example, if there's a brand of shampoo you can't live without, you can make sure your soap and laundry detergent are paraben- and lauryl sulfate-free.) Whenever possible, opt for 100 percent natural products, such as soaps made from goat's milk, oatmeal (my personal favorite), or vegetable oils, or soap that's pure castile. Read the labels, and avoid ingredients with any mention of the word *phthalate* (like diethyl phthalate) or *laureth* in the name. The Environmental Working Group's Skin Deep Cosmetics Database (ewg .org) and the GoodGuide (goodguide.com) are both excellent web-based resources that rate or score products based on their toxicity level. Anything you're curious about or suspicious of, you can look up in a flash.

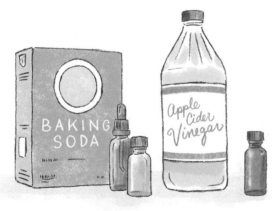

TOSS YOUR TOXIC HOUSEHOLD CLEANING PRODUCTS

I remember cleaning my very first apartment after graduating from college and having to open the windows because I felt like I was going to pass out. Oh, how little I knew back then about those toxic fumes! These days, the link between harsh cleaning products and asthma and respiratory issues is well known, but you'll want to be especially careful if you're expecting: According to a 2010 study by the New York State Department of Health, children born to women who held cleaning jobs while pregnant had an elevated risk of birth defects.

On the plus side, there are now a slew of natural cleaning products on the market. On the downside, they can be expensive. Here are three super-simple, totally natural DIY versions:

ALL-PURPOSE CLEANER

Into a half gallon (64 ounces) of water, mix ½ cup organic apple cider vinegar and ¼ cup baking soda. Excellent for bathroom fixtures, tile floors, windows, and mirrors, but don't use on marble or wood.

MOLD AND MILDEW REMOVER

Into 1 cup of water, add ½ cup of 3 percent hydrogen peroxide. Pour into a spray bottle and squirt over mold or mildew; let stand for up to one hour. Scrub with a sponge or brush. Repeat as necessary.

HAND AND DISH SOAP

Mix eight parts water to one part natural castile soap—we buy Dr. Bronner's Fair Trade & Organic Castile Liquid Soap (unscented) by the gallon. Add in several drops of your favorite essential oil. Works great on hardwood floors, too!

DITCH THE DRYER SHEETS!

You may want to rethink laundry that smells like "fresh meadows." Fabric softeners and dryer sheets are some of the most toxic items we have in our homes. According to a small study published in *Air Quality, Atmosphere, and Health*, scented laundry products contain more than 25 kinds of hazardous air pollutants, including known carcinogens acetaldehyde and benzene.

BEWARE THE LITTER BOX

If you're a cat owner, you now have an excuse not to change the litter box for the next nine months (#sorrynotsorry, husbands and partners). Though occurrences are very rare, the litter box is a possible source of toxoplasmosis, a parasitic disease that can cause birth defects.

If you must change the litter yourself, wear gloves, wash your hands thoroughly, and make sure the litter is cleaned daily. Gardeners also may want to wear gloves; the feces of some wild animals can be a source of toxoplasmosis, too.

JUST SAY NO TO GMOS

Genetically modified organisms, or GMOs, have become a subject of hot debate in politics, public policy, *and* on the interwebs. Some believe they'll end world hunger. Others consider them a threat to our very survival. So what's the *real* deal?

Contrary to what many purists may think, we humans have been "tweaking" our food for millennia, using cross-pollination and selective breeding to produce the tastiest and hardi-est crops possible. The modern banana, for example, is the result of hundreds of years of human tinkering. (Ancient bananas had large seeds, and the insides looked a little like okra—who knew?) To make GMOs, however, scientists splice genes from other organisms—like, say, bacteria—into fruits and veggies, in order to produce crops with a desired trait (such as resistance to pests). The end result is DNA that wouldn't otherwise exist in nature. And while

THE MOST IMPORTANT NUTRIENTS FOR MAMA AND BABY

Vitamin A	Supports eye, brain, heart, and respiratory development.
Vitamin B_6	Helps red blood cell formation and eases morning sickness.
Vitamin. B_9 (folate)	May prevent neural tube defects and supports the placenta.
Vitamin B_{12}	Promotes blood formation and may prevent birth defects.
Choline	Assists in brain formation, liver function, and healthy metabolism.
Vitamin C	Nourishes the amniotic sac and placenta; good for gum health.
Vitamin D	Helps mom utilize calcium and strengthens baby's bones.
DHA	Builds baby's brain and promotes a healthy fetal weight.
Vitamin K	Supports strong bone formation and healthy blood clotting.
Calcium	Aids bone and teeth development as well as muscle function.
Iron	Helps prevent anemia, low birth weight, and premature delivery.
Iodine	Enhances immune system and healthy thyroid function.
Magnesium	Helps with good blood pressure and blood sugar levels.
Zinc	Supports immune system functions and enzyme production.

some believe that GMOs are totally harmless, they have been banned in dozens of countries around the world. Yet they are currently legal and unlabeled in the United States—which makes it *very* difficult to know when you're eating them.

So, what's a natural mama to do? Personally, I seek to limit my exposure by avoiding conventional foods that contain the most common GMO crops, including corn, soy, canola, and sugar beets (usually the source of sugar in processed foods). That means almost all processed and fast foods are out. You might also choose organic foods whenever possible. Better yet, look for foods labeled with the third-party "Non-GMO Project" logo.

If you make most of your food at home and stick with organic when possible, you're probably avoiding most GMOs.

GET ON A PRENATAL

Growing a baby is tough work! All throughout pregnancy, baby will steal the vitamins and minerals he needs from you, whether you've got enough to spare or not. That's why it's important to ensure that you're *both* getting adequate nutrition. In an ideal world, mamas would get everything they need from a diet rich in whole foods. After all, vitamins that exist naturally in food are the most bioavailable (meaning the most easily absorbed by the body). Whole foods also contain a variety of important minerals, phytonutrients, and cofactors that work together in a perfect blend for maximum utilization.

But even mamas who eat a clean diet of organic fruits and vegetables, pasture-raised meats, wild fish, whole grains, and healthy fats might have some deficiencies.

Soil depletion means that many of the foods grown today aren't as nutritionally dense as the food grown decades ago. Plus, most of us lead busy lives. We don't always have the time (or the energy) to make the absolute best choices. If you're prone to lots of takeout or love to snack on processed foods—otherwise known as the "standard American diet"—you're almost certainly not getting enough of what you need.

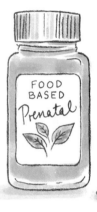

Enter prenatal vitamins, which became a standard form of care after researchers discovered a very strong link between folate and iron deficiencies and certain types of birth defects. Most doctors will tell you that prenatal vitamins are important if not essential during pregnancy. Some will recommend you begin taking them as early as six months to a year before trying to conceive.

Unfortunately, both prescription and OTC prenatals (the kind you can pick up at virtually any drugstore) can be really tough to take—heartburn, indigestion, cramps, queasiness, and constipation are all common side effects. They're also synthetic, highly processed prenatals, where individual vitamins are isolated and separated from their natural cofactors. Synthetic vitamins are less bioavailable than vitamins that exist naturally in food (one reason that prenatals will never replace the need to eat a healthy, balanced diet during your pregnancy). Synthetic vitamins have also been linked, ironically, to a host of health issues. Synthetic vitamin E, for example, has been associated with an increased risk for hemorrhagic stroke and prostate cancer, and in pregnant women, babies born with congenital heart defects. High levels of synthetic vitamin A, meanwhile, have also been linked to birth defects when taken by pregnant women. And that brings us to the synthetic form of folate—folic acid.

Folic acid is arguably the most important nutrient to take in supplement form during pregnancy. The link between low folate levels and neural tube defects (i.e., defects of the brain, spine, or spinal cord) is so strong that in 1998 the US government declared that all refined grains—flour, bread, breakfast cereal, rice, pasta, noodles—had to be fortified with folic acid. (Unless you're 100 percent gluten-free, you've likely been ingesting small amounts of folic acid, unknowingly, for nearly two decades.) Folic acid, however, isn't the same as folate. And while rates of neural tube defects did go down—a 36 percent decrease over the first ten years of the program—there is some concern that too much folic acid, for certain people, might be harmful. Recent research also suggests that up to 50 percent of Americans have at least one mutation in their MTHFR gene, which can make converting folic acid (and even folate) into a usable form incredibly difficult. The unusable folic acid starts to build up in the body, leading to—ironically—a folate deficiency, as well as other health issues.

So, where does all that leave us?

Generally speaking, you'll want a natural, food-based prenatal.

They *are* more expensive, and they often have lower levels of each vitamin and mineral than what you'll find in a purely synthetic version; however, they tend to be gentler on the tummy and more easily absorbed in the body, and they contain fewer unnecessary filler ingredients. Keep in mind that just because the label says "natural" or "food-based" doesn't mean it's 100 percent free of synthetic ingredients. Look for actual food sources listed on the label—like "oranges" or "acerola cherry" as opposed to "vitamin C" (with no explanation of where the vitamin came from). Popular brands include Garden of Life, Vitamin Code, and—the prenatal I took—MegaFood Baby & Me (I like that they include choline in their formulas).

Ideally, the prenatal you choose will fulfill 100 percent of the Daily Value (i.e., recommended dose) for each of the important nutrients you'll need during pregnancy. However, many food-based prenatals will have little to no calcium or magnesium, which is why I made sure to eat plenty of organic, whole-fat dairy products and took supplemental magnesium at night for a restful sleep. Two more important things to look out for when you're browsing the shelves:

VITAMIN A

Many manufacturers started dropping the amount of vitamin A in their prenatals after research linked large doses (more than 10,000 IU, or international units, a day) to birth defects, including malformations of the head, heart, brain, and spinal cord. Some healthcare providers, however, have gone a little overboard, and now suggest little to no supplementary vitamin A—at all—for their pregnant patients. That can be a pretty big problem.

Vitamin A is a vital nutrient for a growing baby, and deficiency has been linked to birth defects, too.

What's important to note is that the research in question focused only on the preformed type of vitamin A known as retinol, and it largely had to do with retinol taken in *synthetic supplement form*. Beta-carotene, on the other hand, is a plant-based precursor to vitamin A (meaning it converts to vitamin A in the human body), which has *not* been shown to cause birth defects. Unfortunately, isolated synthetic beta-carotene isn't so great in supplement form, either—it's been linked to an increased risk of lung cancer in smokers. Ugh, what's a natural mama to do?!

Well, most high-quality, food-based prenatals take a middle-of-the-road stance and contain vitamin A in the form of "mixed carotenoids" or "natural beta-carotene" in a dosage between 3,500 and 5,000 IU. You can also incorporate natural, food-based forms of vitamin A into your diet, but we'll talk more about that in the next chapter.

FOLATE

When it comes to this all-important nutrient, you'll want a prenatal that offers folate rather than folic acid, in a dosage at or very near 100 percent of the Daily Value (800 mcg per day). Women who have the MTHFR mutation, meanwhile, may want to look for a prenatal that offers a "methylated" type of folate (folate that's already been converted to a usable form). It'll be listed as L-5-methyltetrahydrofolate, L-methylfolate, or L-5-MTHF on the label.

We are only just beginning to understand MTHFR defects and their implications. While genetic testing is available, many people who have the mutation are asymptomatic (although some *very* early-stage research indicates that women with a history of recurrent and unexplained miscarriages might have a MTHFR mutation). If you don't know, think you might have the mutation, or have a history of miscarriages, you might want to take a prenatal with methylfolate, just to be safe. It won't harm you, and you'll still get an adequate amount of folate even if you don't have the mutation. Of course, let your midwife or doctor know if you're super-sensitive to supplements, even "natural" ones, and work with him or her to determine the best prenatal support for you.

~ mama-do list ~

- Pick out a natural, food-based prenatal vitamin and get on it.

- Consult your healthcare provider about any medications or supplements you may be taking, prescription, over-the-counter, and nutritional supplements.

- Curb your alcohol consumption (or quit completely), even if you're still in the baby-making stage.

- Consider tossing out some of those old, scratched-up plastic food storage containers and eliminating your exposure to toxic chemicals and endocrine disruptors.

- If you're in the market for a home pregnancy test, know that the more *sensitive* the test is, the *lower* the "mIU/ml" measurement will be. In other words, a 20 mIU/ml test will detect the hCG in your urine sooner than a 100 mIU/ml version. How to tell? Read the box!

what's on the menu

WHAT'S UP WITH *baby*?

Remember, your due date isn't calculated from the precise moment of conception, but rather from the first day of your last menstrual period—which means most women are not actually pregnant at all during Weeks 1 and 2 of pregnancy. Week 3, however, is when the magic happens. Between twelve and twenty-four hours after papa's sperm meets your egg, your genetic material has combined, baby's sex has been determined, and your single-celled zygote has started traveling through the fallopian tube. Once arriving inside your uterus—anywhere from three to five days later—he (or she) will implant into the uterine lining, snuggling deep into the sponge-like tissue, making himself (or herself) a cozy home.

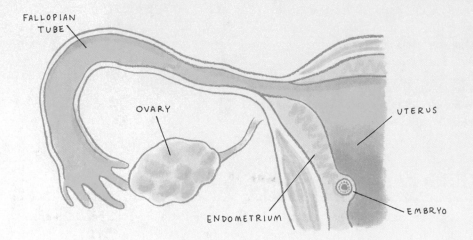

FALLOPIAN TUBE

OVARY

UTERUS

ENDOMETRIUM

EMBRYO

WHAT'S UP WITH *mama*?

In a word (or two): not much. It's still way too early to detect your little guy or gal via a home pregnancy test—your body likely hasn't started producing hCG, and most mamas won't even realize they're pregnant for several more weeks. Some women, however, may experience some *very* early signs and symptoms, including fatigue, nausea, feeling especially hot or cold, a heightened sense of smell, or light spotting. Your breasts might also feel full or tender, and your areolas may seem darker. Let the games begin!

It's no secret that baby is already counting on you to make the best nutritional choices possible. A diet full of fruits and veggies, pastured meats, whole grains, and healthy fats will not only help him grow, but it will also set him up for a lifetime of healthy eating long after he exits the womb. But Mama? Smart pregnancy nutrition isn't all about baby. Nourishing your body with fresh, organic foods will give you more energy, as well as improve your chances for an easy, low-key pregnancy. (Complications like gestational diabetes and preeclampsia—both of which can be caused or exacerbated by poor nutrition—don't usually show up until the third trimester; by then, adjusting your diet may not be enough to turn things around.)

If you're aiming for a natural birth, free from intervention, eating well is one of the most important things you can do.

The problem? There is a mountain of conflicting advice out there.

Eat mostly plants or mostly protein?

Avoid too much salt or salt everything at the table?

Enjoy plenty of fish, or avoid seafood like the plague?

Personally, I don't think any one "diet" is right for *every* woman—how could it be? We all have different nutritional needs, food sensitivities, personal convictions, and tastes, and a one-size-fits-all approach would be rigid and restricting. So let's break it down by major food groups. But first, let's tackle the foremost question on many mamas' minds:

SHOULD I REALLY BE EATING FOR TWO?

Because I used to be 65 pounds heavier, I approached the weight-gain aspect of pregnancy with perhaps a bit more trepidation than the average woman. Once I could see the bigger picture—that I was nourishing *life*—I quickly got over my fears. But it's important to point out that the adage "eating for two" means eating with both you and baby in mind—*not* eating double the calories (which would be both unhealthy and, frankly, pretty tough for most women to do).

Conventional wisdom is that mamas-to-be should aim for an additional 300 calories a day, starting in the second trimester, and a little more than that—around 500—during the final twelve to thirteen weeks before D-Day. (That's delivery day, not the Invasion of Normandy.) I'm not a big fan of counting calories, however.

It's tedious and a little beside the point, since eating an extra serving of chips or cookies isn't doing anything for your health or your baby's. In fact, eating too much of the wrong kinds of foods can be harmful. If you're not flooding your body with nutrients, baby will pull what he needs from your organs, tissues, and even bones, leaving you weaker, nauseous, and fatigued.

So forget counting calories. I think a much better, simpler approach is to count *nutrients*.

Do the foods you eat give you a lot of bang for your buck? White rice, iceberg lettuce, celery, and cucumbers, for example, while not exactly *bad* for you (they're better choices than, say, Hot Pockets) aren't particularly nutrient-dense. Eating them will give you a calorie

EAT FOR TWO? I'M SO NAUSEOUS I CAN BARELY EAT FOR *ONE*. COULD I BE STARVING MY BABY?

During my first pregnancy, I noticed that my morning smoothie suddenly had a kind of plastic-y aftertaste. A week or so later, I figured out why: the frozen fruit I'd been using came packaged in—you guessed it—plastic. My husband joked that my pregnancy "super power" wasn't that I could grow a baby in my belly, but that I could smell kale from 2,000 feet. Speaking of smell, a pregnant friend of mine insisted her husband throw out every ounce of the trout he'd caught and stored in their freezer. (Luckily, they had a second freezer in the garage.)

It's estimated that upwards of 75 percent of women will develop these kinds of heightened senses during pregnancy. There are lots of theories as to why (we know, for example, that high levels of estrogen have been linked to an increased sense of smell), but one of the most popular has to do with basic survival: in the wild, the threat of eating spoiled or poisonous food is real. With a heightened sense of taste and smell, the logic goes, mama-to-be is better able to steer clear of anything that might harm her baby.

Of course, when you can sniff out frozen fish from three rooms away, those intense tastes and smells may be more likely to turn your stomach. That, combined with routine morning sickness (experienced by as many as 80 percent of pregnant women) can make eating much of *anything* in the first trimester a bit tricky—forget loading up on *additional* calories. But, Mama, there's no need to worry.

At this stage, baby is still very, very small. So small, in fact, that there's no medical need to gain any weight at all during the first trimester; some mamas may even lose a pound or two. Sneak in some nutrient-dense foods when you can. Toss an avocado into your smoothie or eat some dry whole-grain toast (rather than snacking on oyster crackers). And hold on—morning sickness tends to calm down (or outright disappear) by the second trimester, so you'll likely have your appetite back soon.

boost, but not the wide spectrum of vitamins and minerals that both you and baby need. Instead, opting for a variety of deeply colored fruits and vegetables (pomegranates, carrots, kale, blueberries), high-quality protein (grass-fed beef, seafood, and seeds), and healthy fats (whole-milk yogurt, organic butter, coconut and olive oils) nets you plenty of nourishment without having to pull out a food scale, total up food points, or keep track of calories.

THE BIG THREE: CARBOHYDRATES, FATS, AND PROTEINS

A closer look at what to eat, what to avoid, and what to indulge in.

HEALTHY CARBS

It's a real shame that carbohydrates have gotten such a bad rap, and it's mostly due to our fast-food culture. More than ever before, we're pounding down highly processed, prepackaged foods, and we're paying for it with sky-rocketing rates of diabetes, cancer, heart disease, and obesity. Our systems just weren't designed to consume instant cereals, soda with high fructose corn syrup, and white bread with each and every meal.

Healthy carbs, on the other hand, boost energy levels, support gut health (by feeding good bacteria), and nourish our adrenal and thyroid glands. It's easy to forget that fruits and vegetables are carbs, too—not to mention an important source of fiber and phytonutrients.

Aim for *at least* six (1 cup) servings of fruits and veggies a day, plus three to four (half cup) servings of starchy carbs or whole grains.

Good Choices

Hearty root vegetables such as potatoes (sweet potatoes, blue potatoes, red potatoes), beets, carrots, plantains, taro, yams, and rutabagas. White potatoes are fine in moderation.

Whole grains such as oats, quinoa, buckwheat, einkorn, spelt, and millet. (If you're gluten-free and craving baked goods, coconut, almond, and cassava flours are all great options.) Rice is good, too, whether brown, red, black, or wild. White rice is fine in moderation.

Fresh fruits such as berries, pomegranates, apples, pears, grapes, melons, kiwi, grapefruit, mango, banana, and pineapple. In other words, just about every fruit in the world earns a big fat seal of approval. Rotate the colors of fruit you eat, however, to ensure you're getting a wide variety of nutrients, and don't skimp on yellow and red fruits, as they're loaded with vitamins A and C.

Fresh vegetables such as leafy greens (kale, spinach, arugula, collards, romaine), broccoli, cabbage, cauliflower, radishes, bell peppers, and zucchini. Veggies should make up a significant portion of your diet. As with fruits, rotate the colors you eat, and make sure you're getting plenty of greens, as they're a natural source of folate.

Not-So-Good Choices

Canned fruits and vegetables, dried fruit with added sulfur dioxide, and agave syrup (it's high in fructose).

HEALTHY CARBS

Starchy Vegetables	Whole Grains
Fresh Fruits	Fresh Vegetables

Avoid Completely

Processed grains (instant rice, instant oatmeal); puffed grains; white flour; unripe or "green" papaya (it may stimulate contractions); raw sprouts, including alfalfa and bean sprouts (they're particularly susceptible to harmful bacteria including *E. coli*); and artificial sweeteners like NutraSweet, sucralose, and saccharin.

HEALTHY FATS

By the time I reached my teens, I was so afraid of fat that I would pour water over my Special K because skim milk was just too *creamy*. Thankfully, I've changed my ways.

Good fats are *vital* for a healthy pregnancy. They're the building blocks of cholesterol and hormone production. Essential fatty acids such as DHA and EPA, meanwhile, are critical for the development of baby's brain while in utero—in fact, studies have shown that mamas who get plenty of DHA in their diet have a reduced risk of preterm labor and deliver babies with healthier birth weights. Unfortunately, our national obsession with fat—in particular, saturated fat—means that modern Americans have been shunning it for years in favor of low-fat and no-fat foods (which are almost always loaded with sugar). After five decades of fat phobia, however, the USDA is finally rolling back some of its earlier, misguided recommendations: newly released Dietary Guidelines, for example, removed a long-standing limit on cholesterol intake. You know what that means, Mama? Eggs—*with* the yolks—are back on the menu.

Aim for *at least* one serving of added fat (like 1 tablespoon of oil or butter, ½ cup avocado, or ¼ cup nuts, seeds, or olives) per meal.

Good Sources

Organic butter, oily fish such as sardines and salmon, coconut oil, extra virgin olive oil, avocados, farm-fresh milk and cream, coconut cream, olives, high-fat nuts (walnuts, macada-

A HEALTHY FAT THROWBACK: COD LIVER OIL

Ask your grandmother (or great-grandmother) and there's a good chance she took cod liver oil when she was pregnant, or gave her kids—ahem, *your parents*—a spoonful of the stuff every day. Cod liver oil is an excellent source of omega-3 fatty acids, in particular DHA; it's also packed with vitamins A, D, and K, which are vital for baby's brain, eye, and bone development. Unfortunately, it fell out of favor back in the mid-'90s, after a study linked high levels of vitamin A (more than 10,000 IU a day) to an increased risk of birth defects.

But here's the thing: the link was strongest in women who consumed large amounts of vitamin A in *synthetic* supplement form—not from food, where the vitamin exists naturally with multiple cofactors in a balanced ratio. Also important to note, vitamin A *deficiency* has been known to cause birth defects, too.

Based on recommendations from the Weston A. Price Foundation, which focuses on nutrition education, I took a teaspoon daily of high-quality cod liver oil (with no added synthetic vitamins) during each of my pregnancies and felt great. And—pardon my bragging—but I think my kids turned out pretty brainy. So ask your healthcare provider if cod liver oil (or cod liver oil capsules, which may be easier to stomach) might be right for you.

mia nuts, pine nuts, Brazil nuts), beef tallow, high-quality duck or goose fat, and lard.

Not-So-Good Sources

High-omega-6 oils, including sunflower oil, sesame oil, safflower oil, and peanut oil.

Avoid Completely

Margarine, industrial oils (canola, soybean, corn, cottonseed), "light" olive oil (which can be mixed with cheap, low-quality oil, so stick with extra virgin), trans fats. The FDA banned trans fats—which are particularly toxic—in 2015, but manufacturers have several years to remove them from their products. In the meantime, you'll want to avoid them at all costs. Examine the ingredient label. Anything with the words "hydrogenated" or "partially hydrogenated" goes back on the shelf.

DO YOUR GRAINS AND BEANS NEED A BATH?

Whole grains (like quinoa, oats, and barley) and beans are packed with protein. Nuts and seeds, meanwhile, are excellent sources of healthy fats. But all of these foods contain anti-nutrients—enzyme inhibitors and phytic acid, for example—which prevent them from sprouting too early, before conditions in the wild are optimal for their survival.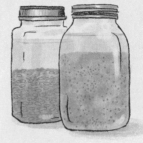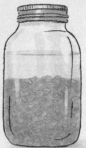
The problem? These anti-nutrients can be hard for our bodies to break down, and the vitamins and minerals that exist naturally in these foods aren't very bioavailable. Luckily, neutralizing them is simple: just add water.

Just as adequate rainfall encourages seeds to sprout, soaking our nuts, grains, beans, and seeds—overnight, in a bath of salty or acidic water—washes away the anti-nutrients, actually *increases* the vitamin content (by activating the production of beneficial enzymes), breaks down gluten, and eases digestion. Soaking is easy, as you'll see below. But you can also purchase pre-soaked, sprouted, or fermented versions.

To Soak Grains: Place your grains in a bowl and cover them completely with warm filtered water. Then, for every cup of water you used, add 1 teaspoon of an acid (try raw apple cider vinegar, lemon juice, or yogurt). Soak overnight at room temperature, rinse and drain in the morning, and cook as usual.

To Soak Legumes: Place your beans in a bowl and cover them completely with warm filtered water. For lentils, black beans, and garbanzos, add 1 teaspoon of raw apple cider vinegar, lemon juice, or yogurt for every cup of water you used. For kidney-shaped beans (like pinto or white beans) use a pinch of baking soda instead. Soak overnight at room temperature (the fridge is okay if you live in a hot climate), rinse and drain in the morning, and cook as usual.

To Soak Nuts and Seeds: Place your nuts or seeds in a bowl and cover completely with filtered water. Add ½ tablespoon sea salt. Soak overnight at room temperature, rinse and drain in the morning, then dry in the oven at the lowest possible temperature (it'll take several hours) or toss 'em in a food dehydrator. If you're soaking cashews, drain them after four hours. (Otherwise, they'll get soggy.) Store your soaked nuts and seeds in an airtight container.

HEALTHY PROTEIN

Protein provides a building block for bones, skin, hair, nails, blood, muscles, and cartilage—in other words, pretty much every single cell in your body. And since you're creating a *new* body (your baby's) you'll need plenty to meet his needs *and* yours.

Aim for three to four 3-ounce servings a day, or at least 75 grams of protein. (Three ounces is roughly the size of a deck of cards. One egg or ½ cup of legumes equals 1 ounce of protein.)

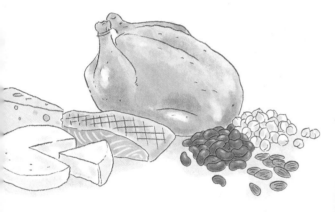

Good Sources

Pastured, free-range eggs; wild, low-mercury seafood; organic grass-fed beef and bison; pastured poultry (chicken, turkey, duck); sprouted or soaked lentils; split peas; beans; chickpeas; legumes; organic, whole-fat dairy products (yogurt, kefir, aged cheeses); organic tempeh and miso; nuts; seeds; nutritional yeast flakes; gelatin/collagen; homemade bone broth.

Not-So-Good Sources

Conventional pork; tofu (unfermented soy is difficult to digest); Spam or canned meats; charred or burnt meats (they're harder to digest and may be carcinogenic).

Avoid Completely

Raw or rare meats; raw eggs; raw fish (think sushi); unpasteurized, soft cheeses; hot dogs; deli meats; high-mercury seafood.

> Pregnant women need at least 1,000 mg of calcium each day. Include 3 to 4 servings of dairy or other calcium-rich foods.

SKIP THE DELI SECTION

Although hot dogs and lunch meats are fully cooked, they're susceptible to a strain of bacteria called *Listeria monocytogenes*, which can trigger a serious infection if ingested. Deli salads—potato salad, ham salad, chicken salad, etc.—are prone to it, too. Because *Listeria* is destroyed by high heat, some sources believe these foods are safe to eat if they've been heated to "steaming hot" (approximately 165 degrees Fahrenheit), but I think it's safest to just avoid them. They aren't that good for you, anyway.

SAFE SEAFOOD DURING PREGNANCY

Wild seafood is some of the most nutritionally dense food on the planet: full of protein; loaded with trace minerals like iodine, selenium, and zinc; and packed with omega-3 fatty acids. The FDA, the American Pregnancy Association, and the Academy of Nutrition and Dietetics *all* recommend moderate fish consumption for pregnant mamas, provided you limit yourself to 12 ounces, or about two to three servings, a week.

The concern about fish during pregnancy—and the reason it was once considered off-limits during pregnancy—has to do with mercury, which collects in oceans, lakes, and streams and accumulates in the bodies of fish over time, where it turns into methylmercury, a potent neurotoxin. High levels of methylmercury can cause nervous, digestive, neurological, and immune system problems in adults. For babies in utero, it's especially dangerous.

In other words: you want to eat fish, you just want to make sure—and this is crucial—that it's the right *type*. Smaller species are best, since bigger fish tend to have higher levels of mercury. To further reduce environmental contaminants, remove the skin and *always* make sure your fish is well cooked.

Seafood to eat during pregnancy
(lowest in mercury)

Wild salmon	Sardines
Herring	Trout
Shrimp	Atlantic and Pacific mackerel
Anchovies	Oysters (cooked)

Seafood to limit during pregnancy
(no more than 6 ounces per week)

Bluefish	Sea bass
Grouper	Albacore or "white" tuna

Seafood to avoid during pregnancy
(highest in mercury)

Swordfish	Tilefish
Marlin	Orange roughy
Mackerel (King or Spanish)	Ahi tuna
	Shark

PROTEIN AND THE BREWER DIET

I didn't up my protein intake much during my first pregnancy. I knew, of course, that protein is essential for baby's development, as well as breast health and the growth of uterine tissue. I'd heard about the benefits of eating a high-protein diet in my childbirth class. I'd even made some light tweaks to my diet, like eating more Greek yogurt and sprinkling nutritional yeast flakes into my smoothies. But I didn't make eating more protein a priority, nor even think about it that much. Fast-forward to the last six or eight weeks of my pregnancy, and my feet and ankles looked like they belonged on the Stay Puft Marshmallow Man.

During my second pregnancy, I craved protein something fierce. A typical breakfast was poached eggs and avocado. Throughout the day, I'd nosh on yogurt, meat (preferably red), nuts, and cheese. And as I neared my due date, even though I was big as a house, I experienced no swelling. Zip. Zero. Nada.

It turns out that a high-protein diet may be a great way to stave off not only swelling but some other not-so-great pregnancy ailments.

Obstetrician and researcher Dr. Thomas Brewer proposed that preeclampsia (dangerously high blood pressure, which typically shows up in the third trimester) is due to abnormal blood volume caused by inadequate nutrition. In the 1950s and '60s, he developed the Brewer Diet in order to treat preeclampsia and gestational diabetes in his patients. (Here's some counterintuitive info: he also advocated salting everything to taste. During pregnancy, the amount of blood pumping through your veins increases by about 50 percent; adequate salt intake helps to support this increase.) For some mamas, however, the Brewer Diet can be tough to follow—among other requirements, it calls for 80 to 100 grams of protein a day, which is a lot. It's also not without controversy. For example, new research indicates that preeclampsia may be linked to abnormal placenta attachment rather than anything diet-related. Brewer also supported unrestricted weight gain during pregnancy, which the vast majority of doctors will tell you is not only unhealthy, but dangerous. Still, I noticed a marked difference between my two pregnancies, and many midwives would agree that pregnant mamas should incorporate more protein into their diets.

HEALTHY BEVERAGES

You already know that staying well hydrated is important for your overall health, but it's essential during pregnancy. You need more fluids than usual to support the formation of amniotic fluid and for breast milk production. Mamas-to-be are also supplying nutrients—and removing waste—for two, and water helps flush that waste from the kidneys and keeps the digestive system moving. Another plus: drinking adequate amounts of water can lower your risk of urinary tract infection (UTI) and constipation, two common pregnancy complaints. So, drink up—especially when the temperature outside starts to rise. Just be sure to use a filter if you're drinking straight from the tap.

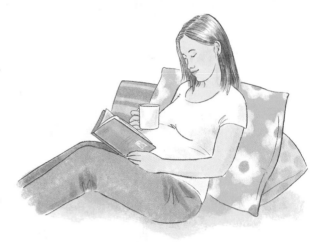

Aim to drink half your body weight in ounces per day, the bulk of which should be filtered or spring water. (Coffee, caffeinated tea, and soda don't count!)

Good Sources

Spring or filtered water; homemade lemonade or limeade; tart cherry or cranberry juice (with no added sugars); coconut water; kefir; additive-free coconut, almond, and other nut milks; ginger, lemon, or peppermint tea in moderation; organic whole milk.

Not-So-Good Sources

Coffee; black, white, or oolong tea (no more than 2 cups a day); natural sodas; orange and other sweet juices (high in sugar); commercial and/or sweetened rice, almond, and coconut milks.

Avoid Completely

Excessive green tea (it's thought to limit folate absorption—no more than a cup or so a day); raw milk; soy milk; condensed milk; skim milk (devoid of nutrition); regular or diet soda; Gatorade and other sports drinks; Red Bull and other energy drinks; Crystal Light and other beverages with artificial sweeteners; unpasteurized, store-bought juices.

CAN I DRINK COFFEE?

I'm not a coffee drinker, but I've seen the love, devotion—*and urgency*—with which many mamas consume their morning cup o' Joe. Caffeine, however, is a stimulant (it boosts your heart rate) as well as a diuretic (it can dehydrate you), so you definitely don't want to overdo it while pregnant. Though numerous animal studies have shown that caffeine can cause premature labor and preterm delivery, the science in humans is much less clear: some studies show a correlation between increased risk for miscarriage and consumption of caffeine in excess of 200 milligrams a day (the equivalent of about 12 ounces of coffee). Others didn't identify any adverse effects in women who consumed less than 300 milligrams. I think your safest bet, however, is to limit yourself to one cup a day. Consider having less—or none at all—during the first trimester (when the risk of miscarriage is higher). No need to go cold turkey, however. The last thing you need is a caffeine withdrawal headache!

Are you a soda lover? For an occasional fizzy treat, stick with natural sodas or stevia-sweetened sodas like Zevia and Virgil's Zero Soda. Kombucha can also curb soda cravings—read more about it on page 206.

And if you think doubling down on green or black tea might make for a good coffee substitute, think again. Some studies suggest these teas—particularly green tea—may inhibit folate absorption. Best to limit yourself to no more than a cup a day, and to avoid it entirely during the first trimester.

WHAT ABOUT JUICING?

Unpasteurized store-bought juices—including most cold-pressed juices—are out due to contamination risks, but you can safely make your own juice at home. Just be sure to wash your fruits and veggies well, especially your leafy greens. Here's a not-so-fun fact: leafy greens are the second most common source of E. coli outbreaks in the United States (beef is the first). In 2012, the FDA actually rated them No. 1 on its "riskiest foods" list. So give your veggies a quick spritz with a three-parts-water to one-part-vinegar mixture—it's more effective at removing bacteria and pesticide residue than water alone. You'll also want to balance out fruits and sugary vegetables (like beets and carrots) with non-starchy ones like lemons, limes, lettuce, cucumber, and celery to keep your blood sugar nice and steady.

A WORD ABOUT WEIRD PREGNANCY CRAVINGS

The idea that our bodies crave what they need—that menstruating women lust for red meat, for example, to compensate for a temporary loss of iron—has been around for ages. And everybody knows that pregnant women can get some pretty weird cravings: pickles and ice cream, lemons straight up, hot sauce on everything. During my second pregnancy, I was suddenly desperate for milk. I *hate* milk, but I guzzled roughly a quart a day all throughout the first tri-

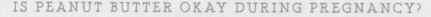

IS PEANUT BUTTER OKAY DURING PREGNANCY?

Due to sharp increases in allergies among young children, the American Academy of Pediatrics began urging pregnant women—two decades ago, now—to refrain from eating peanuts and tree nuts. However, studies have since shown that (a) this is not effective in reducing nut allergies, and (b) may even be a culprit of *more* allergies. So, in 2008, the AAP reversed its position. Bottom line? If you aren't allergic, consume these nuts freely. In fact, I *made* myself eat a little peanut butter (not a fan) just in case it might be protective. Call it a coincidence, but neither of my kids has a nut allergy.

TIPS FOR VEGETARIANS AND VEGANS

FROM NURSE/DOULA *Maura*

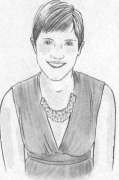

I was following a vegetarian diet when I got pregnant with my first child, but I soon found myself craving protein. At first, I just ate tons of eggs, but eventually juicy burgers started to look *amazing*. Since I was struggling to put on much weight, I decided it was best to listen to my body and go back to eating meat—and I continue to eat meat to this day.

Lots of mothers-to-be face a similar dilemma, and I would encourage them to listen to their bodies, too. (After all, we get pregnancy cravings for a reason!) If you're feeling fine with your current diet, though, just know that you'll still need to make a few adjustments. You'll need the same amount of extra calories each day as a meat-eating mother (around 300 more per day during the second trimester, around 500 more a day during the third), but pay particular attention to the following vitamins and nutrients:

Protein: Traditionally, protein (and iron) are highest in meat, particularly red meat. To make sure you're getting enough—between 60 and 80 grams per day, at minimum—eat plenty of eggs, high-quality dairy, tempeh, pea protein, nuts and seeds, beans and legumes, and whole grains. You might want to consider adding some fish or seafood to your diet, too, if that's tolerable.

Iron: In addition to legumes and nuts and seeds, incorporate lots of dark green vegetables, dried fruit, and even blackstrap molasses into your diet. Vitamin C (particularly high in citrus fruit) can further enhance iron absorption from plant sources.

Calcium: Vegetarians may want to focus on whole-fat dairy products and seafood with bones (if you're a pescatarian, that is), while vegans may prefer to stick with leafy greens, beans, peas, and fortified non-dairy milk.

Vitamin D: This important vitamin boosts calcium absorption. Eggs are a good source for vegetarians. Vegans, meanwhile, should try spending 10 to 15 minutes a day in direct sunlight or supplement according to blood test results.

Vitamin B_{12}: You don't need much more than usual during pregnancy, but vitamin B_{12} is found only in animal products. Eggs and dairy foods may be appropriate sources for vegetarians. Vegans, however, absolutely need to supplement. Luckily, most prenatals include vitamin B_{12}. You can also add fortified nutritional yeast to your diet for added insurance.

DHA: This essential fatty acid is vital for baby's brain and eye development, but it's most abundant in oily fish and egg yolks. The only vegan source is algal oil, which isn't quite as effective as fish oil. Talk to your midwife about your supplementation.

mester. (By the second trimester, I didn't want it anymore and never drank it again. Strange.) Some women even crave nonfood items, including clay, dirt, and—scary as it sounds—laundry detergent. There's actually a medical term for this: pica.

There is no medical consensus as to the cause of these cravings, but plenty of people believe it's your body crying out for what baby needs. Cravings for clay and laundry detergent, for example, are thought to be a sign of iron deficiency, while a hankering for dirt could signal a need for more soil-based probiotics, which can aid in digestion and boost good bacteria in the gut. Obviously, you never want to eat harmful substances during your pregnancy—or ever (if you think you have pica, give your doctor a call and don't be embarrassed; it's surprisingly common). But generally, I find that if we listen to our body's promptings, it won't be telling us to eat Froot Loops and Twinkies, but rather whole, unpro-

THE POWER OF
BIRTH AFFIRMATIONS

During my first pregnancy, I occasionally listened to "birth affirmations"—positive, inspirational statements to promote relaxation and dispel fear during childbirth—although truthfully, I thought the whole idea was sort of hokey. After a twenty-seven-hour labor to deliver my son, however, I changed my tune. (It turns out that pain is an excellent motivator!) During my second pregnancy, I decided to train my *mind*, as well as my body. I listened to natural childbirth affirmations during the weeks preceding the birth, on the way to the hospital, and during labor, and I truly believe it made all the difference.

My daughter was born within an hour of our arrival, and her birth was nearly pain-free!

That's why you'll find a positive affirmation at the end of each chapter going forward. I encourage you to ruminate on the affirmation—say it aloud to yourself, or write it down and post it in a place you'll see regularly. It could make all the difference for you, too, Mama!

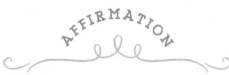

AFFIRMATION

My body is open and accepting of the new life within.
Giving birth is a natural, normal experience.
I am strong. I am able.

cessed foods, rich in nutrients and straight from nature.

So go ahead and eat that burger (high in zinc and iron), that peanut butter and jelly sandwich (high in folate) and, yes, even that half jar of pickles (sour flavors stimulate digestion). Trust that it's all part of the glorious design—because it is!

CONFESSION TIME: *MY PREGNANCY CRAVINGS*

My hardest "vice" to give up during pregnancy wasn't coffee or margaritas—and it certainly wasn't processed deli meat. No, it was salmon sushi. In fact, I *did* indulge a few times, but I only got my sushi rolls from a highly reputable restaurant. (Sure, there were *cooked* rolls I could have ordered, but none of those fit the bill.) I also ate runny eggs, put raw egg yolks in my smoothies, and drank raw milk. I know. I'm a food rebel.

Raw milk—something our grandmothers certainly drank during pregnancy—has been growing in popularity in part due to its high nutritional content (pasteurization destroys important enzymes). A number of studies have suggested that raw milk also has wide-ranging health benefits and may even protect against asthma, allergies, and certain immune diseases. Consuming raw foods, however, comes with a risk of bacterial contamination, which is why the CDC, the FDA, and the American Academy of Pediatrics do *not* recommend doing so during pregnancy—in fact, they consider it dangerous. Some people would argue that I was irresponsible or even jeopardizing the health of my unborn baby.

So why do it?

First, my body was craving milk, and I believed in the validity of those cravings. Second, I did my research and made an *informed* decision—I felt the rewards outweighed the potential risks. Most important, I went to a local farmer I knew and trusted—*not* a conventional confinement dairy. I know plenty of natural-minded mamas who are interested in the benefits of raw milk. But understand that if you choose to consume foods on the "no-no" list, you do so at your own (and baby's) risk. If you're thinking about eating raw, unpasteurized, or uncooked foods, I'd also recommend doing plenty of your own research.

mama-do list

- Make the commitment to eat a clean diet of whole, natural foods—the best to nourish you and your growing baby.

- Up your protein. Consider purchasing a gelatin protein powder to toss in smoothies and shakes; choose one that doesn't "gel" (like Vital Proteins Collagen Peptides) if you plan to use it in smoothies and cold beverages.

- Talk to your healthcare provider about taking cod liver oil or any supplements you're just not sure about.

work that body

WHAT'S UP WITH *baby*?

Exciting things are happening this week, Mama. Now that baby has officially arrived inside your uterus and implanted into the uterine lining, she'll begin transitioning from a blastocyst to an embryo. (Which is a fancy way of saying your little one is growing up!) Meanwhile, the amniotic sac is forming and filling with fluid—the sac will rupture roughly 36 weeks from now (when your water "breaks"), but from now until then it will serve some important purposes: to cushion baby from bumps, to regulate her temperature, and to encourage her lung formation. Because, yes, she will swallow and "breathe" the amniotic fluid while in utero. The "yolk sac" has started coming together now, too. Not entirely unlike the yolk of a chicken egg, the yolk sac will nourish baby until the placenta is fully formed, nearer the start of the second trimester.

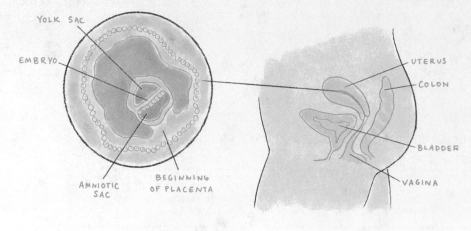

WHAT'S UP WITH *mama*?

Your body has (finally!) started producing hCG, but it's still a wee bit early to detect via a home pregnancy test. About one third of women, however, will experience a bit of bleeding or spotting this week. (During implantation, baby may disrupt a few blood vessels in the endometrium, causing some of your uterine lining to shed.) Though implantation bleeding is typically very light—potentially as light as a drop or two—many women may mistake the sight of blood for their regular menstrual period. How to tell the difference? Implantation bleeding will start light and remain light, whereas menstrual flow typically gets heavier over the first day or two of your period. The blood may also appear darker and/or more brownish in color than a regular menstrual cycle. Light cramping during implantation is fairly common, too.

Before I had kids, back when I had all the free time in the world (enjoy it now, Mama!), I stayed in shape by taking a brisk four-mile walk most mornings, a routine I continued through the bulk of my first pregnancy. By my second trimester, however, I noticed that runners and bikers along my regular route had started doing double takes at the sight of my ever-expanding belly. Perhaps I was paranoid, but it seemed as though the majority of people I passed were trying to figure out why I wasn't at home, sitting on the couch with my feet propped up, eating bonbons.

You'd think that in our pro-workout world, those fellow fitness buffs would've been cheering me on, but cautionary tales and myths about the "dangers" of exercising while pregnant persist. After all, it really wasn't all that long ago when mamas-to-be were thought to be so frail and fragile that they were discouraged from doing much of anything physical. A pamphlet distributed by the Canadian government in the 1940s, for example, warned that even *watching* sports might prove too strenuous for pregnant women—forget playing them. (Also dangerous, according to *The Canadian Mother and Child*? Listening to the radio too loudly, because "real harm may be done to the nervous system.")

Whoa.

Of course, we can chuckle at this kind of advice now. (Here's another gem, from a book written in the 1920s by an American doctor: Pregnant women who want to deliver beautiful children should "avoid thinking of ugly people.") But even much more recent guidelines still treated mamas-to-be with kid gloves: In the 1980s and early '90s, we were told not to let our heart rate exceed 140 beats per minute, because it was thought that strenuous exercise would divert blood and oxygen away from the baby. Turns out, that's not true, either—the

American College of Obstetricians and Gynecologists removed the recommendation from their guidelines back in 1994.

These days, despite all those old-school worries and warnings, we know that regular exercise is actually one of the best things you can do for your body *and* your baby. Starting or maintaining a workout routine can:

♡ Lower your risk of developing complications like gestational diabetes and preeclampsia (dangerously high blood pressure).

♡ Boost and regulate your mood, thanks to all those feel-good endorphins.

♡ Increase the likelihood that you'll stay within a healthy weight range—and get back to your old self more quickly after giving birth.

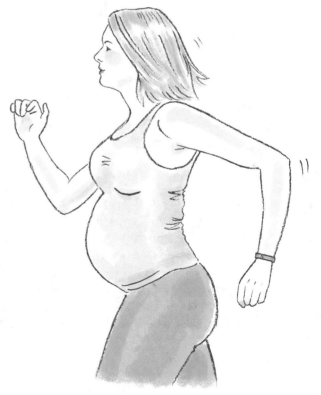

WHEN *NOT* TO EXERCISE DURING PREGNANCY

While the vast majority of women can benefit from working out during pregnancy, there are some instances where mamas-to-be should *not* break a sweat. Your doctor may advise you to take it easy if you have medical complications like heart or lung disease, if you're at risk for preterm labor, or have placenta previa (when the placenta grows in the lower part of the uterus and covers the cervix; more on that later). Women carrying multiples are sometimes advised to limit their workouts, too—strenuous exercise can put too much strain on the already stressed-out pelvic muscles holding those babies in utero.

If you're thinking that women who are put on "bed rest" will have to forego the gym, too, it may surprise you to know that "activity restriction"—the idea of restricting a mama's movement to avoid going into preterm labor—is largely a thing of the past. In fact, the American College of Obstetricians and Gynecologists doesn't recommend strict bed rest *at all* anymore; it turns out there are no research-based benefits to the practice, but there are plenty of side effects, including loss of muscle and bone mass and an increased risk of blood clots. Unfortunately, some doctors still prescribe it—although bed rest can have a range of meanings, from getting off your feet for a few hours every day to virtually zero physical exertion. If your doctor recommends bed rest, of course, you should follow that advice, but discuss the details with him or her; ideally, you can find a way to keep baby safe without being rendered completely immobile.

And the best news is that you don't have to join CrossFit or sign up for high-intensity spin classes to reap the benefits: just 30 minutes a day of moderate exercise is enough for most women.

Newbies can start with as little as 10 minutes a day, gradually building up to a half hour.

But what if you've never worked out before? If you're overweight or obese, or haven't moved a muscle in years, surely now is *not* the time to get moving, right?

Wrong-o, Mama.

The idea that sedentary women shouldn't work out during pregnancy is a myth, too. While you should always consult your midwife, doctor, or healthcare provider before getting started (obligatory medical disclaimer here), the vast majority of women will benefit enormously from even a little bit of light aerobic activity and strength conditioning. So grab your yoga mat, dumbbells, or walking shoes, and let's work that body!

Pepper Salad

Since your bag of waters and placenta are forming as we speak—well, as you read—support them both by boosting your intake of vitamin C. You might think oranges are the best source of this important nutrient, but did you know that bell peppers contain three times as much? That's why this week's recipe isn't citrus-based, but instead features an array of vitamin-packed veggies!

INGREDIENTS

1 large organic red bell pepper

1 large organic yellow bell pepper

1 large organic green bell pepper

2 organic cucumbers

1 pint organic cherry tomatoes

1 avocado

VINAIGRETTE

¼ cup olive oil

2 tablespoons raw apple cider vinegar

1 clove garlic, crushed

Sea salt and cracked black pepper to taste

Start by washing your veggies well, then chop peppers and cucumbers into bite-sized squares and slice the cherry tomatoes in half. Toss your veggies into a large bowl and set aside. In a smaller bowl, whisk together the vinaigrette ingredients. Pour the dressing onto your salad and toss. Garnish with fresh avocado. Serves four to six.

WHICH WORKOUT IS RIGHT FOR YOU?

Mamas-to-be who were regulars at the gym, were avid cyclists, or who spent lots of time pounding the pavement can more or less continue their normal routines. Fears that intense activity or running might jostle the baby or "shake him loose" are holdovers from an earlier time; there's virtually no medical evidence to back up those claims. What you'll want to avoid, however, are contact sports—soccer, basketball—since it's possible you could take a hit to the abdomen, as well as any activity with a high risk of injury. (I hate to break it to you, but your downhill skiing, base-jumping, and roller derby days are over, at least for the next eight or nine months.) Keep in mind, though, that even very active women will likely need or want to alter their workouts, especially as their bellies increase in size. In fact, you may find that you don't have to exert yourself as much as before to get a good sweat going.

Over the course of your pregnancy, the blood flowing through your veins will increase in volume by as much as 50 percent.

Since your heart has to work harder to pump all that blood around, you may feel tired earlier into a workout than ever before. You may find yourself getting winded sooner, too. That's because mama has to supply oxygen not only to herself, but also—via her bloodstream—to the placenta and her baby. In other words, you are "breathing for two," because baby's lungs are nowhere near fully developed yet. (Even when they *are* fully developed, they still won't be functional. Remember, they're filled with amniotic fluid.) During the first trimester, rising hormones will trigger your lungs to begin breathing more deeply (although not more frequently).

Speaking of hormones, one called relaxin will begin to loosen or "relax" the ligaments supporting your joints. This makes it easier for the pelvic bones to expand (making room for a growing baby, as well as her eventual delivery), but it also makes you more prone to strains and sprains. Carrying more weight around your middle will also change your center of gravity, which can affect your balance.

For these reasons and more, low- and no-impact exercises are best for expectant mamas, especially those who haven't been very active. Some of the best include:

WALKING

It may be as simple as putting one foot in front of the other, but walking can keep your whole body in shape as you approach the big day, without putting undue stress on the knees, hips, and ankles. Mamas who were already active can aim for 30 minutes or more five days a week, preferably outdoors in the fresh air and sunshine. (If it's super-hot outside, a treadmill works, too. An air-conditioned shopping mall is another great option for mamas who don't have gym memberships.) To avoid straining your back, especially as that belly

DID YOU KNOW? EXERCISE MAY BOOST BABY'S BRAIN POWER

According to a study from researchers at the University of Montreal, just 20 minutes of moderate exercise three times a week can boost your baby's brain development. Wonder how in the world they determined that? Starting in the second trimester, women in the study were randomly assigned to one of two groups: those who exercised regularly during pregnancy or those who remained sedentary. Once the babies were born, researchers attached 124 soft electrodes to each baby's head to measure electrical activity in the brain (via a process called electroencephalography). The results, according to lead researcher Élise Labonté-LeMoyne, showed that babies born to women who exercised had more mature cerebral activation, "suggesting their brains developed more rapidly." Interesting, right? Although, I can't get that image of a baby with 124 electrodes strapped to her head out of my mind. Ah, science.

gets bigger, be sure to focus on your posture: head up, shoulders relaxed, arms bent. During your second and third trimesters, you may want to avoid rough paths or uneven terrain, since you're more likely to stumble or lose your balance. An outdoor track (try your local high school) can provide all the stability and support you need.

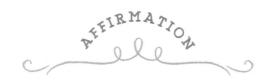

*My body is beautifully and wonderfully made.
My body is strong and resilient. My body is
more powerful than I know.*

For mamas who *aren't* in shape, walking is one of the best—and certainly easiest—ways to get moving. All you need is a decent pair of shoes! The American College of Obstetricians and Gynecologists recommends starting with as few as 5 minutes a day, and adding an additional 5 minutes a week until you can comfortably walk for 30 minutes.

YOGA

If you're already an accomplished yogi, feel free to keep rolling out that mat—but you may want to skip Bikram or hot yoga. Although there is virtually no research concerning the effects of hot yoga on pregnancy, we do know plenty about the dangers of excessive heat, including an increased risk of birth defects. (This is why you've likely heard that pregnant mamas should avoid saunas and hot tubs.)

An excellent alternative is prenatal yoga, which (as the name suggests) is tailor-made for mamas-to-be. Since yoga teaches focused breathing (in addition to stretching and meditation), it can be incredibly helpful as women begin to experience shortness of breath—caused by the uterus pushing against

the diaphragm—during the second and third trimesters. Advocates of mindful yoga will tell you that a regular practice can decrease pain and facilitate labor. Prenatal classes are emotionally supportive, too. If you can't find a local prenatal yoga class, look for a "gentle" or "restorative" class instead.

SWIMMING

You've probably heard countless stories about pregnant women struggling with lower back pain. No matter how big a mama-to-be may feel on land, however, we all feel virtually weightless in water, so swimming and aquatic exercises can provide huge relief for tired, aching joints and sore muscles. Taking a dip has surprising benefits on the cardiovascular system, too.

Water exerts pressure on everything submerged within it—just think about the increasing pressure you feel, or the need to pop your ears, as you dive deep into a lake or a pool. When you're standing in water, that hydrostatic pressure is greatest at your feet and ankles, so it forces blood upward toward your heart. This is called "venous return," and improving it helps to reduce swelling and—get this—*increase amniotic fluid.* (After a jog or a run, on the other hand, gravity pulls all that blood down to your feet, which can leave you feeling dizzy or light-headed.) Hydrostatic pressure's

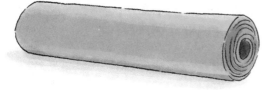

upward force also helps to support the pelvic floor muscles and abdominal region.

If you're a super-crunchy mama who's worried about chlorine exposure, applying a bit of coconut oil mixed with a quarter-teaspoon of non-GMO ascorbic acid to your skin can help to offset exposure. (Interesting to note: vitamin C has been used by the U.S. Forest Service to dechlorinate municipal water before discharging it into lakes and streams.) Better yet, find a saltwater pool or a clean natural body of water to swim in.

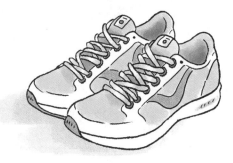

CARDIO

Whether you're a fan of Zumba or boot camp, you can continue attending your favorite classes, provided you don't compare today's squat thrusts and lunges to your pre-pregnancy performance. After all, the goal now isn't losing weight or besting personal records—it's about *maintaining* your health for you and baby. When it comes to intensity, the newest rule of thumb is that you should be able to carry on a conversation while exercising; if you're too winded to get a word out, you're likely pushing yourself too hard. Make sure to give yourself plenty of time to warm up and cool down, and if you need to skip a move or two, step down your intensity level, or transition to an easier class, do it!

No matter what kind of exercise routine works for you, the most important part of maintaining your physical fitness during pregnancy is to listen to your body.

Some women feel great running or doing aerobics or lifting weights throughout their pregnancies. Other mamas? Not so much. Headaches, feeling dizzy or light-headed, or experiencing extreme fatigue after exercise are all signs that you're pushing yourself way too hard. If you experience bleeding or swelling, chest pain, or light contractions, stop what you're doing and call your doctor immediately.

mama-do list

- Talk to your midwife, doctor, or healthcare provider about what type of exercise is right for you.

- Consider signing up for a prenatal yoga or water aerobics class. It's a great way to stay accountable and meet other mamas-to-be.

- See if your partner wants to get in on the action. Working out together keeps you comitted and close during this special time.

location, location, location

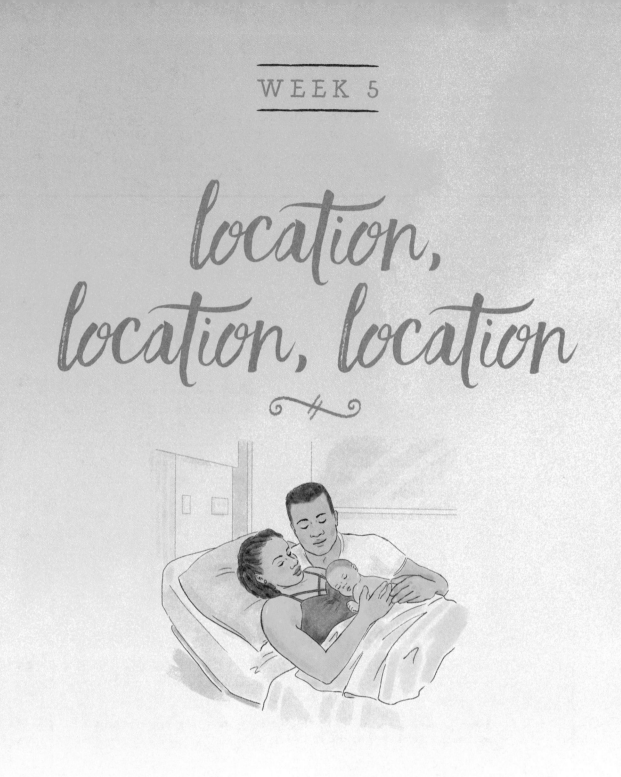

WHAT'S UP WITH *baby*?

Welcome to the official start of the embryonic period! For the first time since conception, baby's rapidly multiplying cells are taking on specific functions—some are destined to become blood cells, while others will soon blossom into kidney or nerve cells. Baby's major organs, including his brain, heart, and spinal cord, have started to develop, and his body is beginning to elongate. He may still be teeny-tiny—only a millimeter or so tall, in fact—but this is a monumental phase in his growth; this week and next he is most at risk of birth defects caused by external factors, including excessive drinking, drug use, and exposure to certain medications.

WHAT'S UP WITH *mama*?

If you didn't know before, you likely do now—because this week, Mama, you've officially missed a period. Congratulations! (If you've just confirmed your pregnancy, make sure to go back and read through Weeks 3 and 4—there's some info about eating and exercising for two that you won't want to miss.) While the majority of mamas won't experience many *physical* symptoms for another few weeks, you may already be feeling some *emotional* side effects, like a delirious mix of joy, gratitude, anxiety, and maybe even fear. (Totally normal, by the way, especially if you're a first-timer.) Some mamas may wish to document their baby's unique "creation story," so consider picking up a journal or scrapbook now to begin recording your ideas, thoughts, and feelings. As exciting as this time is, however, it's important that you take care of yourself: eat a balanced diet, take your prenatal vitamins, and get some extra rest.

Though it's awfully early in your pregnancy, chances are you've already started to think about your birth experience—what it'll be like, who will be there with you, and how long it'll take to push that baby out! You may have even started thinking about (or worrying about) the pain. But have you considered *where* you want to give birth yet?

It might seem like a bit of an odd question. After all, the vast majority of American women—around 98 percent—will deliver in a hospital.

Mamas these days, however, have more choices than they often realize, and *where* you give birth may play a part in determining *who* will assist you during delivery.

For me, deciding where I wanted to give birth was a bit of a Goldilocks experience.

I knew that I didn't want to deliver in a traditional hospital. The harsh fluorescent lighting, the constant *beep-beep-beep* of an electronic fetal monitor, the cold metal stirrups . . . None of that sounded very appealing to me. But I also knew that I didn't want to have my baby at home. As beautiful as home birth sounded, Michael and I lived in a small, urban condo near Chicago at the time. We didn't have tons of open space or a big bathtub, and we certainly didn't have any special birthing equipment. That's why I landed on a birth center. It had some of the comforts of home (a queen-size bed, soft lighting, a whirlpool bath; okay, it was *better* than my home) combined with some of the medical resources of a hospital. Not too clinical, not as cramped as my own apartment. For me, a birth center was just right.

SO, WHAT'S A BIRTH CENTER ANYWAY?

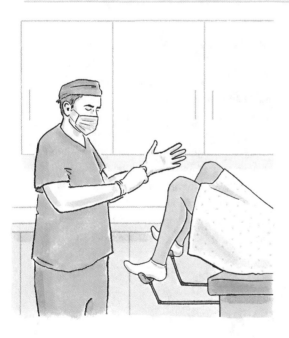

Birth centers are cozy, homelike facilities that place a particular emphasis on low-intervention, natural childbirth. Care that's often considered standard at a hospital, including continuous electronic fetal monitoring, IV fluids, epidurals, and Pitocin drips, are *not* standard at a birth center—in many cases, those interventions aren't performed or available at all. Unlike a traditional maternity ward, where ob-gyns are in charge, midwives are the primary caregivers.

And though it may surprise you, birth centers are, in many respects, *safer* than hospitals when it comes to childbirth.

According to a study by the American Association of Birth Centers, for example, out of 15,500 women who intended to deliver at a birth center, less than 6 percent ended up having a C-section—compare that to the 24 percent of similarly low-risk women who go on to have C-sections when laboring in a hospital setting, or the 30-plus percent of pregnancies that end in a Cesarean overall. A 2013 study published in *Health Services Research* found that women who delivered at birth centers were less likely to have an instrument-assisted birth (like forceps or vacuum extraction), as well as less likely to deliver a preterm baby. A third study of more than 75,000 low-risk births in Oregon, published in the *New England Journal of Medicine*, found similar results:

Women delivering at birth centers were less likely to be induced, had less vaginal tearing, and were less likely to have a Cesarean, and their babies were less likely to be admitted to the neonatal intensive care unit (NICU).

Outside the United States—where midwifery care and birth centers are even more common—women can expect similar results. In fact, Britain's National Institute for Health and Care Excellence issued new guidelines in 2014, urging low-risk women to consider delivering at home or at a birth center, where they may be less likely to experience surgical intervention, infection, and other complications.

Aside from ensuring the health and safety of both mama and baby, birth centers can provide loads of other benefits, too:

GREATER COMFORT

Birth centers are typically outfitted with the creature comforts of home: televisions, stereo systems, cushy furniture for guests, kitchens, and a queen-size bed for mama (rather than a twin-size hospital gurney), which means

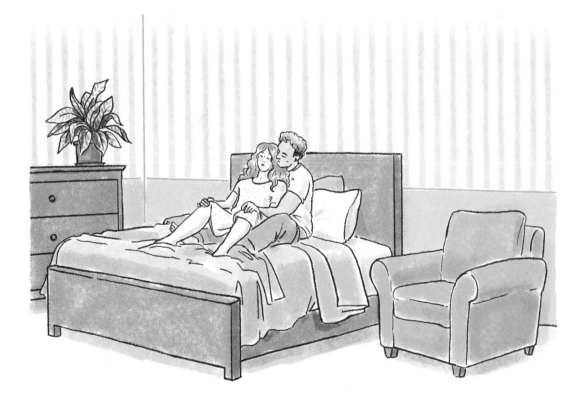

there'll be plenty of room for Papa to rest and recover next to you. And forget laboring or recovering next to total strangers—at a birth center, you'll always get your own room. Most birth centers will also allow you to choose the length of your stay, which means you may be able to go home the day-of if you want to.

FAMILY-CENTERED ATMOSPHERE

When giving birth at a hospital, you may be separated from baby at least some of the time—potentially overnight, if policy doesn't allow for "rooming in" and you're forced to send him off to the nursery. Hospitals often impose pretty strict visiting hours, too. But at a birth center, baby will stay with you from the moment he comes into the world until the moment you take him home. Your friends and extended family won't be turned away, either.

TOP-NOTCH CARE THAT WON'T BREAK THE BANK

As you can probably imagine, the cost of delivering at a hospital varies widely—which state you live in, which hospital you birth at (public or private, for example), and how the birth goes (vaginal versus C-section) all factor in when determining how much you'll pay to have your baby. Unfortunately, no matter what kind of birth you end up having, prices are climbing. According to an analysis by the *New York Times*, the costs associated with having a baby *tripled* from 1996 to 2013.

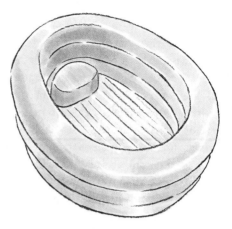

American women pay far more to give birth than women in most other developed countries around the world.

So, just how much are we talking?

According to the American Pregnancy Association, the average hospital birth ranges from $6,000 to $8,000—but the figures can (and often do) go much, much higher. A 2013 report by Truven Health Analytics put the average price of a vaginal delivery at $30,000. A study from UC San Francisco found that California women were billed anywhere from $3,200 to nearly $40,000 for an uncomplicated vaginal birth in 2011. Rates went as high as $70,000 for a routine C-section.

A birth center delivery will likely cost substantially less. The American College of Nurse-Midwives and the American Association of Birth Centers both put the average price right around $2,000. The fact that *you* can determine the length of your stay affects the overall cost too—the shorter your stay, the less you'll pay.

IS A BIRTH CENTER RIGHT FOR YOU?

Perhaps you've never before considered delivering outside of a hospital, but I wouldn't be surprised if a birth center was starting to sound like a pretty attractive option right about now. It's important to point out, however, that birth centers are intended only for

meredith: When I toured the local hospital-affiliated birth center, I knew immediately that was where I wanted to have my baby. It was wonderful—peaceful and quiet, and they had large, deep birthing tubs in the rooms. It was also nice that my husband was able to sleep in the bed with me.

tiffany: There was only one birth center near me, and I was uncomfortable with the midwife at that location, so I delivered at a hospital, but I'd prefer not to do that again. I was unable to get out of bed, to eat, or to fully relax. Every 5 minutes, I was asked if I wanted an intervention.

nicki: I had gestational diabetes, so I chose a hospital based on their support of the natural process and kangaroo care. I caught my daughter, pulled her onto my chest, and then she never left my arms (or my husband's) the entire time we were there! We felt heard and respected, so we chose the same place for the birth of our son.

samantha: The first time around we were new to the area and didn't feel like our rental was appropriate for a home birth, so we chose a birth center. I had a wonderful experience, but I really wanted to be at home for baby #2. It ended up being a great call, since my second was born at 10:30 p.m. I ate a sandwich, got into bed, and went to sleep!

low-risk, uncomplicated pregnancies. Though nurse-midwives are highly trained medical professionals—we'll talk more about their certification and licensing next week—they are not able to perform surgical deliveries (so no C-sections). Mamas with medical and/or pregnancy complications including gestational diabetes and preeclampsia, who are expecting multiples, or who are otherwise deemed "high-risk" are typically advised to give birth at a hospital.

If a birth center still sounds like it might be right for you, you need to know that there are actually two different types:

FREESTANDING BIRTH CENTERS

These stand-alone facilities are usually owned and operated by a midwife or team of midwives—signing up to deliver at one typically means choosing one of those midwives to be your primary healthcare provider (as opposed to finding a doctor or midwife on your own). You'll come to the center for all of your prenatal needs, including regular checkups, ultrasounds, and genetic testing. (Keep in mind that if you've already seen your regular doctor, you can still transfer to a birth center; some will even admit you in your third trimester.)

Although freestanding centers don't typically have an ob-gyn in-house, your midwife may consult with obstetric and pediatric professionals as necessary, or even refer you to a physician if you develop a complication that bumps you to the high-risk category. One more important thing to point out: epidurals are almost *never* offered at freestanding facilities, because they require the care of an anesthesiologist. If you decide that you want one, you'll be required to transfer to a hospital.

HOSPITAL-AFFILIATED BIRTH CENTERS

A hospital-affiliated birth center will offer similar accommodations to a freestanding facility (think: queen-size beds and whirlpool tubs). It may be housed in a stand-alone building or

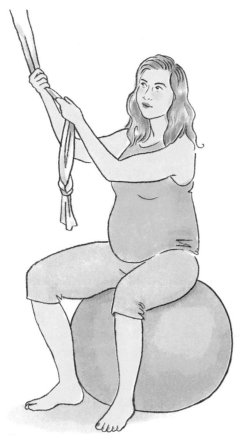

located within the hospital itself, but it will *not* be part of the regular maternity ward.

In terms of who will care for you at a hospital-affiliated center, it varies. Some ob-gyns will agree to deliver your baby at the birth center. Some centers are affiliated with multiple midwifery practices, so you may have lots of options when choosing your healthcare provider. Even if you're being attended by a midwife, however, hospital-affiliated centers typically have physicians and/or RNs on staff who will be involved with the birth in some way, however loosely. (At my daughter's birth, for example, I was attended by my midwife, my doula, *and* a hospital nurse.) While your chances of having a natural delivery here are definitely higher than in the labor and delivery wing, know that some hospital-affiliated centers will have higher intervention rates than freestanding facilities, in part because they must adhere to the hospital's policies, protocols, and standards.

No matter which type of facility you choose, both freestanding and hospital-affiliated birth centers are equipped to transfer your care should a complication arise. If you're wondering what happens in the event of an *emergency*, you're not alone—it's probably the most common question mamas-to-be have when deciding where to give birth, especially those who are skeptical of anything alternative or nontraditional.

Emergencies at birth centers, however, are pretty rare.

Over the course of your pregnancy, your midwife will be tracking your overall health and documenting the growth of your baby, of course, but she'll also be monitoring whether a birth center continues to be the safest and best option for you. Should a complication arise— perhaps you develop high blood pressure late in the third trimester—she'll transfer you to the care of a physician long before the big day arrives.

In the event of an unexpected situation during labor, birth centers and the midwives who run them have hospital transfer agreements and arrangements in place. Birth centers are equipped with oxygen, infant resuscitation equipment, and certain medications, and midwives are trained to use them. The vast majority of in-labor transfers, however, happen for nonemergency reasons: either mama decided that she wanted an epidural after all, or her labor stalled (many birth centers can't or won't administer Pitocin or other labor-inducing medications, so transfer to a hospital becomes necessary in those cases).

In the American Association of Birth Centers study mentioned above, only 1.9 percent of in-labor transfers were due to emergency medical situations.

If your midwife has hospital privileges and you're transferred for a nonemergency, she may still be able to treat you—and deliver your baby—even at the hospital. In the event of an emergency, she may be able to work in collabo-

> ### BEWARE THE HOSPITAL-BIRTH CENTER BAIT-AND-SWITCH
>
> As a more natural approach to having babies becomes increasingly popular, some hospitals have started calling their regular labor and delivery wings "birth centers." A birth center that is not run by or in collaboration with midwives, however, will not offer you the same standard of care—you'll usually be subjected to the intervention-friendly, medical management view of birth, albeit in a prettier, "homier" package.

ration with a physician, depending on the care you need. (Midwives can't perform Cesareans, but some may assist during a C-section should you need one.) Keep in mind, too, that if you selected a hospital-affiliated center, the regular maternity ward—even the operating room—may be just an elevator ride away.

HOW TO FIND A BIRTH CENTER IN YOUR HOMETOWN

To meet the growing demand for natural birthing options, more freestanding and hospital-affiliated centers have started popping up around the country—more than one hundred have opened since 2010. However, some areas of the country—especially rural areas—are still underserved, so your options may be limited depending on where you live. You'll also want to look at your medical insurance. Both freestanding and hospital-affiliated birth centers are often

covered, but policies vary widely. Know that if you have a high deductible, you may actually pay less for uninsured midwifery care at a birth center than what you'd be responsible for out-of-pocket (after insurance) at the hospital.

To find a birth center near you:

♡ Visit the American College of Nurse-Midwives webpage (midwife.org) and click on their "Find a Midwife" tool. Even if you're undecided on seeing a midwife versus an ob-gyn, this is a great way to get a sense for what's available in your area.

♡ About one third of birth centers across the country are accredited by the Commission for the Accreditation of Birth Centers, which uses standards set by the American Association of Birth Centers. Be aware that hospital-affiliated centers—including the one I gave birth at—are rarely accredited, in part because they must follow hospital policy. To search for an accredited birth center in your area, visit the Commission for the Accreditation of Birth Centers website (birthcenteraccreditation.org).

♡ Finally, don't underestimate the power of recommendations from your friends and family. Send out an email blast, post a message on your Facebook page, or try an old-fashioned Google or Yelp search. You can always work backward to see if the center your friends gave birth at is licensed and accredited.

Once you've found a birth center (or two) that looks promising, the next step is to call and arrange a tour. This will give you a chance to learn more about the facility, meet the staff, get answers to your most pressing questions, and—most important—get a gut feeling about the place. No matter how lovely a birth center seems online, nothing can compete with that first impression you get in person. If you can't see yourself delivering there, keep looking!

WANT TO DELIVER AT A HOSPITAL?

If you're expecting multiples, or if you have a chronic medical condition or a pregnancy-related complication, the labor and delivery wing of a hospital is where you want to be; this is the best place to ensure your and baby's health and safety. A hospital may also be the right choice for you if you'd prefer to stick with your regular doctor (provided he or she will not deliver at a birth center), or if you're just more comfortable in a standard maternity ward.

Wherever you feel the most safe and supported, Mama, is exactly where you should give birth.

But just because you've settled on a hospital doesn't mean you don't still have some choices to make.

Okay, a *lot* of choices.

Though it's common to select your physician first—especially in the event of a high-risk pregnancy—it's also possible to pick your preferred hospital and then work backward to find an affiliated healthcare provider. After all,

the care you can expect to receive from one hospital to the next, even at hospitals located within the same zip code, can vary widely.

Some hospitals, for example, will allow you to deliver with an ob-gyn *or* a midwife, even in the regular labor and delivery wing. Some hospitals also offer private birthing rooms—in an LDR, for example (short for "labor, delivery, and recovery"), you'll leave only in the event that you need a Cesarean. (C-sections, of course, are *always* performed in an operating room—not as cozy, but the only appropriate setting for a surgical procedure.) Once baby is born, you'll be moved to a semiprivate postpartum wing. If the hospital offers LDRPs (*P* for postpartum), you'll stay in the same spot from the time you're admitted to the minute you pack up and go home.

Hospitals have wide-ranging policies in terms of the number of people allowed in your room, the length of your stay, and "rooming in" (some mandate that baby sleep in the nursery). If you think you might want or need *some*

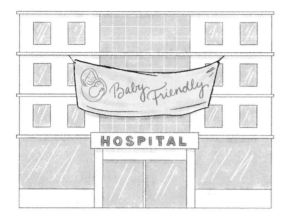

for amenities like private rooms or may require you to stay a certain number of days to receive full coverage.

Finally, if a natural birth is your top priority, know that hospitals with high intervention rates may be more likely to mandate things such as continuous electronic fetal monitoring and IV fluids, or may encourage you to labor on your back, all of which can increase the likelihood that you'll end up needing a C-section.

If you're planning on sticking with your regular ob-gyn, find out where he or she delivers now. Some mamas, unfortunately, don't figure out which hospital they're destined to go to until the second or even third trimester; by then, you've likely developed a close relationship with your doctor, and switching providers can be, at minimum, a hassle. If there are multiple hospitals in your area, consider touring several of them. (In fact, if you're still undecided about where you want to give birth, I'd recommend touring hospitals *and* birth centers. Know your options, Mama!) Some hospitals will arrange private tours, while others will provide tours in a group setting. You'll get a chance to view the triage/registration area, family waiting rooms, the labor and delivery wing, and the postpartum floor—if the hospital offers both LDRs and LDRPs, ask to see both.

interventions (like pain-relief drugs), you'll want to keep in mind that not all hospitals have an anesthesiologist on call 24/7, which may affect your ability to get an epidural, as well as influence what type of anesthesia you'll receive in the event of an emergency C-section.

Not all hospitals have neonatal intensive care units (NICUs), which may likewise affect your decision about where to deliver, especially if you've had complicated deliveries in the past or are facing issues with this pregnancy.

You'll want to consider the price: the range of fees from one hospital to the next can be exorbitant. (In the California-based study referenced earlier, the difference between the cheapest and most expensive vaginal delivery was $35,000!) You'll also want to check your insurance. Some plans may charge extra fees

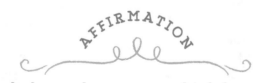

AFFIRMATION

My body knows how to grow this baby, and my body knows how to birth this baby. I walk with the billions of mamas who have birthed before me.

HOME BIRTH: IS IT SAFE?

Though home births account for less than 2 percent of all US deliveries—around 35,000 births or so every year—the numbers are rising; in fact, there's been a 56 percent bump in the last decade alone. This shouldn't be all that surprising. After all, there's just no place like home.

Like delivering at a birth center, a home birth allows for more intimacy, greater privacy, and increased comfort, since you'll have access to your own bed, your own food, and as many friends and family members as you want—even your own bathroom. You're also looking at fewer birth interventions, less likelihood of complications (including tearing), a lower chance of eventual C-section, and in the case of low-risk and uncomplicated pregnancies, equal or perhaps even better safety.

Yes, safety.

For years, quality research about home births in the US was hard to come by. Too often, large-scale studies and reports relied on data collected from birth certificates, which made no distinction between unplanned, unassisted home births and *planned* home births attended by highly trained, highly qualified physicians or midwives. (Obviously, delivering at home with an unqualified provider—or no provider—increases your risk of a negative outcome.) Other studies have been highly questionable or flat-out biased, and were used to scare people away from the practice. Thankfully, that's starting to change, partly due to the release of a large-scale, first-of-its-kind 2014 report published in the *Journal of Midwifery & Women's Health*, using data from the Midwives Alliance of North America (MANA). In reviewing nearly 17,000 women who planned to give birth at home between 2004 and 2009, researchers found that only 5.2 percent ended up having a Cesarean, and an exceedingly low number of

women needed an epidural and/or Pitocin to augment labor (4.5 percent). Only 11 percent of women were transferred to a hospital, almost always for nonemergencies. Further, 86 percent of babies were exclusively breastfeeding at six weeks postpartum (nearly 97 percent were breastfeeding at least some of the time).

Overall, researchers concluded that the majority of women had "excellent" outcomes.

As amazing as the experience can be, however, home births are still controversial. The American College of Obstetricians and Gynecologists does not outright recommend or support it, although it acknowledges that the "absolute risk of home births is low" and believes that mamas should have the option to deliver at home if they want to. The American College of Nurse-Midwives, on the other hand, believes that home birth is a safe alternative to hospital birth for low-risk women and aggressively supports the practice. Still, it's not unusual for mamas who choose home birth to face concern (or even disapproval) from friends and family. One thing that's definitely true, if you're considering giving birth at home, is that it will take a serious level of commitment. You'll need to be diligent about your health (since eating well and getting regular exercise lower the risk of pregnancy-related complications). You'll need to choose an appropriate licensed and credentialed healthcare provider. (We'll talk more about that next week.) You should definitely take a natural childbirth education class. And—most important—do your research.

Good home birth candidates must:

♡ Be in excellent health. Just about everyone in the birthing world agrees, mamas who are considering having a baby at home should have no chronic medical issues or pregnancy-related complications, including diabetes, gestational diabetes, hypertension, or preeclampsia, nor be at risk for a preterm delivery or have a history of complicated pregnancies. Additionally, the College recommends that mamas who are post-term (more than 42 weeks), expecting multiples, whose babies are in the breech position, or who are attempting a vaginal birth after Cesarean (VBAC) deliver at a hospital. While many women are able to deliver breech babies and attempt VBACs at home, the fetal death rate is higher than what we'd see in a hospital setting (5 out of 222, and 5 out of 1,052, respectively, according to a report published in the *Journal of Midwifery & Women's Health*).

♡ Be committed to a natural birth. Obviously, delivering at home means you're foregoing epidurals and virtually all other pain relief drugs, as well as most other interventions—unless you transfer to a hospital.

♡ Live near a quality hospital. There's a popular saying in obstetrics: "Thirty minutes from decision to incision," meaning that all hospitals and medical centers should be able to perform an emergency Cesarean within 30 minutes of deciding that mama needs one (although

in certain emergency situations, doctors agree that surgery should commence even sooner). The point is, where you live matters—a commute longer than 30 miles may indicate that home birth is not the best option for you. You'll also want to take into account traffic patterns in your town (heavy congestion means longer drive time), and even weather—are you due to deliver in the middle of winter in a part of the country that gets heavy snow? Be conservative with your estimates in order to play it safe.

♡ Finally, check your insurance plan. Home births aren't always covered, though lack of coverage doesn't mean home birth is off the table. In many cases, it may still be less expensive than what you'd pay out-of-pocket at a hospital.

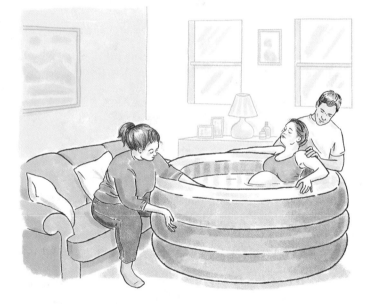

WHAT ABOUT WATER BIRTH?

Although the idea of delivering a baby while submerged in water isn't exactly *new*—the first documented water birth popped up in the medical literature way back in the early

1800s—the practice didn't really take off in the US until the 1990s. Part of the appeal was (and is) that warm water provides a relaxing environment for the mother, as well as a great

Semi-Tolerable Sardines

Baby's major organs are developing this week, which makes now a great time to eat a few servings of fatty fish. They're high in omega-3s, a nutrient our bodies can't manufacture. (In other words, they must come from food.) Wild salmon is delicious when baked with lemon and garlic. Cod liver oil is easy enough to choke down if you mix it with a little OJ. Sardines, however . . . Now those are a little harder to saddle up to. And that's a shame. Canned sardines are not only inexpensive and environmentally friendly, but they are high in omega-3s, calcium, selenium, and vitamin D. Which is exactly why I'm gonna share with you three ways to mask their flavor:

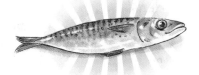

- Try sauteeing sardines with onion and Dijon mustard, and serve over brown rice.

- Cook some sardines in tomato sauce and serve over whole wheat pasta.

- Make a sardine salad (think: tuna salad, just with sardines) with plain yogurt, mustard, raw apple cider vinegar, and scallions.

For all you vegetarian mamas, great plant sources of omega-3s include flaxseed oil, chia seeds, and hemp hearts.

---

deal of pain relief during labor. And since baby spends nine months floating in amniotic fluid, it's long been thought that a water birth might make for a gentler entrance into the world. But are water births *safe?*

Like so many aspects of childbirth, the answer you'll get largely depends on whom you ask.

In 2014, the American College of Obstetricians and Gynecologists and the American Academy of Pediatrics released a rather surprising joint statement, sounding the alarm about the potential dangers of water birth and suggesting the procedure be limited to "appropriately designed clinical trials" *only*. And there *are* some risks: One is the potential for infection in the newborn, particularly if the birthing tub hasn't been properly sanitized and the baby was to breathe contaminated water; another is the potential for drowning. Even though a newborn generally won't take his first breaths until emerging from the water, it is possible that a baby might aspirate water into his lungs on his way to the surface.

But is that likely? Not hardly. And therein lies the controversy.

The statistics and studies cited by the College and the AAP in their joint statement have been pretty rigorously contested, in particular by the American College of Nurse-Midwives. In fact, the ACNM not only supports water birth as a safe and reasonable choice for low-risk women, but cautioned that the College/AAP statement "does *not* accurately reflect the large and growing body of research" highlighting the safety or benefits of the practice. When it comes to the possibility of infection, for example, the overall risk is extremely low; plenty of studies, including a 2005 study published in the *Journal of Maternal-Fetal & Neonatal Medicine*, found no increase in the risk of infection at all. (What the study *did* find? A shorter first stage of labor, a lower episiotomy rate, and less need for pain relief drugs.) A 2016 study published in the *Journal of Midwifery & Women's Health*, meanwhile, found no evidence that water birth poses harm to newborns.

So . . . what does all this *mean*?

In short, if you're interested in a water birth, discuss your options with your midwife or doctor. Know that not every birthing facility is equipped for water birth, nor is every mama an appropriate candidate. If you're considering a water birth at home, make sure you'll be attended by a skilled provider who can ensure that your set-up is clean and safe.

Looking for a middle-of-the-road option? Talk to your provider, too, about *laboring* in a birthing tub but delivering on land—immersion during labor is something the College, AAP, *and* the ACNM support.

mama-do list

- Take a peek at your insurance plan to get a sense of your options. Are you covered for special amenities (like a private room) at a hospital? Are you covered at both hospital-affiliated and freestanding birth centers? What about home births?

- Start researching birthing locations in your hometown. Some cities may have lots of hospital-affiliated birth centers but no freestanding facilities. Some may have a mix of both public and private hospitals. Find out what's available in your part of the world.

- Then, when you're ready to tour your local hospital or birth center, flip over to Part Five. I've included lots of specific questions to ask about intervention rates, available pain relief methods, and amenities.

- Not sure which type of healthcare provider you want to hire? We'll talk about midwives—training, certification, level of education—next week. I'll give you some tips for finding a natural-minded obstetrician, too.

meet your midwife

WHAT'S UP WITH *baby*?

Your lil' sweet pea has grown so much, Mama—she's now the size of, well, a pea! This week, little buds for her arms and legs have started to sprout. (She's got a tail, too, but don't worry—that'll disappear in another few weeks.) Although you can't hear it, her little heart is already pumping away at nearly 100 beats per minute. Her "neural tube," a.k.a. the earliest form of the nervous system, is coming together—one of many reasons those folate-packed prenatal vitamins are so important right now. Last but definitely not least, her brain has begun to develop into three distinct parts: the forebrain, midbrain, and hindbrain. Pretty smart!

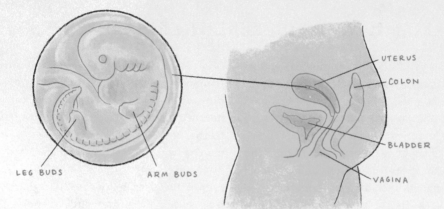

LEG BUDS　　ARM BUDS

UTERUS

COLON

BLADDER

VAGINA

WHAT'S UP WITH *mama*?

There's a lot going on in that body of yours, too, even if you don't have the belly to show for it yet. One thing—make that two—that may have *already* increased in size? Your boobs. Many women will need to buy a few new bras—and yes, even this early on in a pregnancy, some women's cups may already runneth over. If that sounds like you, consider picking up a package of bra "extenders"—they can give you an extra inch (or three) in bandwidth, which may tide you over until you're ready to spring for a proper nursing or maternity bra. Other breast-related changes you may notice include: the appearance of prominent blue veins running from the top of the breast down toward the nipple (due to increased blood flow and blood volume), darkening of the areolas (to help baby hit the bull's-eye when breastfeeding), and little flesh-colored bumps on the areola—these are called Montgomery glands, and they secrete an oily fluid to protect and lubricate the nipple while you're breastfeeding (something you'll appreciate down the road, I promise).

I was sitting quietly in the waiting area, scanning the room to see if the place was really *for me*.

Natural living magazines strewn about—check.

Another mama drinking water out of a Mason jar—check.

Then I noticed some big photo albums stacked up on a coffee table, and decided to flip through one. That's when I got an unexpected eyeful: boobs hanging out, newborns covered in birth, uh, *secretions* . . . and picture after picture of mamas looking positively euphoric from the afterglow of delivering their babies. I'll be honest—the images scared me, but they also called to me. I knew that I wanted to give birth like that, too, in the most natural way possible. I also knew my ticket for the ride would be a midwife.

HOW ARE MIDWIVES DIFFERENT FROM DOCTORS?

Obstetrician-gynecologists are medical doctors (MDs)—or in some cases, doctors of osteopathy (DOs)—which means they've completed four years of medical school, plus an additional four years, if not more, in a residency program before applying for certification from the American Board of Obstetricians and Gynecologists. (Specialists, including maternal-fetal medicine specialists, a.k.a. perinatologists, undergo even more training.) Ob-gyns may work in private practice, or in hospital or clinical settings. Aside from offering prenatal care and delivering babies, they're able to serve as primary care doctors—you probably see one for your annual Pap smear. But it's easy to forget that ob-gyns are *surgeons*. This makes the field of obstetrics unlike most others (after all, you probably wouldn't visit a brain surgeon to treat, say, strep throat or the flu). Most ob-gyns also hold a "medical management" view of childbirth, and tend to be dependent on technology, relying frequently on continuous electronic fetal monitoring, IV fluids and medications, and labor induction. Across the board, ob-gyns are the most likely of healthcare providers to use interventions during birth.

Midwives, on the other hand, are trained to focus on wellness, whole-body health, and prevention. They are ardent supporters of natural, vaginal birth, provide individualized (rather than routine) care, and empower mamas to make informed choices.

Across the board, midwife-attended deliveries result in fewer interventions and equal or better care for mama and baby. Like ob-gyns, they also receive extensive medical training, although there are three different types of credentialed midwives (see opposite page).

In your search for a healthcare provider, you may come across yet another term: the "Direct-Entry Midwife."

Until 1994, the CNM was the only nationally recognized certification available; all other non-nurse midwives, regardless of their training or educational background, were referred to as "direct-entry." These days, a direct-entry midwife might be licensed to practice in your state but may or may not be certified. Depending on state law, direct-entry midwives may sometimes refer to themselves as a "Licensed Midwife" or a "Registered Midwife."

Certified Nurse-Midwife (CNM)

Certified nurse-midwives are trained in both nursing and midwifery—they are licensed registered nurses (RNs) who have gone on to a graduate-level nurse-midwifery education program and received certification from the American College of Midwifery Certification Board. CNMs are licensed to practice in all fifty states. They may work in private practice, in freestanding or hospital-affiliated birth centers, or in hospitals or clinics alongside physicians and nurses. Some CNMs also perform home births. Like ob-gyns, they may serve as primary care providers, and can usually prescribe some medications (though that varies from state to state).

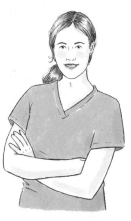

Certified Midwife (CM)

Certified midwives do not have nursing degrees but attend the same graduate-level nurse-midwifery education programs and take the same certification exam as CNMs. Certified midwives are legally allowed to practice in five states: they are licensed in New York, New Jersey, and Rhode Island, allowed to practice by permit in Delaware, and authorized to practice in Missouri. Only in New York, however, may CMs write prescriptions.

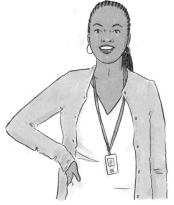

Certified Professional Midwife (CPM)

So, this third category gets a little more complicated. Certified professional midwives obtain certification from a *different* governing body—the North American Registry of Midwives (NARM)—than CNMs and CMs do. They may or may not have a high school diploma, bachelor's degree, or graduate degree. Their training varies, too. CPMs graduate either from an accredited midwifery program or complete an apprenticeship program (though *all* CPMs must pass written exams and skill-assessment tests). The CPM is the only midwife certification that requires knowledge of and experience with out-of-hospital and home births.

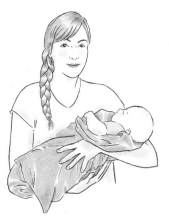

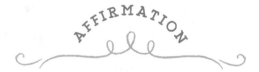

AFFIRMATION

I am safe. I am secure.
I can navigate the unexpected if need be.
I am prepared for whatever comes my way.

Finally, a "lay midwife" (sometimes called a traditional midwife) may have graduated from a midwifery program or completed an apprenticeship, but it's more likely that he or she is self-taught. Lay midwives are generally not licensed *or* certified.

Wondering why there are so many different titles, laws, rules, and regulations to wade through? After all, hiring a midwife these days may seem as trendy as quinoa and juice cleanses. Why must it be so confusing?

The answer is that many states still have archaic and discriminatory laws in place, holdovers from a time when doctors and midwives were pitted against one another—when midwifery fell out of favor and doctors began to advertise their more "modern" and "sophisticated" techniques. Some laws haven't been updated since the first half of the twentieth century. Midwifery care is not as strongly integrated into the American health system as it is in other countries, particularly those in Europe. In Sweden, for example, midwives oversee virtually *all* pregnancies, and the country is consistently ranked as one of the best places in the world to have a baby by nonprofit and advocacy groups, including Save the Children. In the Netherlands, where midwifery care is likewise respected and prioritized, around 30 percent of women give birth at home (compared to less than 2 percent of American women); another 10 percent deliver at birth centers.

Slowly, little by little, we are changing all that. Several states currently have pro-midwifery legislation pending, and a number of advocacy groups are pushing for inclusion and reform. (If you're interested in reading more, check out the Big Push for Midwives Campaign at pushformidwives.com.)

FINDING A MIDWIFE WHO'S RIGHT FOR YOU

The type of midwife you choose will in some ways depend on *where* you want to give birth. Hospitals and hospital-affiliated birth centers employ nurse-midwives (CNMs) almost exclusively. Freestanding facilities, on the other hand, may be staffed by nurse-midwives, CPMs, or direct-entry midwives (who may or may not be certified). Choosing a midwife for a home birth can be a little trickier.

Both the American College of Obstetricians and Gynecologists and the American Pregnancy Association recommend choosing a certified nurse-midwife or a physician if you're planning to deliver at home. Certified

SAFE ESSENTIAL OIL USE

Essential oils are suddenly all the rage, and they can be a nice tool in your natural remedy kit. But it's important to use them safely, especially when pregnant, as they're very concentrated and potent plant oils. For example, one drop of pure peppermint essential oil is equivalent to about 25 cups of peppermint tea! So as a good rule of thumb, limit your use in the first trimester—no more than one to two times a week—when baby is most vulnerable. And when you do use them, stick with the following guidelines:

- *When applying topically, you'll want to dilute your oil to a 1 percent dilution rate. Try adding 1 drop of essential oil per teaspoon of carrier oil (i.e., a cold-pressed vegetable oil, such as olive oil) and see how that works for you. The feet, by the way, are a great place to apply oils, since the skin is thick and far removed from delicate mucous membranes.*

- *Diffusing essential oils is another great way to reap the benefits, since aromatherapy stimulates the limbic system, which regulates mood, memories, and feelings of well-being. Choose a quality diffuser, add some water and a few drops of oil, and diffuse for 20 to 30 minutes in a well-ventilated room.*

- *Never ingest essential oils when pregnant.*

When it comes to which oils you choose, plenty should be safe for occasional use during pregnancy, including bergamot, cedarwood, coriander, frankincense, grapefruit, lavender, lemon, rosewood, sandalwood, and tea tree (and that is by no means an exhaustive list). Always check the list of ingredients in oil blends, however, since they may include oils that may not be safe during pregnancy. And, of course, get the green light from your midwife or doctor.

nurse-midwives, however, don't always attend home births; CPMs and direct-entry midwives, on the other hand, are the most likely to offer the service, but they're regulated to practice in only twenty-eight states. You can see how this can be a bit of a catch-22. To find out if non-nurse midwives are regulated where you live, visit the Midwives Alliance of North America homepage (mana.org) and click on their "State by State" tool. You can read about registration and licensure, get a list of which bodies provide licensure, and see which professional

midwife organizations may be operating in your area. You can also check out the Big Push for Midwives website (pushformidwives.com) and read through their "CPMs Legal Status by State" page.

It's up to you to determine what level of training and education you're most comfortable with, but don't forget that you want to choose a midwife you connect with on a personal level, too. As inherently crunchy as the role may seem, I've known some midwives to recommend Tylenol, Benadryl, and the flu shot—things *this* mama would prefer to avoid. Don't just assume that she'll share your same philosophy about birth or be as natural-minded as you are; you want to work with someone who will honor your choices as much as possible. Remember, you're *hiring* this person. Midwives work for you!

To find a midwife:

♡ Remember that you can search for a free-standing or hospital-affiliated birth center *first* and work backward to select a health-care provider. Some birth centers work with multiple independent midwifery practices; in other words, lots of different midwives may operate out of the same facility.

♡ Visit the American College of Nurse-Midwives homepage (midwife.org) and click on their "Find a Midwife" tool. Keep in mind that this website only lists CNMs and CMs, not CPMs or direct-entry midwives.

♡ Check out the Midwives Alliance of North America's public education program, Mothers Naturally (mothersnaturally.org) and click on their "Find a Midwife" tool. This directory lists CNMs, as well as CPMs and direct-entry midwives, who are more likely to offer home birth.

♡ You can also contact your state midwifery association for a listing of midwives in your area. Visit your state government's website, or log on to the nonprofit Citizens for Midwifery homepage (cfmidwifery.org) and click the "State by State" tool.

Once you've found a few different midwives to choose from, you'll want to set up an interview (just as you will arrange to tour your prospective hospital or birth center). Be sure to turn to page 472 for a thorough list of midwife interview questions.

FINDING A NATURAL-MINDED PHYSICIAN OR OB-GYN

No doubt about it, a midwife can be a huge asset when planning a natural childbirth. In some cases, however, hiring a midwife just might not be possible or preferred. Not to worry! It's still possible to have a natural childbirth with an ob-gyn, but you'll need to find one who prioritizes low-intervention, vaginal deliveries and will attempt, as much as possible, to honor your feelings, wishes, and birth plan.

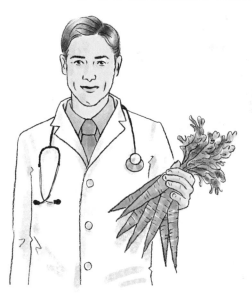

Collard Greens and Bacon

We probably hear more about folate than any other nutrient during pregnancy—and for good reason. Adequate folate levels can reduce your baby's risk of neural tube defects, such as spina bifida. And since the neural tube is forming this week, now's a great time to supplement what you're already getting from your prenatal vitamin with some collard greens (naturally high in folate) and bacon. Mmmm, bacon. Not a pork-eater? Omit it and top your greens with a dollop of avocado; the fat will improve mineral absorption.

INGREDIENTS

4 strips pastured bacon, cut into ½-inch pieces

1 small yellow onion, chopped

2 cloves garlic, minced

Pinch of sea salt

½ teaspoon freshly ground black pepper

¼ cup raw apple cider vinegar

1 large bunch collard greens (about 16 oz.), stems removed, chopped

1 cup chicken broth

Cook bacon over medium heat until slightly browned. Then add onion and cook until translucent, about five minutes. Add garlic, salt, and pepper, and cook for an additional minute. Add the apple cider vinegar, and simmer until the amount of liquid in the pan reduces by half. Finally, add the collard greens and chicken broth, reduce heat to medium-low, and simmer until the collards have wilted and turned dark green, about 15 minutes. Serves four.

TIPS ON FINDING THE RIGHT PROVIDER
FROM MIDWIFE *Cynthia*

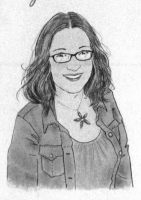

Generally speaking, any practice that offers consultation visits, meet-and-greets, or open houses really tends to have their clients' best interests at heart. And as a healthcare provider, I *want* mothers-to-be to choose the midwife or doctor who best fits their particular needs! Over the years, I've seen the full spectrum in terms of where clients are "at" in their searches. Some families come to my office, for example, without actually knowing what a certified nurse-midwife is or what role he or she might serve during childbirth; others are on the hunt for a provider whose values and beliefs more closely match their own. During these visits, I'm often quoting practice stats (i.e., our epidural or C-section rates) or explaining standard care practices.

What rarely gets discussed, however—and what I secretly love finding out—is what drew mama to a midwife in the first place. This info provides a snapshot of the patient, and helps give me a clearer understanding of her expectations for prenatal care. It also allows me to get a sense for her mental and spiritual needs, the kind of support that exists in her day-to-day life, and it clues me in to any preexisting health conditions. There are times when it's obvious that I am *not* a good fit—like the majority of CNMs, I don't attend home births, for example. But in these situations, I do my best to direct her to groups in the area that could provide the type of service she needs.

Another thing to keep in mind during your search: while it's important to know how many births a potential provider has attended, I strongly encourage mamas not to discount a newly graduated midwife on the basis of this info alone—she may not have as many births under her belt, but she may have worked as a doula or lactation consultant previously, or she might have life or work experience that even more seasoned midwives can't claim. At the end of the day, it's the full package you're looking for. Knowing you've found the right provider often comes down to gut instinct.

To find a physician who values natural child-birth:

♡ Get a referral. Your regular doctor (either your ob-gyn or your general practitioner) may know of someone who could be right for you, but cast a wide net—local child-birth educators, lactation consultants, and doulas are all *great* sources of information. Ask the other mamas at your prenatal yoga or aquatics classes, too. Keep in mind that DOs and family practice physicians some-times take a more holistic approach than MDs.

♡ Look for a hospital-affiliated birth center. Regardless of where *you* intend to give birth, ob-gyns who support labor and delivery at hospital-affiliated birth centers, as well as in the regular maternity ward, tend to be more natural-minded than their colleagues. Find a birth center that looks promising and work backward.

♡ Search for a midwife. Huh? *Why would I search for a midwife when I'm looking for a doctor?* you may be asking yourself. Because *some* midwives work in partnership with ob-gyns in private practice; doctors who employ midwives are likely to be respectful of the midwifery model of care and priori-tize natural childbirth.

Once you've found a few promising candi-dates, use the interview questions in Part Five as a starting point for your interview. Good luck, Mama!

mama-do list

● Read up on the legal status of midwives in your home state. Certified nurse-midwives (CNMs) are licensed to practice in all fifty states; direct-entry midwives may or may not be regulated.

● If you haven't started touring birth centers and/or hospitals and interview-ing healthcare providers, now's the time. Midwives will typically schedule your first prenatal appointment between Weeks 8 and 10 of your pregnancy, whereas ob-gyns may want to see you sooner than that (between 6 to 8 weeks, in some cases).

● Planning on delivering at a hospital with an ob-gyn? I would encourage you to hire a doula; she can be an amazing advocate for your choices in the delivery room. We'll talk more about doulas in Week 16.

natural remedies
for morning sickness

WHAT'S UP WITH *baby*?

This is a massive growth week for baby. Last week he was the size of a pea; this week he'll double in size, to something more like a blueberry. Your little Einstein is undergoing a serious mental workout, too; he's adding about one hundred new brain cells each and every minute. His little face is slowly starting to resemble mama's and papa's—well, at least it's starting to look a little more *human*: the tip of his nose, eyelids, mouth, and tongue are all forming. Some important internal organs have started to develop, including the kidneys, liver, appendix, and pancreas. The little buds for his arms and legs are more pronounced now, and the earliest signs of his hands and feet are appearing—but no precious, kissable fingers and toes yet.

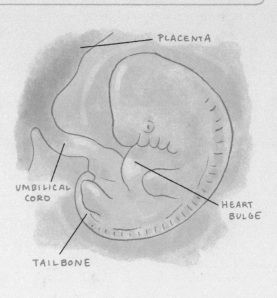

WHAT'S UP WITH *mama*?

It's possible that your weight will fluctuate a little this week: you might gain a pound or two, or you might actually lose a little, because—and I hate to break this to you—now's the time when many mamas get hit with their first bout of morning sickness. If you're feeling dizzy or queasy, or the mere thought of, say, tuna casserole sends you running for the toilet, don't worry. You're right on schedule. Other symptoms you might be experiencing include fatigue or exhaustion, sore breasts, and an overall sense of feeling "hormonal." But what if you have *no* symptoms? Should you worry? Is that a sign that something's wrong with the baby?! No, Mama. Not everyone gets saddled with morning sickness. Yay! So be thankful and let go of any fears.

How could something (or some*one*) the size of a blueberry make me feel so . . . terrible? That was a question I frequently pondered during my pregnancy with baby #2. You see, my first pregnancy was pretty smooth sailing: a little queasiness here, a little nausea there, but nothing to get too worked up about. But my second? Ha! Big difference. I warned my husband—repeatedly—that he was *never* to let this happen again. (And by "this," of course, I meant pregnancy.) I didn't actually puke, thankfully, but the nausea lasted all day long. The intense fatigue didn't help much, either.

As many as 80 percent of expectant mamas will experience some form of *nausea gravidarum*, the more scientific—and much more accurate—term for morning sickness, since the sudden urge to vomit can strike at virtually any time, day or night. Some mamas might get sick in the middle of the afternoon, while others may feel unwell at various points throughout the day. Dizziness, sour stomach, acid reflux, and sensitivity to certain smells are common during this time, too.

Lovely.

Unfortunately, morning sickness may just be—for most women—one of the many joys of pregnancy. The good news is that it's usually manageable, and typically subsides by the end of the first trimester.

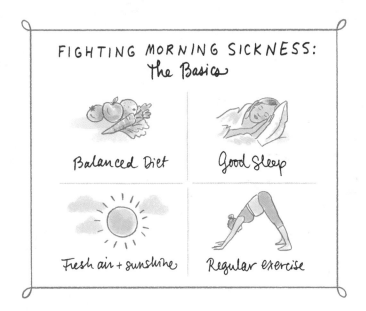

FIGHTING MORNING SICKNESS: The Basics

Balanced Diet

Good Sleep

Fresh air + sunshine

Regular exercise

WHAT CAUSES MORNING SICKNESS? THREE WORKING THEORIES

Why *do* so many of us barf up breakfast—especially now, when baby is at such a critical stage of development? The truth is that we don't know what causes morning sickness, at least not with any certainty. Here are three of the most common theories:

THEORY #1: BLAME IT ON THE HORMONES

When you're creating a new life, Mama, your body is *flooded* with hormones. Remember that hormone you needed to get a positive reading on your home pregnancy test? That's human chorionic gonadotropin (hCG). While you have lots of hormones swirling around in your system right now, hCG in particular is often blamed for making women feel queasy, perhaps because it peaks—to as high as 300,000 mIU/ml of urine—when morning sickness symptoms are typically at their worst, during Weeks 9 through 12 of your pregnancy. (By comparison, the pregnancy

WHEN MORNING SICKNESS SEEMS TOO EXTREME TO BE NORMAL

In rare cases—less than 2 percent of all pregnancies—morning sickness is more than an inconvenience; it becomes debilitating. *Hyperemesis gravidarum*, which translates literally as "excessive vomiting while pregnant," can lead to weight loss and dehydration, malnutrition, and even kidney trouble, which is why it's so important to seek treatment. Severe cases may require a hospital stay for IV fluids.

How to know if you have it? Hallmark symptoms include continuous vomiting (as in, twenty to thirty times *a day*), nausea that won't go away, weight loss of more than a few pounds, the inability to keep any food down, and signs of dehydration (dark urine or an infrequent need to pee). No matter how awful you might feel, however, the condition is unlikely to affect your baby, and symptoms usually clear up around 20 weeks. If you think you may have *hyperemesis gravidarum*, speak with your doctor or healthcare provider.

test you bought likely registered positive at just 20 mIU/ml!)

Then again, it could be that rising levels of hCG trigger your ovaries to produce more estrogen. Women who use hormonal contraception or undergo hormone replacement therapy, both of which increase estrogen levels, often experience nausea, too.

You're also producing more progesterone, which relaxes not only the muscles in your uterus—discouraging early contractions—but also the muscles of the stomach and intestines. This makes digestion less efficient, which can lead to heartburn and acid reflux (not to mention burping and flatulence). Good times!

THEORY #2: CHALK IT UP TO SURVIVAL OF THE SPECIES

Back in Week 3, we talked about the fact that mama's heightened sense of smell might be all about survival—if she's better able to smell spoiled, rotten, or poisonous food in the wild, the logic goes, she may be better able to pro-

tect her growing baby. According to a couple of biologists at Cornell University, morning sickness may provide a similar protection, encouraging mama to avoid or regurgitate potentially harmful foods.

During the first trimester, your immune system is suppressed—this makes your body less likely to label and attack baby as a "foreign intruder," but renders you more susceptible to foodborne illness. That may explain why Japanese women experience morning sickness at the highest rates of any industrialized society in the world (at least, according to the Cornell researchers)—raw fish, highly susceptible to contaminants, is a Japanese dietary staple. Societies with the lowest rates of morning sickness, on the other hand, eat a diet composed primarily of "safer" plant products like beans and corn. Interestingly, women who experience morning sickness are significantly less likely to miscarry and more likely to deliver healthy babies, another indication that nausea and vomiting may be protective measures.

THEORY #3: CONSIDER IT A SIGN OF A NUTRITIONAL DEFICIENCY

Some experts believe that morning sickness is caused, at least in part, by low blood sugar, although there are no studies to support this theory. (Nausea can definitely be worse on an empty stomach, however, so you'll want to try and eat *something*, even if dry toast is all you can keep down.) Others believe that mamas-to-be are often deficient in key vitamins and minerals, which may contribute to or exacerbate that queasy feeling.

There are eight different vitamins that make up the B family—if you read the earlier chapters, you're already familiar with one: folate,

---

NOM OF THE WEEK

Morning Sickness Smoothie

When nothing sounds good to eat (or nothing will stay down), it may be time to try some liquid nutrition. Broth, natural ginger ale, and pureed soups are all good options. Smoothies, however, can be especially great, since the blender does some pre-digesting for you, which may ease your tummy troubles. (Some mamas also find that cold or frozen foods are easier going—and staying—down.) This smoothie is specifically designed to replenish some of the nutrients lost during vomiting. Added bonus: your partner will probably think it's pretty tasty, too.

INGREDIENTS

1 frozen banana (rich in potassium)

¾ cup coconut water (high in electrolytes, including potassium and magnesium)

½ cup cooked, chilled oats (the fiber and complex carbs steady blood sugar)

1 to 2 tablespoons all-natural almond butter (high in protein and healthy fats)

½ teaspoon organic ginger powder or 1 teaspoon grated ginger (for its anti-nausea effect)

1 tablespoon raw honey (for sweetness)

Ice (optional)

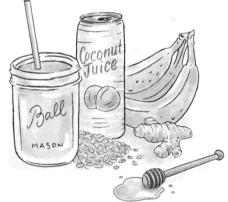

Combine in a blender and puree. For added minerals and protein, add a dash of sea salt and a scoop of protein powder. You can also empty a probiotic capsule into your smoothie to boost gut flora.

otherwise known as vitamin B_9. However, several studies have shown that taking supplemental B_6 can significantly reduce the symptoms of morning sickness. I can vouch for this. At the recommendation of my midwife, I took 50 milligrams of B_6 with each meal throughout the first trimester of my second pregnancy. It not only helped squash the nausea, but on days when I *forgot* to take it, I noticed that queasiness coming back.

There's also some evidence to suggest that the majority of Americans, pregnant or not, have some level of magnesium deficiency.

We talked a little about soil depletion in Week 3, the idea—backed up by plenty of research, including a landmark 2004 study from the University of Texas at Austin's Department of Chemistry and Biochemistry—that the fruits and veggies grown today aren't as nutritionally dense as those grown decades ago. Combine that with a stressful lifestyle and a high-sugar diet (two more things that deplete magnesium stores), and it's no wonder that many of us are in desperate need of a mineral boost.

You can find magnesium in supplement form—magnesium glycinate is well tolerated by most people. But an easy way to get this calming mineral is directly through the skin. I used topical magnesium oil, which you can rub on the insides of your arms and legs (thin-skinned areas) just like lotion. Magnesium is also great for the bowels. I found that it kept things, uh . . . *moving*.

WHY IS MY THROAT ON FIRE?

Ever seen one of those street performers who "eat" fire? You know, the guys who stick flaming swords down their throats for the sake of entertainment? I think that image accurately describes the severe heartburn that can accompany pregnancy (although, as anyone who's experienced it can attest, ain't nuthin' *entertaining* about it). And while heartburn doesn't exactly cause morning sickness, it certainly won't do anything to help your queasiness. It feels a bit like hot lava flaring in the chest, and it leaves a nasty taste in the mouth. What gives?

Progesterone not only relaxes your muscles but also the little valve that separates your stomach and esophagus. This makes it easier for stomach acid to migrate uptown, which causes that burning, irritated feeling. While heartburn can rear its head in the first trimester, it often intensifies in the third, as baby begins to compress your digestive organs and your diaphragm, pushing the stomach contents due north. This is a fairly routine aspect of pregnancy, and many mamas will experience some level of heartburn at some point.

The good news is that what and how you eat can make all the difference
(and may help quell some of your morning sickness, too).

Try to avoid acidic foods that trigger irritation: raw onions, fried foods, refined sugar, and caffeinated or sparkling beverages. Instead, opt for more soothing foods, like yogurt, soft fruits like mango and melons, broth, and sprouted brown rice. When it comes to *how* you eat, try making lunch your main meal of the day—in other words, don't eat right before going to bed or taking a nap, and refrain from lounging or lying down immediately after a meal, since that can push the stomach contents back up into the esophagus.

Some mamas also may find great relief from digestive aids. Ripe papaya, pineapple, and avocado, for example, are naturally high in enzymes that help break down hard-to-digest proteins found in meat, wheat (gluten), and dairy (casein). Naturally fermented foods, meanwhile—think: sauerkraut, yogurt, miso—can boost good bacteria in the gut, further easing indigestion. (Beware of faux-fermented products, though, which won't have these beneficial properties. How to tell? Real fermented foods are usually kept in the refrigerated section and shouldn't contain any vinegar.) You can also talk to your midwife or doctor about taking a hydrochloric acid supplement—ironically, heartburn can sometimes be caused by too little stomach acid.

Still breathing fire? Try adding some crushed fennel seed, mint leaves, or a teaspoon of grated ginger to hot tea—these have all been used to calm digestive issues for centuries. I found that the same peppermint lozenges I used to soothe morning sickness—Zand Menthol Herbalozenges—worked wonders for alleviating heartburn, too.

TAKE THE QUEASY WAY OUT

Now that we know what causes morning sickness—well, *sort of*—let's get to work soothing those symptoms, Mama. First, you'll want to start with the basics. As best you can:

♡ Eat a balanced nutrient-rich diet.

♡ Stay hydrated. Sometimes morning sickness can be caused by something as simple as dehydration. Aim for half of your body weight in ounces of fluid per day. Adding fresh lemon to water can help, and be sure to flip to page 137 for major drink inspiration!

♡ Get adequate sleep (at least eight hours a night).

♡ Exercise regularly (even if that means just walking around the block).

♡ Get loads of fresh air and sunshine. (Fun fact: Your body produces vitamin D, which is essential for magnesium absorption, when exposed to direct sunlight.)

If you find that certain smells or aromas—your husband's cologne, for example—are suddenly turning your stomach, consider switching to unscented toiletries and household products (or asking *him* to switch) for the next few weeks. And even though it may be difficult to keep food down, try not to let yourself get too hungry.

Nausea + an empty stomach = a greater chance of losing your lunch.

If bland foods are the most palatable right now, try to choose nutritionally dense options, such as brown rice with sea salt, avocado on whole-grain toast, bone broth, or bananas and natural almond butter. You may find that eating a late-night snack or nibbling on some crackers before getting out of bed in the morn-

ing helps, too, in part by keeping your blood sugar stable.

Of course, even when you're being diligent about your health, nausea, dizziness, or the urge to purge can strike out of nowhere. Here are some of the most effective, all-natural remedies that got me through:

PEPPERMINT

The entire peppermint plant contains menthol, a numbing agent with a cooling sensation, which is just one reason that peppermint has been used as a remedy for nausea, upset stomach, vomiting, headaches, and menstrual cramps for centuries. I searched high and low for peppermints that didn't contain sugar or NutraSweet—Zand Menthol Herbalozenges (available online and at many health food stores) have neither; I usually popped one after each meal. Peppermint tea is another great option (and safe to drink during pregnancy, in moderation).

GINGER

Think back to your childhood. Did you sometimes sip Canada Dry to soothe an upset tummy? Ginger is another ancient remedy for nausea; it works, in part, because it contains gingerol and shogaol, two naturally occurring chemicals that relax the digestive system. While the herb is safe during pregnancy, you'll want to stick with the food-based form only, since large doses can lead to uterine cramping. A cup of ginger tea or homemade ginger ale are great to have on hand when queasiness hits. Natural ginger ale and ginger chews are also available at most health food stores, including Whole Foods.

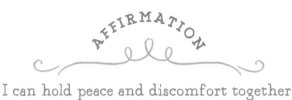
I can hold peace and discomfort together
with grace. What if the contractions
aren't pain, but *power?*

COCONUT OIL

Helicobacter pylori (*H. pylori*) is a type of bacteria that's often found in the gut—approximately two-thirds of the world's population is infected, according to the CDC. While most people will never suffer any symptoms, the bacteria can cause gastritis and stomach ulcers over the long term. More recent research, however, including a 2014 study published in the *American Journal of the Medical Sciences*, suggests a strong link between the presence of *H. pylori* infection and *hyperemesis gravidarum*.

One way to fight the infection—and perhaps get some relief from severe morning sickness? Coconut oil. It's one of the richest dietary sources of lauric acid, an antimicrobial fatty acid (also present in breast milk) and proven bacteria killer. Try using extra-virgin coconut oil instead of olive oil when cooking, or add some to smoothies and shakes—shoot for two

WHAT OTHER *natural mamas* SAY

christina: I was nauseous during my first trimester, but it wasn't unbearable. I had a very small appetite, and at times nothing sounded palatable besides pineapple, mango, or watermelon!

cortney: I was sick day and night from the sixth to sixteenth week. When I got hungry I felt sick, so I tried to eat every one to three hours. Ginger hard candies were very helpful. I also tried the wristbands that help with seasickness.

emily: Sipping on a cup of water mixed with a teaspoon of apple cider vinegar worked wonders!

nicki: Psi Bands were amazing. And crystallized ginger bits are hidden gems!

to three tablespoons a day. You might also want to speak with your midwife about taking a monolaurin supplement. Lauric acid converts to monolaurin in the body, and monolaurin in particular has been shown to actively kill *H. pylori*.

ACUPUNCTURE

Acupuncture is an ancient method of stimulating various points on the body—usually by inserting teeny tiny needles into the top layer of the skin—which may improve energetic function and balance. Studies have also shown, however, that it can help to ease morning sickness, particularly when focused on what's known as the P6 acupressure point.

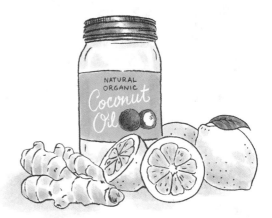

To find the P6, place three fingers on the inside of your wrist—the P6 lies just beyond your pointer finger, directly on top of two (often visible) tendons. Research indicates that stimulating this point for five minutes every two hours is the most effective way to relieve nausea. But an easy (zero-effort) way to do this 'round-the-clock? Seek out a product called Sea-Bands, which are elastic wristbands with little plastic studs that put constant (painless) pressure on the P6. I wore these during pregnancy—they're available at most drugstores and on Amazon—and they *did* help, but be warned: they're a dead giveaway that you're preggers. You can also visit an acupuncturist in your area for more personalized care.

mama-do list

- Headed to the grocery store? Stock up on lemons, fresh ginger or natural ginger ale, coconut water, and peppermints; that way, you'll have them on hand should sudden queasiness hit.

- Talk to your midwife or healthcare practitioner to see if supplemental vitamin B_6 might be right for you. You could ask about supplemental magnesium, too, or just stick with a topical lotion or spray.

- Morning sickness may be a drag, but it's also a sign that everything is progressing as it should. If the symptoms have you completely sidelined or if you're vomiting 'round the clock, however, you could have *hyperemesis gravidarum*. Don't hesitate to give your midwife or doctor a call.

feeling testy?

PART I

FIRST TRIMESTER
CHECKUPS AND SCREENINGS

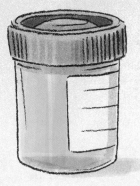

WHAT'S UP WITH *baby*?

Wait. Are those actually . . . ? Let me count them. One, two, three . . . Yes! We officially have ten fingers and ten toes here, Mama (webbed though they may be). We've also got movement. For the first time, baby will begin moving in small, spontaneous fits and starts, though you almost certainly won't feel any of this yet, since she's still quite small and well cushioned inside your uterus. (Baby's first movements, it's worth pointing out, are frequently mistaken for gas bubbles.) Her tail is almost gone now—whew! Her features are becoming more refined, and her eyes have started to migrate toward the center of her face. Elbows have formed, her arms will start to bend and curl toward her body, and her legs are lengthening and extending. Just how tall is baby now? A whopping half an inch!

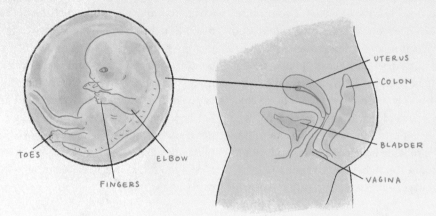

WHAT'S UP WITH *mama*?

At this point in my first pregnancy, I was working a full-time office job, and it was tough. By the end of the day it was all I could do to crawl home, shovel down some food, and collapse into bed. So if you're feeling knackered, know that fatigue is totally normal. Your body is working overtime now as it ramps up to create this new life. Meanwhile, rising levels of progesterone tend to lower blood pressure and blood sugar, which can make an already sleepy mama feel practically comatose. And Mama, if you find yourself crying over a pickle jar that won't open or at the sound of an Adele song (*any* Adele song—she's just so . . . *deep*), that's normal, too. Hormonal fluctuations—combined with the exhaustion—can render even the steeliest of mamas a little weepy. This will pass, but you may want to strategically place some tissue boxes around the house.

From the time you hold that positive pregnancy test in your hand until the moment you arrive for your first prenatal appointment can feel like an absolute *eternity*. I told you already that I remember phoning my midwife, giddy with the news, and balking when she said, "See you in ten weeks." *Ten weeks?!* Was she *crazy?* What if something happened to the baby before then? What if I messed something up? What if my baby *needed* something? But then I reminded myself: there wasn't much she—or anyone—could do to "save" my child during those first few months. So I surrendered. And waited. And wondered. Until finally, it was time.

BUILDING A RELATIONSHIP

If you've already interviewed several practitioners and officially chosen your healthcare provider, you likely have a sense for your midwife's experience, educational background, and philosophy as it relates to natural childbirth. (If you haven't pre-interviewed candidates, now's the time. Check out the interview questions on page 472. You'll want to know where he or she stands on labor induction, pain management, and reliance on interventions, at a minimum.) You'll also probably have some questions about the symptoms you've been experiencing or the food you've been eating. But remember, midwives (unlike ob-gyns) specialize not just in monitoring your physical health but also in caring for your emotional well-being, so don't hesitate to bring up any anxieties or fears you might be having, too. The two of you are building a partnership, and the more open and honest you are with her, the better able she'll be to support you during your birth. Expect her to counsel you on nutrition, holistic wellness, and natural remedies for everything from morning sickness to constipation. She can also direct you to various specialists such as doulas or chiropractors.

EATING DISORDERS AND YOUR PREGNANCY

Gaining weight, upping your calorie intake, and frequent vomiting (*hello*, morning sickness) can all be triggers for mamas who have or have had anorexia, bulimia, and binge eating disorders. Now more than ever, it's imperative to be honest and open with your midwife or doctor. If you're struggling with body image issues, weight gain, laxative use, or the like, seek out a compassionate counselor. A nutritionist, meanwhile, can help you come up with a healthy eating plan for you and baby. There's nothing wrong with staying fit during pregnancy (in fact, it's encouraged), but you don't want to overdo it in an attempt to control weight gain or for self-worth purposes. On the other end of the spectrum, you also don't want to binge on junk food with no nutritional value. Know that you're not alone. Thousands of mamas with eating disorders (myself included!) go on to have wonderful pregnancies and births. The most important thing you can do is get some support.

ASSESSING YOUR HEALTH

Your midwife will also have plenty of questions for *you*. Be prepared to talk at length about your medical history, as well as your family's medical history. In fact, you may want to ask your parents or relatives about any pregnancy-related conditions that might run in the family. You should also take note of your partner's family history, especially as it relates to genetic conditions. As for me, my mother had two C-sections, so I wanted to get my midwife's thoughts about my chances for having a vaginal delivery.

Make sure to mention any gynecological issues you've had in the past, such as an abnormal Pap smear, problems with a previous pregnancy, including miscarriage, as well as any prior surgeries. Don't forget to mention any medications you may be taking. Write down the start date of your last menstrual period, as this will be used to help determine baby's due date. You'll want to let your midwife or doctor know if you have a history of anxiety or depression, since these can sometimes up your risk of postpartum depression (but can be managed and treated before you give birth). Based on your medical history and the specifics of your pregnancy, your midwife will assess whether a birth center or a home birth—if that's what you're aiming for—is right for you.

> Got fibroids? No problem—in almost all cases, fibroids will *not* prevent you from having a vaginal birth.

GETTING A PHYSICAL EXAM

Aside from the standard aspects of any routine checkup—documenting your height and weight, taking your blood pressure, etc.—your midwife may want to conduct a pelvic exam, as well as do a Pap smear to check for abnormal cervical cells. (You can decline this, however, if you're uncomfortable with the procedure, as well as delay a routine Pap until after you've delivered the baby). She may also palpate your abdomen to check the *fundal height*, a way of measuring the size of your uterus to assess fetal development.

WADING THROUGH A *MILLION* ROUTINE TESTS AND GENETIC SCREENINGS

Okay, maybe not a million. But the number of tests you'll be offered from now until the end of your pregnancy is enough to make any mama's head spin. These days, we can screen for chromosomal abnormalities such as Down syndrome and Edwards syndrome; we can detect genetic conditions from Tay-Sachs disease to cystic fibrosis. We've got blood tests and DNA screenings. We've got ultrasounds and placenta samples. And that's just during the *first* trimester.

Some of these tests are necessary; for example, your midwife needs to know your blood type, as well as establish a baseline to monitor you for conditions such as anemia, preeclampsia, and gestational diabetes. But

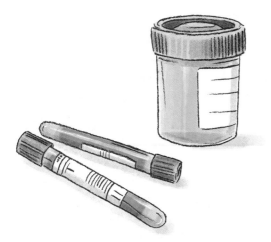

Give your practitioner a heads-up if you've got genital herpes. Active outbreaks just before or during labor can sometimes necessitate a Cesarean (to prevent baby from contracting the virus). Just discovered you've got HPV? Know that human papillomavirus—the most common STI, affecting around 79 million Americans—rarely has an effect on pregnancy.

know that other tests are entirely optional. In fact, the most overwhelming part of the prenatal testing process isn't *taking* the tests—most don't require much more than a blood draw—it's deciding whether or not you *want* to take them. Some mamas want to know about any potential health issues with baby right away, to prepare emotionally or to plan logistically (perhaps by lining up specialized care both during and after the birth). Others feel that testing for genetic disorders in particular would only cause anxiety and so opt to skip them. Still others want to limit the number of ultrasounds or invasive tests their baby is exposed to while in utero.

The point is: you have choices.

Keep in mind that all the tests you'll be offered can be broken down into one of two types: screening and diagnostic. Screening tests determine the likelihood that baby *might* have certain genetic disorders. Diagnostic tests, on the other hand, are much more definitive; they also tend to be more invasive, which is why they're often ordered only after an initial screening has indicated a potential health issue. Here's a rundown of the tests you'll be offered:

BASIC BLOOD WORK AND URINE SAMPLE

Without question, the least invasive of all prenatal tests is the blood draw and urine screen. Your midwife will order the blood test to check your blood type and "complete blood

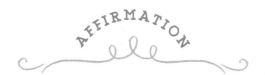

My baby is healthy and well.
Everything is going exactly as it should.

count" (which measures your red blood cells, white blood cells, hemoglobin, hematocrit, and platelet levels). She'll screen you for a range of sexually transmitted diseases, including HIV, syphilis, chlamydia, and gonorrhea, all of which could be harmful to baby if left untreated. She'll also check you for something called the Rhesus (or Rh) factor, a type of protein found in the blood.

Most people in the world have the protein; in other words, they're Rh-positive. If you are,

too, you've got nothing more to do. Rh-negative mamas, however, may require some additional treatment. Since the Rh factor is an inherited trait, it's possible that the baby you're carrying is Rh-positive (assuming his papa is, too), and your blood types are incompatible. As scary as that sounds, this won't matter much during your *current* pregnancy; your blood and baby's blood rarely mix while he's in utero. When and if your blood does mix, however— say, during birth (which is likely, especially

PREPPING FOR YOUR FIRST PRENATAL VISIT

TIPS FROM MIDWIFE *cynthia*

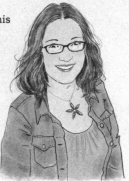

Most physician and midwife practices will schedule a first prenatal visit sometime between 8 and 10 weeks' gestation. Exceptions to this rule do exist, however. If a patient has a history of miscarriage, an unknown last menstrual period, active vaginal bleeding, intractable nausea or vomiting, heightened anxiety or emotional stress, or ambivalence about finding out that she's pregnant, I'll want to see her before eight weeks. During that first appointment, my goal is to answer any and all questions to the best of my ability—and, yes, it is *always* helpful if a mama has written her questions down in advance. This allows the visit to be more patient-centered. I'll also want to know about any and all medications, herbs, and supplements she might be taking, as this can help me identify potential nutritional imbalances (and, of course, educate mamas about the safety of those medications and supplements). After a review of the patient's medical history, I'll conduct a head-to-toe assessment of her physical health. I may or may not perform a pelvic exam. Finally, I'll order some blood work. Understand that most state health departments have recommendations—or in some cases, laws—related to blood tests that should or must be completed during a pregnancy evaluation or "new OB visit." From my perspective—and from the perspective of most midwives I know—these blood-based screenings are essential. There are plenty of other tests, however, that are not mandatory. The best providers will not hesitate to discuss with you the pros and cons of optional genetic screening and can provide you the resources you need to help make your decision about testing, which might include putting you in touch with a genetics counselor.

if you need interventions)—your body will begin to produce Rh antibodies. Then, if you get pregnant with another Rh-positive baby in the future, those antibodies can cross the placenta and attack the fetal blood supply, and that can present a *serious* problem. Luckily, this is all treatable. Rh-negative mamas will be offered a RhoGAM shot (also called Rh immunoglobulin) at 28 weeks, which prevents your body from producing those antibodies. You

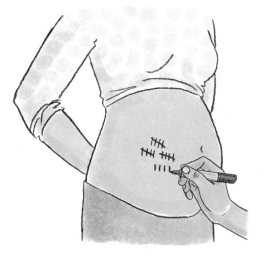

may also be offered a shot after a miscarriage, amniocentesis, chorionic villus sampling, or at any other point when your blood and baby's blood are likely to mix. If your baby is, indeed, Rh-positive, you'll get an additional shot after the birth.

As for the urine test, your midwife will check for signs of a urinary tract infection (UTI), which is quite common during pregnancy. She'll also check for the presence of:

♡ protein in your urine, a potential sign of preeclampsia

♡ sugar, a sign of gestational diabetes

♡ bacteria, a sign of Group B Strep

IS THIS TEST RIGHT FOR YOU?

Definitely. Blood type and Rh status in particular are vital pieces of information to have, and there's virtually zero risk to you or baby. If you're Rh-negative and concerned about the RhoGAM shot, you can discuss the potential risks and rewards of the treatment with your midwife. A less invasive course of action, however, is to test *papa's* Rh status first. If he's negative, too, you're in the clear, since it's not

---

WHEN WILL I HEAR BABY'S HEARTBEAT?

Although baby's heart starts beating around the sixth week of pregnancy, you might not be able to *hear* it for a while. That's because the Doppler—the handheld ultrasound device midwives and doctors use to listen to the fetal heartbeat—doesn't pick up much sound at all until weeks 9 to 12, and isn't totally reliable until weeks 12 to 14. (The position of your uterus and placenta—as well as baby's position *inside* the uterus—can make finding the heartbeat this early difficult, if not downright impossible.) And as glorious as that fluttering *whomp-whomp* sound is, you don't have to consent to use of the Doppler at all. In fact, there are a few reasons you might want to forego use of the Doppler entirely. We'll talk more about that next week.

crown-to-rump length—the distance from the top of his head to his bottom—can give pretty accurate data for how far along you are.) The ultrasound may be performed transvaginally (by inserting a probe into the vagina) or abdominally (using the wand on your belly). You'll likely be asked to drink a certain amount of water beforehand; when baby is this small, a full bladder can push the uterus up, making it easier to see what's inside. If there's a discrepancy of more than five days between the due date as determined by your last menstrual period and what's indicated by the ultrasound, your provider may change your due date.

IS THIS TEST RIGHT FOR YOU?

You may want to skip this one—as I did—especially if you're concerned about radiation (more on that soon) and want to limit the number of ultrasounds you receive. In fact, some providers will offer it only if mama is unsure of the date of her last menstrual period, has very irregular periods, or if the pregnancy was a total surprise, since these scenarios can make it harder to pinpoint the date of conception. One thing to keep in mind: having an early dating ultrasound *may* lessen the chance that you'll be unnecessarily induced if you go postterm.

possible for two Rh-negative people to make an Rh-positive baby. You might also want to ask about fetal RHD genotype testing, a simple blood test that can reportedly determine baby's Rh status with 99 percent accuracy.

DATING ULTRASOUND

As the name implies, the dating ultrasound—which is typically performed between 8 and 12 weeks—can help zero in on your baby's due date. (All babies of this gestational age are about the same size, so measuring the

FIRST TRIMESTER SCREEN

Sometimes called the "nuchal translucency" or "sequential one," the First Trimester Screen is actually three separate tests that, when combined, reflect the chances of having a baby with a chromosomal abnormality, specifically trisomy 21 (Down syndrome) and trisomy 18 (Edwards syndrome). The test is usually performed between 10 and 13 weeks, and includes:

Beta hCG: This is a blood test to measure hCG levels, the same hormone that was present in

WHAT'S UP WITH THE FLU SHOT?

If you're pregnant during cold and flu season—October through April—your midwife or doctor may suggest getting the flu shot, and she won't be alone. Virtually every major medical organization, including the CDC, the American College of Obstetricians and Gynecologists, *and* the ACNM recommends the flu vaccine for mamas-to-be. Partly that's because your immune system is suppressed during pregnancy, leaving you more vulnerable to illness, and partly it's because pregnant women are more likely to develop severe complications from the flu. Getting the flu shot may also provide immunity to your baby for the first six months or so of her life.

It's no secret, however, that vaccinations of all kinds are controversial, especially in the natural world. And in fact, plenty of natural-minded practitioners choose to focus instead on lifestyle factors—in particular good hygiene, clean diet, and adequate rest—as it relates to warding off illness and boosting immunity.

Isn't that *less* effective than getting a flu shot, you may be wondering? Welp, it kind of depends on how you look at it. There are literally hundreds of strains of influenza, for example, and the effectiveness of the vaccine differs (often significantly) from year to year. Meanwhile, a 2014 Cochrane review of more than 116 studies determined that the vaccine had only a "very modest effect" in reducing symptoms in the general population. There are staunch advocates on either side of the debate, so as with all healthcare decisions, you should do your own research, talk to your midwife or doctor, and together decide what's the best course of action for you.

If you do opt for the vaccine, be sure to stick with a "thimerosal-free" version. Thimerosal is a mercury-based preservative present in multi-dose vials. Single-dose vials and prefilled syringes should not contain thimerosal, although some brands may contain trace amounts. Also important to point out: the nasal spray vaccine is *not* considered safe for pregnant women, as it contains a live form of the virus.

For mamas looking for more targeted natural options, you might want to explore homeopathic medicine, which is gentle and generally safe to take during pregnancy. For flu prevention, check out Influenzinum 9C, which is updated each year based on recommendations from the World Health Organization. Some crunchy mamas take it in combination with Thymuline 9C (an immune system booster) for natural protection all winter long, and add Anacoccinum 200C (an acute flu relief remedy) if and when symptoms appear.

Wondering about the Tdap shot, too? We'll talk more about it in Week 12.

your urine to give you a positive pregnancy test. Very high hCG can sometimes indicate Down syndrome.

PAPP-A: This is a blood test to measure pregnancy-associated plasma protein A (or PAPP-A) levels. Very low PAPP-A levels can sometimes indicate a chromosomal abnormality.

Nuchal Translucency: Using ultrasound, a sonographer evaluates the "nuchal fold" at the base of baby's neck; large amounts of fluid at the fold can sometimes indicate a chromosomal abnormality. The sonographer can also screen for congenital heart defects.

IS THIS TEST RIGHT FOR YOU?

For women at risk of having a baby with a chromosomal abnormality (risk factors include advanced maternal age, a family history of chromosomal abnormalities, or a previous baby

NOM OF THE WEEK

Nourishing Bone Broth

As baby begins building connective tissue, it's a great idea to increase your broth consumption. You heard me right. Chock-full of alkalizing minerals, chicken stock (a.k.a. bone broth) has nourished societies for thousands of years. When made from scratch, it's also loaded with gelatin-based protein, a digestive aid and healer. To make bone broth, toss the bones from a roasted chicken into a large stockpot. (To supercharge your broth, add a few pounds of chicken necks, backs, or feet—ask your local farmer or butcher. Alternatively, you could use lamb or beef shanks, oxtails, or other bones.) Cover the bones with cold, filtered water and a few teaspoons of raw vinegar or lemon juice, then let sit for an hour or so in the fridge; this extracts more minerals from the bones. Next, place the stockpot on the stove and bring the broth to a boil. Let cook for 10 or 15 minutes, skimming off any scum that floats to the surface with a slotted spoon. Then reduce the heat to the lowest setting and let it gently simmer for anywhere from 4 to 24 hours. (Don't worry—you have to do this only once. When you're done, you'll have pints and pints of broth, and it freezes beautifully.)

When the broth has finished cooking, remove the bones and let it cool completely. Store in the fridge for another 24 hours, so the fat can rise to the top. Skim off the fat and discard. Portion your broth into several glass containers or Mason jars, and enjoy it in soups, stews, sauces, or even on its own. It can be stored in the fridge for 3 to 4 days or in the freezer for up to 3 months. FYI: when you heat it up, it'll no longer be gelatinous.

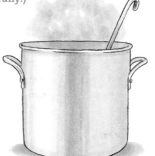

with a birth defect), this test *may* provide reassurance that the chances of a genetic problem with this pregnancy are low. If the results are positive, on the other hand, you can decide if you want to move forward with more invasive diagnostic testing. If you'd like to minimize the number of ultrasounds you receive during pregnancy, you may want to skip this test altogether or combine this test with the dating ultrasound; your sonographer can verify your due date, as well as let you hear baby's heartbeat during the NT screening.

CELL-FREE DNA SCREENING

Sometimes called the MaterniT21, Verifi, or Harmony prenatal test (or other brand names), this is a blood test that can determine the risk of having a baby with a chromosomal abnormality, specifically Down syndrome, Edwards syndrome, or trisomy 13 (Patau syndrome). It's fairly new to the market and very accurate—between 91 percent and 99 percent of the above defects are detected; false positives are reported in less than 1 percent of cases.

DYING TO KNOW THE SEX OF YOUR BABY?

Well, do yourself a favor and do not buy one of those sex-predictor urine tests from your local drugstore. They're expensive and notoriously inaccurate. And I should know—I was the sucker who bought one when I was pregnant with Paloma, and it said I was having a boy. Hmm . . .

Results may be reported as positive, negative, or as a fraction indicating the risk of a particular defect, such as 1/1,000. The test also determines the sex of the baby.

IS THIS TEST RIGHT FOR YOU?

Mamas who want to know the sex of their baby used to have to wait for the "anatomy ultrasound," which is typically performed around

---

CAN I CONTINUE BREASTFEEDING MY TODDLER?

If you're a mama to an older infant or toddler, you may be wondering if you can continue to breastfeed now that you're pregnant again. In a word? Absolutely. Plenty of mamas continue nursing right through pregnancy and even postpartum (a practice known as "tandem nursing," since you'll be nursing for two). Just know that surging hormones may affect the taste and quality of your breast milk during pregnancy—while some children don't mind this at all, others may wean themselves naturally. You may also need to get a little creative with breastfeeding positions as your belly grows, but that's nothing you and your flexible toddler can't figure out. When your newborn finally does arrive, however, you'll want to be sure that he or she gets dibs on your colostrum, a super-potent, nutrient-dense pre-milk that serves as baby's food for several days after birth. We'll talk more about the benefits of colostrum in Week 33.

20 weeks. Cell-free DNA screening, on the other hand, is available much earlier—I had the test done at 10 weeks, because I wanted to know the sex right away. (Yes, I'm impatient. But let me tell you, it was wild to know I was having a girl even before hearing her heartbeat!) The test can be costly, and your insurance may cover it only if you have certain risk factors. The test is not appropriate for women who are expecting multiples, since it can't distinguish between one baby's DNA and another's in the maternal bloodstream.

CHORIONIC VILLUS SAMPLING (CVS)

This is a diagnostic test, not a screen; while the results are much more accurate—CVS detects virtually any chromosomal abnormality, including Down syndrome, Tay-Sachs disease, and sex chromosomal disorders such as Turner syndrome with 98 percent accuracy— the test is considerably more invasive and thus carries more risks. CVS is performed by inserting a small tube into your uterus through the vagina, or by inserting a needle into your uterus through the skin of your lower abdomen to obtain a very small piece of the placenta.

The tissue collection may involve some discomfort but shouldn't be painful. If the tissue is collected vaginally, you may experience a small amount of bleeding afterward. The risks, although rare, include infection, rupture of the amniotic sac, limb reduction of the baby, and miscarriage (in 1 percent of cases). If mama is Rh-negative (and her partner is Rh-positive), she'll likely be given a RhoGAM shot, since it's possible that her blood and baby's blood could mix during the procedure. CVS also requires use of an ultrasound to guide the needle or tube during insertion.

IS THIS TEST RIGHT FOR YOU?

Since CVS testing is by far the most invasive of all the first trimester tests, you likely won't want to move forward until or unless you've received an abnormal result from a First Trimester Screen and/or cell-free DNA screening. If you do decide to get the procedure done, be sure you understand all the risks and discuss your options with your healthcare provider. Know that CVS testing cannot detect problems with the baby's brain or spinal cord, such as spina bifida.

mama-do list

- Before you head in for your first prenatal appointment, remember to write down the date of your last menstrual period, any medications you're taking, any unusual symptoms you're experiencing, and any family history of pregnancy complications or birth defects. Between the nerves and the excitement, it's likely you'll forget *something* without a reminder.

- If you're planning on limiting the number of ultrasounds you'll receive, you prefer not to use a Doppler, or you intend to decline most genetic screenings, let your midwife know now so the two of you can get on the same page.

from
iPhones to ultrasounds

SMART TECHNOLOGY USE

WHAT'S UP WITH *baby*?

Baby hits a major milestone this week, Mama: he's officially graduating from an embryo to a fetus! But the name change isn't the only big news. This week, he's getting a bumper crop of new internal organs, including a liver, spleen, and gallbladder (important components of the digestive and lymphatic systems). Teeny, tiny muscles are developing in his arms and legs. His eyelids have fully formed, too, and are tightly shut. They'll stay closed until about the seventh month of pregnancy, but even when they do open there won't be much to see in there. After all, it's pretty dark inside your uterus. (He will be able to sense bright lights *outside* your body, though.) Speaking of baby's

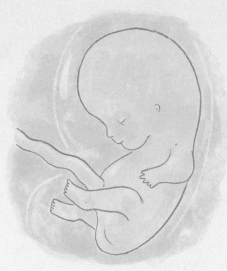

BABY'S LIVER, SPLEEN AND GALLBLADDER ARE DEVELOPING THIS WEEK.

eyesight, one of the best things you can do for him right now, besides eating a balanced diet with plenty of vitamin A, is to get some sunshine. According to recent research in *Ophthalmology*, preterm infants born to women who got pregnant during the darkest months of the year—a.k.a. the dead of winter—have an increased risk of developing certain eye disorders.

WHAT'S UP WITH *mama*?

Congratulations are in order, Mama! Why? Because you've made it to month three, the final month of your first trimester. Right about now, however, you might be starting to wonder what happened to your waistline. It's common to start feeling thicker through the middle at this point, even though you're still weeks away from developing a true baby bump. (If your clothes are getting snug, you may be ready to invest in what I consider a crucial component of any mama's wardrobe: *yoga pants*. Or, if you need a more polished look: *leggings*. Seriously.) Now, let's talk about some good news: Since baby has entered the fetal stage of development, he's safer from certain developmental disorders and less susceptible to external factors that could damage his health or lead to birth defects. Woot!

When my mother went into labor with my older brother, things progressed pretty normally, at least initially. She breathed through her contractions without much fuss. Her cervix dilated slowly but surely. And soon enough, she was ready to push. Which was right around the time her doctor discovered that the baby (my brother) still hadn't "dropped" into her pelvis, the first essential step toward making his way through the birth canal. Since babies usually drop as early as a few *weeks* before delivery, there was some concern that she might have something called cephalopelvic disproportion, an extremely rare condition in which mama's pelvis isn't big enough to accommodate the size of her baby. So, her doctor ordered a pelvic x-ray.

Nowadays, x-raying a pregnant mama would almost *never* happen. Back then, however, it wasn't so strange. X-raying pregnant women to determine the position of their babies in utero was increasingly common starting from the 1950s on, even though evidence was already floating around about potential risks to the unborn baby. (Namely, an increased risk of developing childhood cancer. Eek!) The practice wasn't really phased out until the mid-1970s, a few years after my brother was born.

The problem with x-rays, of course, is that they're a form of radiation, specifically high-energy, ionizing radiation, which is powerful enough to affect our cells and mutate our DNA.

X-rays are actually classified as a known carcinogen by both the US government and the World Health Organization. If you're wondering why we use them *at all*, it's because the rewards—in certain cases—far outweigh the risks. After all, misdiagnosing an injury or illness, or missing the presence of an injury or illness altogether, can be far more dangerous to your health than the small hit of radiation you'd get from a single x-ray. That's why doctors do what they can to limit exposure (read: they avoid unnecessary imaging). It's also why you'll be asked to wear one of those charming lead vests at the dentist's office (to protect your vital organs). And since babies in utero are at a higher risk of developing radiation-related health issues, x-rays—especially of the abdominal area—are typically avoided during pregnancy.

Problem solved, right?

Except, x-rays aren't the only form of radiation in the world. In fact, we're exposed to different types of radiation *all the time*. The sun, for example, emits ultraviolet radiation. Highly radioactive radon gas exists naturally in the earth's atmosphere, soil, and groundwater. A portion of all potassium atoms are radioactive—fun fact: eating 600 bananas is the radiation equivalent of getting a chest x-ray. Even humans emit radiation, of the thermal and infrared kind (which is why we "glow" when photographed by infrared cameras).

For years, we've known that high-energy ionizing radiation, the type emitted by x-rays and gamma rays, can be dangerous. We also know the dangers of high-energy, *non*-ionizing radiation: too much UV light can cause sunburn.

But there are concerns in the natural world about our increasing exposure to electromagnetic fields (EMFs), a form of *low*-energy, non-ionizing radiation emitted from household appliances and tech gadgets, in particular mobile phone signals and wireless internet connections.

Even though EMFs exist naturally (the build-up of charges in the air during a thunderstorm, for example, creates electric fields, while the earth's magnetic field causes a compass needle to point north), there's no doubt that we are exposed to considerably more manmade, nonnatural EMFs now than at any other time in human history. This growing network of radiation that surrounds us all is sometimes referred to as electrosmog, electrical pollution, or dirty energy.

What everyone's trying to figure out is: are EMFs actually dangerous?

THE POTENTIAL DANGERS OF EMF EXPOSURE

That's the $10,000 question. And to be frank, the answer you'll get depends on whom you ask.

The World Health Organization (WHO) and its affiliated International Agency for Research on Cancer (IARC) say no. After an exhaustive review of the existing scientific literature, the WHO couldn't identify any health risks associated with low-level exposure. It has acknowledged that "gaps" in the knowledge exist, however, and that more research is needed. It also hasn't been able to prove that EMFs *aren't* harmful, which is why "radiofrequency electromagnetic fields" were classified as a Group 2B carcinogen (a substance that *might* be cancer-causing in humans) back in 2011. Other 2B carcinogens include known bad guys like engine exhaust, lead, and gasoline, but also coffee and—strangely enough—pickled vegetables.

About that scientific literature. Yes, there have been many studies to suggest that EMFs are plenty dangerous. A 2011 study published in the *Archives of Pediatrics & Adolescent Medicine* suggested that exposure to high levels of EMFs during pregnancy can increase baby's risk of developing asthma. A 2012 study published in *Epidemiology* found a link between high EMF exposure and miscarriage. The American Cancer Society acknowledges that there is some evidence—across multiple studies—that children at the highest levels of exposure may have an elevated risk of leukemia.

The problem with these studies, however, is that the results have not been easily replicated. In some cases, larger, more comprehensive studies have directly conflicted with such findings. There are some people who have reported physical symptoms—headaches, fatigue, muscle pain, trouble sleeping—but in double-blind studies were unable to detect the presence of EMFs when exposed to them. (I'm not saying those symptoms don't exist, mind you, just that some studies have been inconclusive.)

And yet, some groups—particularly those outside the United States—are taking sweeping steps to limit and regulate exposure.

In 2011, a committee from the Council of Europe, a policy advisory group with forty-seven member states, recommended banning *all* mobile phones and wireless networks in classrooms and schools due to EMF-related health concerns. That same year, Health Canada, a department of the Canadian government, recommended limiting the length of cell phone calls and lessening the use of cell phones by children. The German government has recommended that its citizens limit their exposure to Wi-Fi from cafés, schools, and private homes. The French government has banned Wi-Fi in nursery schools. In May 2015, EMFscientist.org sent an appeal to the United Nations and the WHO—signed by 220 scientists from forty-one countries around the world—pleading for the development of more protective guidelines, precautionary measures, and public education about the dangers of exposure, particularly as it relates to children and pregnant women.

So you see, concern about EMFs isn't exactly a fringe movement.

To be honest with you, though, I wasn't thinking too much about any of this during my first pregnancy—until one night, when I had my laptop perched atop my growing belly, and I noticed the computer fan switching on. It felt hot against my body, too. Wait a minute. Was I overheating the baby and inadvertently cooking my womb?!

I started doing some research (as I am prone to do in times like these), which is when I realized that most of us are using our electronic devices all wrong. And before you start thinking I'm some crazy lady who's about to tell you to throw your cell phone out the window, consider this: all wireless communication devices sold in the United States have to meet minimum guidelines for radiofrequency exposure set by the Federal Communications Commission (FCC). But if you peek at the user manual for, say, the Apple iPad (or virtually any Wi-Fi-enabled device), you'll see that in order to meet those guidelines, you're supposed to hold the thing *away from your body*. So if you're resting your laptop or tablet in your lap or talking with a cell phone pressed directly against your ear—the way these gadgets are *designed* to be used—then you may be exceeding the FCC's limit on EMF exposure.

Yikes.

The thing is, we may be years—or even decades—away from knowing the true toll that our reliance on technology is taking on our health and our bodies. The Council of Europe, however, is one group that thinks a "wait and see" approach is not in our collective best interest. As written in their 2011 report: "waiting for high levels of scientific evidence and clinical proof can lead to very high health and economic costs, as was the case in the past with asbestos, leaded petrol, and tobacco." They have a point. It wasn't so long ago, after all, when cigarette smoking was thought to have health *benefits*, even for pregnant women.

SO . . . DO I NEED A TINFOIL HAT NOW OR WHAT?

Most of us live in homes with the Wi-Fi turned on 24/7, a utility company "smart meter" attached to the exterior wall of our living rooms, and we sleep with our cell phone on the nightstand. Our children play with our devices, too, using tablets and other devices to learn (via kid-friendly games and apps) or to distract them long enough to give mama and papa a much-needed break.

EMF-emitting technology has become, for almost all of us, a way of life, and it isn't going away.

But the truth is, I wouldn't want it to. I *love* my iPhone. My husband and I run an internet-based company. And I don't know about you, but I'm not quite ready to go back to candles and lanterns to light up my house at night. Even that wouldn't totally eradicate the daily dose of EMFs to which we're all exposed. *Limiting* your exposure, however, is a great idea—especially during your pregnancy. As a general rule, we know that children (and certainly babies in utero) are more susceptible and vulnerable to the effects of radiation. The good news is that you can take simple steps to ramp up your safety without switching to a landline, moving off the grid, or living in the Dark Ages. Here are some things you can do for a start:

MINIMIZING YOUR DIRECT CELL PHONE EXPOSURE

Did you know that just about every cell phone and smartphone on the market comes with a warning about using it too close to the body? (Seriously. Read your owner's manual.) One thing that's not up for debate when it comes to EMFs is that the intensity of radiation is dependent on how close you are to the source; levels fall off dramatically when you put just a little distance between yourself and the device in question, even mere inches. When using your cell, avoid talking with the phone pressed directly to your ear whenever possible. Instead, use a wired headset, earbuds, or the speaker

function. There are special low-EMF headsets on the market, too. Texting is always a great alternative. You'll also want to:

♡ Avoid carrying your cell directly on your body. I've seen men store their phones in their pants pockets—hello, family jewels!—as well as their front shirt pocket, directly over their hearts. I've even known some women to carry their phone around in their bras. Please, do not do this. If you absolutely must carry your phone on your body, put it in airplane mode.

♡ Avoid making calls when your signal is low; the fewer bars you have, the harder the phone has to work to communicate with the nearest cell tower.

♡ Disable Bluetooth when you're not using it, or quit using it altogether.

♡ Consider purchasing a phone with a low "specific absorption rate" (SAR); in other words, a low-radiation cell phone.

KEEP TABLETS AND COMPUTERS AWAY FROM YOUR BELLY

Despite the name, laptops should *not* be placed directly on your lap and certainly not balanced atop your growing baby bump. Rest your laptop on a table instead. When you're not actually surfing the web, turn off the Wi-Fi feature.

CONSIDER PROTECTING YOUR DEVICES WITH EMF SHIELDS

There are loads of protective cases available for virtually every type of gadget you own. We have an EMF-blocking case on our iPad (specifically for when my son Griffin uses it), as well as a shield on my phone. Be warned, however, that not all companies that offer such products are reputable. I've seen

Mom, it's getting hot in here!

some seriously questionable claims and supposed "evidence" on certain websites, so don't just shell out money for whichever case you clap eyes on first. Do your research. DefenderShield, Pong, and Belly Armor make good products.

TURN OFF YOUR WI-FI AT NIGHT

It's as easy as flipping a switch (or pulling a plug). Turning your Wi-Fi off in the evening will save you eight or nine hours—if not more—of exposure. Michael and I have a router with an actual on/off button, which makes it easy to enable the Wi-Fi only when we need it. When we're working in our home office, we stick with a wired connection. Speaking of wired connections, you may want to rethink installing other wireless systems in your home, especially those you would intend to run 24/7 (like a wireless security system). Same goes for baby monitors—opt for a wired monitor, and/or place the monitor as far away from baby's crib as possible. You'll still be able to hear him cry, even if the monitor is resting just outside the door of his nursery.

BE SMART ABOUT YOUR SMART METER

Smart meters are just updated versions of those old-school analog electric meters affixed to the outside of your home. These devices measure your electricity usage and report back to the utility company for billing purposes. The big difference is that smart meters communicate wirelessly (and constantly). Depending on where yours is located, you may be unknowingly blasting yourself with an extra helping of EMF radiation, so walk the perimeter of your house and find yours. If it's outside a high-traffic area (a living room or bedroom, for

JUST SAY NO TO AT-HOME FETAL HEART MONITORS

It's now possible to purchase at-home fetal heart monitors to listen in on baby whenever you like. While that may sound like a lovely idea, there are risks—and not just the extra dose of EMFs. According to the FDA, fetal heart monitors are intended as prescription devices, *only* to be used by trained healthcare professionals. Unless you happen to be a sonographer, you may not be able to "read" the sounds you are hearing correctly. This can lead to unnecessary worry and stress (not good for you or the baby)—or worse, you may think everything is "fine" after hearing what you *think* is a heartbeat, when in fact you need to seek medical attention. Resist the urge to buy one, Mama, and leave Dopplers to the pros.

example), you may want to consider purchasing a protective shield. You could also call your electric company and request an older analog meter, though that'll cost you.

Sweet Potato Custard

Vitamin A—crucial for the development and long-term health of baby's eyes—is our star performer this week. Of course, if you're taking your daily cod liver oil, you're already getting a decent dose. Other good sources include egg yolks, cream, and butter . . . Are you noticing a theme, here? Animal-based sources of vitamin A are the easiest to assimilate, but I like adding in some plant-based sources, too, since they're rich in phytonutrients. This cozy sweet potato custard combines both.

INGREDIENTS

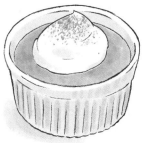

2 medium organic sweet potatoes

2 organic, pasture-raised eggs

½ cup organic cream (or substitute coconut cream)

¼ cup coconut sugar or 30 drops stevia

1 teaspoon vanilla extract

1 teaspoon pumpkin pie spice (or a mix of ground cloves, nutmeg, cinnamon, ginger, and allspice)

Preheat the oven to 350°F. Wash the sweet potatoes and pierce them a few times with a fork. Place in the oven and let cook for 45 minutes or until soft. Remove from the oven. Once the sweet potatoes have cooled slightly, scoop out the flesh and place in a bowl. Combine all remaining ingredients and mix with an immersion blender. Pour into small ramekins and bake for 30 minutes or until slightly browned. Serve with a dollop of whipped cream. Serves 4 to 6.

TO ULTRASOUND OR NOT TO ULTRASOUND? THAT IS THE QUESTION

Ah, the ultrasound. It is perhaps *the* defining moment on the journey to motherhood, isn't it? The first ultrasound constitutes a major scene in virtually every movie that in some way features a pregnancy, and it always plays out the exact same way: the friendly sonographer guides a wand across mama's belly, the strange, underwater, alien sound of the Doppler fills the room, and soon enough mama is weeping tears of joy at the sight of her precious little baby up on the screen. Is it any wonder that so many of us believe getting an ultrasound is vital to ensuring a healthy pregnancy?

It would perhaps surprise you to know, however, that ultrasounds are not mandatory, nor do they provide any proven medical benefit to mama or baby.

Wait, what?

That's right. Multiple studies have shown that ultrasounds do not improve neonatal outcomes. Mamas who have repeat imaging are not any more likely to deliver healthy babies than those who forego the procedure. There's even some evidence to suggest that ultrasounds may lead to more interventions during birth. (A doctor may be more likely to recommend a Cesarean, for example, if he thinks a post-term baby is too big for a vaginal delivery. Unfortunately, size estimates based on ultrasounds can be off by as much as a pound or two.)

Ultrasounds are also a form of—you guessed it—radiation.

Much like the concern about EMF exposure from cell phones and wireless networks, we lack solid, definitive proof that ultrasounds are harmful. The American College of Obstetricians and Gynecologists, however, does recommend that ultrasounds be performed *only* for medical reasons and *only* by qualified healthcare providers. There is some evidence that the heat from ultrasounds can be an issue; the College also acknowledges that negative side effects may be identified in the future. For these reasons, you might want to limit baby's exposure.

Which happens to be what I chose to do. Some mamas, myself included, want confirmation that everything is progressing as it should.

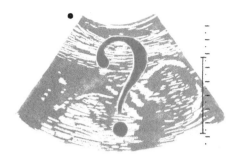

Some—also like me—want a glimpse of their child because it bonds them on an emotional level. This is an important benefit of ultrasounds for many parents—an increased sense of connection with baby. It's worth mentioning, too, that a friend of mine discovered her baby only had one kidney during an ultrasound in her 20th week; the news didn't change much about the pregnancy itself, but she was able to enlist a specialist to be on call for her son's birth. Ultimately, the choice to ultrasound is entirely up to you, but you may want to consider the following:

♡ Skip imaging in the first trimester. Most mamas will be offered at least two or three ultrasounds, or one during each trimester. I elected to have only one during my entire pregnancy—the "anatomy ultrasound" (typically performed around the halfway point) just to make sure my baby was developing normally.

♡ Cut the small talk. Some sonographers, bless them, can be chatty, and they'll want to take lots of pictures to give you as souvenirs. Politely ask yours to get right to checking anatomy and taking measurements in order to lessen baby's exposure as much as possible.

♡ Choose a fetoscope. The handheld Doppler that midwives and doctors use to hear the fetal heartbeat is another form of ultrasound, and it actually emits more radiation

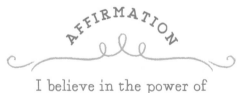

AFFIRMATION

I believe in the power of positive thinking. I let go of fear. I am calm and confident.

than the machine used for imaging. You can avoid the Doppler altogether and opt for a fetoscope, which is basically a fancy stethoscope that emits zero radiation. This will, however, require some patience on your part—the Doppler typically picks up the heartbeat around 12 to 14 weeks, whereas the fetoscope won't until Weeks 18 to 20. Personally, I couldn't wait that long. I used the Doppler once around Week 12 but stuck with the fetoscope for the remainder of my pregnancy.

♡ Avoid 3-D and 4-D ultrasounds. There's no doubt about it: 3-D ultrasound technology is incredible, and it's understandable that many mamas would jump at the chance to see a detailed picture of baby's sweet face. My advice, however, is to skip them. These types of ultrasounds are considered "recreational" and are often performed by people who are not registered sonographers, perhaps with little to no radiology education or certification. The procedure can take longer, too, as much as an hour by some estimates. The FDA "strongly discourages" these types of ultrasounds due to concerns about overheating tissue and cavitation (the formation of small bubbles in baby's tissue).

mama-do list

- Do you use your cell phone as an alarm clock? Consider switching to a battery-powered alarm, and charging your phone somewhere outside your bedroom. In fact, think about relocating all your electronic devices away from your snooze area. You may get a better night's sleep if your bedroom is tech-free.

- Locate your home's smart meter. If it's affixed to the exterior wall of a bedroom or high-traffic area, you may want to look into purchasing an EMF shield.

- Go outside and get some sunshine. You'll get more than a healthy dose of vitamin D; a bit of direct sun exposure, especially during the first trimester, may be protective for baby's developing eyesight.

let the cat out of the bag

WHAT'S UP WITH *baby*?

Your little peanut is the size of, well, a walnut now. There's a lot going on inside that little body—teeth and fingernails have started to form—but there's a lot going on *outside* her body, too. This week, the placenta is gearing up to take over the very important job of supplying baby with the nutrients she needs to keep growing. (The yolk sac will start to diminish in size and will disappear completely between Weeks 14 and 20 of your pregnancy.) Baby's digestive system has come a long way, too. Her stomach is already producing digestive juices, and her kidneys are making urine. Wait a minute. Where does all that urine . . . *go?* Yup—you guessed it. Baby is able to pee now, right into her amniotic fluid, which she'll proceed to "drink" for the next 30 weeks or so. Thankfully, babies don't typically poop while in utero!

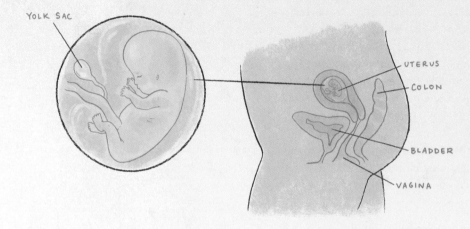

WHAT'S UP WITH *mama*?

Mama, you are one tough cookie. First, there's the morning sickness. Don't even get me started about the extreme fatigue. What else might be coming your way? Dizzy spells. See, even though your blood volume has increased, your blood pressure has gone down. In other words, your heart must work harder to pump that blood all the way up to your brain. So if your head starts spinning when you sit up, know this is probably the cause. Give yourself time when transitioning from lying to sitting, or sitting to standing. Make sure you're drinking plenty of fluids and getting enough protein in your diet, which can reduce dizziness. Aim to eat some strategic snacks throughout the day, like toasted pumpkin seeds with sea salt or celery with salted almond butter. And if you're still feeling lousy, check in with your midwife or doctor.

The morning I finally confirmed my first pregnancy—you remember the story, it only took me five home pregnancy tests, two trips to Walgreens, and a near nervous breakdown to do it—was New Year's Day. Six thirty in the morning on New Year's Day, to be exact. I had leapt out of bed at the crack of dawn to take advantage of my "first morning urine" and was aching to tell somebody the news, but Michael was sleeping so soundly—we'd been out late celebrating the night before—that I didn't have the heart to wake him. I picked up the phone and called my parents instead. Sure, I felt a little guilty about spilling the beans, but my folks had been in a horrific car accident a year earlier, and my dad had spent many months in the hospital. I knew that my announcement, with its promise of new life, would give them a much-needed boost. Dad celebrated with a Champagne toast, and I celebrated (quietly) with dry toast.

Poor Michael. He wasn't the first to know when I got pregnant the second time around, either. Our two-year-old Griffin was the first to get that news.

If you're anything like me, you were ready to shout, "I'M PREGNANT!" the moment you got that positive result, too.

But when is it appropriate to share the news with extended family, friends, and coworkers? Conventional wisdom has always been to wait until the second trimester, since the likelihood of miscarriage drops significantly after the first three months. But the truth is there are no rules. Some mamas think the ol' wait-three-months guideline is old-fashioned, or worse: that it stigmatizes miscarriage. Others value their privacy and would prefer to wait until they're officially "in the clear." Still others would just like to minimize the amount of unsolicited advice they'll have to

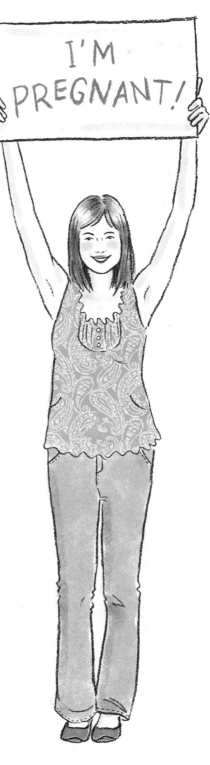

endure—because, yes, every person you have ever known is gonna have *something* to say about the food you're eating, the rest you're getting, and how your kid should be raised. (Don't say I didn't warn you.) No matter which camp you fall into, it's your pregnancy. You can tell whomever you want, whenever you want, however you want.

But if you're thinking about shouting it from the rooftops at work, you may want to pump the brakes.

As you may have heard, the United States ranks pretty much dead last when it comes to maternity rights. We're one of only three developed countries in the world that don't mandate paid time off for new moms. You may

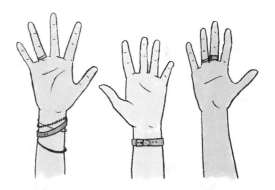

still be entitled to some benefits, however, so before you break the news, you'll want to get clear on company policy and, most important, understand what you are entitled to.

WHAT'S UP WITH THIS TINGLING IN MY HANDS?

As your pregnancy progresses, keep an eye out for a tingling pins-and-needles feeling or numbness in your fingers, hands, wrists, and arms, particularly when working at your computer. These are telltale signs of carpal tunnel syndrome.

What's that got to do with pregnancy?

The carpal tunnel is a small space in your wrist—a tunnel, if you will—between the carpal bones and the transverse carpal ligament. Running right up the center of that tunnel is the median nerve, which gives feeling to your fingers. When we swell during pregnancy—thanks to the increase in fluids and blood volume—the tunnel narrows, squeezing the nerve. Hello, pain and numbness.

The good news is that the symptoms of carpal tunnel syndrome should clear up all on their own in the weeks after birth. But until then, you may want to:

⚜ *Switch to an ergonomic keyboard, which will lessen the strain on your wrists. (Most employers will cover the cost of special equipment like this.)*

⚜ *Take breaks from typing throughout the day to give your wrists, hands, and arms a rest.*

⚜ *Consider wearing a splint or brace, which can help with wrist alignment and keeping the muscles relaxed and in a neutral position. You can find both daytime and nighttime braces, the latter of which is more immobilizing in order to provide greater relief.*

⚜ *Stretch daily to strengthen the muscles surrounding the median nerve.*

KNOW YOUR RIGHTS

I dreaded telling my boss about my pregnancy. Two of my coworkers were on maternity leave, a third had just announced that she was expecting, and I was sure that he was not going to be, shall we say, *excited* to find out that I was going to be out of the office, too. Luckily, he was genuinely pleased and incredibly gracious; I also happened to work for a company with decent benefits. I so wish that was the case for every woman, but the majority of us who work outside the home just aren't eligible for a whole lot of perks. The benefits you can expect are dictated by federal law, state law, the company you work for, and the kind of work you do.

Let's start with the federal laws first.

There are two pieces of federal legislation on the books related to pregnancy in the workplace.

THE PREGNANCY DISCRIMINATION ACT OF 1978

It's illegal to pass you over for a promotion, to fire you, or to otherwise discriminate against you solely on the basis of your pregnancy. Keep in mind, however, that this law does *not* apply to companies with fewer than fifteen employees, nor does it apply to employees who become unable to do the job they were hired to do.

It's that last bit that gets interesting. Imagine for a moment that you broke your foot or were recovering from a major illness. Some companies might offer to lighten your workload until you healed—by putting you on desk duty, for example, if you're a police officer. According to the Pregnancy Discrimination Act (PDA), your employer must treat you as it would treat any employee with a temporary medical disability. In other words, if your employer makes accommodations for someone with a non-pregnancy-related medical condition but fails to make them for you, you've got a claim. In fact, a case just like that—*Young v. United Parcel Service*—made it all the way to the Supreme Court in 2015, after UPS prevented a pregnant woman from working because she could no longer lift the seventy pounds required of drivers. (The pregnant woman won her case, by the way.) Actors have repeatedly fought for their rights under this law, too. In the mid-1990s, for example, a popular soap star was fired from her job on *Melrose Place* when producers argued that she couldn't convincingly portray a "vixen" while pregnant. The actress sued, in part because the show had accommodated a different actress during her pregnancy, and was awarded nearly $5 million in emotional distress and lost wages. The PDA doesn't grant you any maternity leave or paid benefits, but at least you know you've got some level of job security.

THE FAMILY AND MEDICAL LEAVE ACT OF 1993

This second law—the only one regarding maternity leave in the United States—gives you the right to twelve weeks of *unpaid* time off, provided you've worked at your current job for at least one year and logged at least 1,250 hours during that year (meanwhile, the company you work for must employ at least

STAY-AT-HOME MAMAS HAVE RISKY JOBS, TOO

I can attest that staying at home full-time and caring for a toddler is incredibly hard work, especially when you're pregnant. There were plenty of days when sitting at an office for eight hours sounded positively *divine* in comparison (the grass is always greener!). If you're a stay-at-home mama, don't forget that you have work-related risks, too:

❖ *standing on your feet for hours at a time,*

❖ *getting too much activity chasing a toddler,*

❖ *carrying a 20- to 40-pound child or too many grocery bags,*

❖ *caring for a sick child, and*

❖ *not finding the time to eat three square meals a day.*

And the list goes on. Mama, be sure to take good care of yourself. Sit down and honor your mealtimes, even if your toddler is having a fit. Encourage your child to walk herself instead of carrying her (this is the time to use a stroller if need be). When the bagger at the grocery store offers to help you to your car, take him up on it! I also would encourage you to nap when your toddler naps. While it's tempting to get caught up on email or lose yourself in a novel, sleep is so much more restorative. If your child gets sick, be sure you're keeping an appropriate distance from her nose and mouth, since illnesses can spread like wildfire. (Easier said than done, I know.) You also want to wash your hands frequently and boost your immunity (as well as your toddler's)—use the tips in Week 12. It's perfectly fine to get honest with your toddler or older child—in an age-appropriate way—about how you're feeling. I remember explaining to Griffin that Mommy was more tired because her body was changing rapidly to build a new life. These kinds of discussions help to keep the channels of communication open for when baby comes.

> If you're in a committed partnership, now may be a good time to discuss the "division of labor" at home. Will your honey do diaper duty while you handle feedings? Will you share meal prep responsibilities, or divvy up the cooking and cleaning? Becoming parents will *increase* your workload, while *decreasing* the time (and energy!) you'll have to get things done. Make a plan for how you'll handle this new chapter together. It's also a good time to start looking into childcare, daycare, or nanny-care if you plan on returning to work soon after the baby is born. Give yourself plenty of time to get things lined up so you can feel calm and supported when baby arrives.

fifty people within a 75-mile radius). Papas, same-sex partners, and adoptive parents are eligible for FMLA leave, too; however, if you and your partner work for the same company, you'll have to split the twelve weeks between the two of you. Barring an unforeseen medical complication, you must give thirty days' notice before taking your leave.

Of course, the FMLA does you no good if you can't afford to go without a paycheck. You can also be denied benefits if you're among the highest paid 10 percent of employees and your employer can demonstrate that your absence would cause the company serious financial harm. If you cannot return to work after twelve weeks, or if you tell your employer that you don't plan on coming back, you can lose your benefits and your job.

So, yeah. There's really no two ways about it: the federal laws governing maternity leave just aren't all that great. There is hope that the FMLA will be expanded soon. One proposed bill, for example, the Family and Medical Leave Insurance Act, or FAMILY Act, would offer twelve weeks of *paid* leave, funded by contributions from workers and employers, not unlike Social Security. Until then, you may catch a break depending on the state in which you live.

STATE AND LOCAL LAWS

Maternity leave laws vary widely from coast to coast. Nearly half of all states expand on the FMLA by allowing for longer (unpaid) absences from your job, or by extending coverage to employees working for smaller companies— i.e., those with fewer than fifty workers. Some states offer a version of paid maternity leave in the form of short-term disability insurance, which you can claim in the same way you'd seek, say, unemployment benefits. As of this writing, only four states provide true paid leave for qualified workers: California, New Jersey, Rhode Island, and New York (starting in 2018). To learn more about maternity leave laws in your state, contact your local Department of Labor or check out the nonprofit A Better Balance (abetterbalance.org).

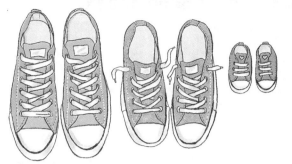

making the announcement

In the age of Pinterest, Instagram, and YouTube, pregnancy announcements aren't just more creative than ever before—they're going viral. In 2015, for example, a Dallas-based couple revealed the news to their folks during family game night and watched the (totally adorbs) video explode on the internet, racking up nearly 6 *million* views. Whether you're planning to go big or keep it simple, here are some ideas to spark your creativity.

The Classic

A postcard or magnet with your picture and a simple message—think: "And baby makes three [due date]"—is timeless and elegant, but don't be afraid to interject some humor. One of my all-time favorite announcements features a sweet pic of Mama and Papa and this message superimposed over the photo:

Photo Paper: $5, Postage $0.41, Envelope: $0.05

The look on your face when you realize there are three of us in this photo: PRICELESS

The Shoes

There is a universal truth we can all agree upon: there is nothing cuter than baby shoes. Showcase the most adorable pair you can find, or line up a pair of Papa's, Mama's, and baby-to-be's in descending order according to size. Bonus points for matching shoes: Top-Siders for the sailing enthusiasts, cowboy boots for a Southern brood, or Tevas for out-doorsy types. Swoon.

The Coming Attraction

A "Coming Attractions" movie poster is sure to create lots of excitement surrounding the "premiere" of your new baby. It's also how Michael and I chose to announce Paloma's birth—*Big Bro* featured our son Griffin in the "role of a lifetime."

Loving these announcement ideas? Find loads more at mamanatural.com, including "The Superhero Sidekick" (for big brothers- or sisters-to-be), "The Jersey" (for devoted sports fans), and "The Double Trouble," for parents expecting—you guessed it—twins.

(Non-Alcoholic) Hot Toddy

Baby's chompers are developing now, so be sure you're getting plenty of calcium every day. Of course, whole-fat dairy products are a great option. But so are bone broth, canned salmon and sardines, almonds, white beans, and—bet you weren't expecting this one—blackstrap molasses (which also happens to be rich in iron, potassium, and magnesium).

Try this velvety delicious take on a hot toddy (non-alcoholic, of course). Since it's full of calcium, it'll lull you right to sleep.

INGREDIENTS

1 cup organic milk (or almond milk)

1 tablespoon organic blackstrap molasses

Pinch of nutmeg (optional)

Pinch of sea salt

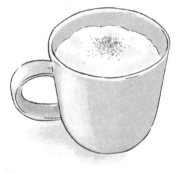

To make, gently warm your milk on the stove. Add your molasses and mix well. Finish with a pinch of nutmeg and sea salt. If you're feeling fancy, you can even "froth" the sweetened milk in a blender or with the steam wand of an espresso machine.

GET FAMILIAR WITH COMPANY POLICY

Now that you know what you're legally entitled to, it's time to pull out the company handbook and find out everything you can about your employer's maternity leave policy. As the issue of paid family leave becomes increasingly politicized, some companies have begun taking huge steps in the right direction all on their own. Netflix, for example, made national news in 2015 when it announced that salaried workers could take up to twelve months of maternity *or* paternity leave—at full pay—following the birth or adoption of a child. (Wow!) Other companies are following suit: Apple offers egg freezing for mamas who aren't quite ready to board the baby train. Facebook shells out a $4,000 bonus it calls "baby cash" and offers breastfeeding rooms in its California headquarters. If you happen to work for a company with such family-friendly policies, however, you're one of the lucky few; only 12 percent of US workers have access to paid leave through private employers. Some companies may require you to use up your (paid) vacation days, sick days, and personal days before your (unpaid) FMLA benefits kick in. On the other hand, even if the state you live in doesn't provide short-term disability insurance, some private companies and unions do. It's important to understand company policy *before* you break the news.

Once you've done your research, look over your finances and determine how many weeks you can afford to stay home. You'll want to balance that number, whatever it is, with a plan that makes the most sense for you. Some mamas, for example, choose to start their maternity leave a week or so before their due date; others prefer to work right up until their water breaks in order to maximize the amount of time they'll have with baby.

Know, too, that you may be able to use part of your FMLA leave *during* your pregnancy if, say, *hyperemesis gravidarum* has you in its grip or if you're put on modified bed rest. Finally, spend some time thinking about how your workload might be handled while you're gone; your supervisor will likely have some questions, and being proactive can go a long way toward alleviating his or her concerns. Just remember: you're not asking for permission to take maternity leave; you're claiming a benefit. You've earned it. Good luck, Mama!

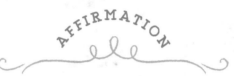

AFFIRMATION

I am never alone. I am surrounded by people who love me. I feel the love they have for me and my baby. I am grateful.

mama-do list

- If Week 10's got you feeling dizzy, aim to incorporate a bit of high-quality sea salt into your diet; the sodium will help support your body's increased blood volume. Chat with your midwife or doctor if high blood pressure is a concern.

- Check out your state's maternity leave laws as well as your employee handbook to get clear on your maternity benefits.

- You probably won't be surprised to hear that papas who take paternity leave tend to play a more active role in childcare duties. Talk to your husband or partner about how much time he can afford to be out of the office. Paternity leave isn't just good for babies—there are loads of benefits for new mamas, too.

take care of
You

WHAT'S UP WITH *baby*?

Whoa! Baby had a bit of a growth spurt this week—he's now more than 2 inches long from crown to rump. Hair follicles have started to develop, though if your child is anything like mine, those follicles won't see a whole lot of action until somewhere around his first birthday. (I was a bald eagle until the age of two.) Nipples are present now, too. Here's something to ponder: If baby's sex was determined at the moment of conception—and it was, based on which chromosome, X or Y, he (or she) inherited from papa—then why do boy babies have nipples? Turns out that male and female embryos develop more or less identically during those first few weeks in utero. By the time testosterone production kicks in (around Week 9) the early mammary structures have already formed. It seems it's just easier for Mother Nature to leave 'em be.

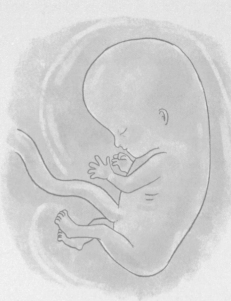

BABY IS MORE THAN TWO INCHES LONG FROM CROWN TO RUMP.

WHAT'S UP WITH *mama*?

I had an infected molar when I was expecting Griffin, and it ached like crazy; I also knew it wasn't great for my pregnancy. (Studies have shown that oral bacteria can find its way into the amniotic fluid, which may contribute to premature childbirth.) Off to the dentist I went, only to discover that the tooth had to be yanked. Turns out that old wives' tale—"Gain a child, lose a tooth"—has some truth to it. Rising hormones can wreak havoc on your gums and the way they respond to plaque, too. Common complaints during this time include tooth sensitivity, overall swelling, and bleeding of the gums, not to mention the arrival of cavities. Make sure to give your teeth a thorough brush twice a day (if not after every meal), floss regularly, and see your dentist *at least* once during your pregnancy. You might also want to get yourself a tongue scraper, since it helps remove harmful bacteria from the mouth. Trust me: having major dental work while you're pregnant is no fun, so keep those pearly whites healthy, Mama!

As soon as you announce that you're expecting, well-meaning friends, family members—even total strangers—are going to tell you the same thing again and again and again: "Enjoy [fill in the blank] while you can. Life as you know it will be over the *instant* you have that baby." I figured the warning was at least partially true. I certainly expected some sleepless nights, some spit-up on my clothes, and I was still feeling apprehensive about our decision to go the cloth diaper route. (Do you just scrape them off or . . . ?) But I also couldn't help rolling my eyes, because surely everyone was exaggerating. Was my world *really* going to change all that drastically overnight? I mean,

all newborns really do is eat, sleep, and poop, right?

Oh, how I wish someone would've sat me down during my pregnancy, looked me straight in the eyes, and said, "Genevieve, you need to take some time out for *you*." Because all those well-meaning friends, family members, and total strangers? They were totally right.

Don't get me wrong. Having children is the best thing I have ever done. Motherhood takes a lot out of you, but it gives back more than you could have dreamed.

Still, it's normal to grieve the loss of your child-free life, especially if you weren't prepared for how all-encompassing the change

WHAT I THOUGHT BEFORE BECOMING A MOM	WHAT I KNOW NOW
Michael and I will make "date night" a priority. That's what grandparents and sitters are for, right?	Good luck finding a sitter on short notice.
Just because I'll be a mom doesn't mean I'll have to dress like one.	Most days, you'll be wearing "Mommy's Eau de Toilette," a charming blend of spit-up, breast milk, snot, and poop.
No yoga pants or grubby T-shirts for me!	Your "fancy" clothes will move to the back of the closet.
I'll be able to sleep in *sometimes*. There are two of us, after all. Michael and I can tag-team it.	HAHAHAHAHAHA.

would be. That's why I'm giving you full permission to indulge in some much-needed—and well-deserved—TLC. The more we can appreciate these moments now, the more we can embrace the new and exciting life that awaits. Here's everything I wish I'd done more of before baby:

LISTEN TO SOME LIVE MUSIC

Let's face it: bars, clubs, concerts, and music festivals aren't exactly child-*friendly*. Neither are loud noise and big crowds, and it's not easy sidling up to a bar stool when you're carting around a baby carrier, diaper bag, toys, nipple cream, and a breast pump. Now is a good time to put on your party boots and hit the town, even if you won't be doing any drinking.

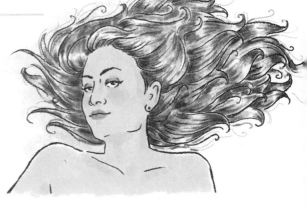

GET YOUR HAIR DONE . . .

I used to get my hair trimmed religiously every three months, now I'm lucky if I make it to the salon twice a year. But aside from the obvious indulgence—is there anything more relaxing than a mid-shampoo scalp massage?!—you may find that pregnancy is an *excellent* time to lavish some attention on your locks. Elevated estrogen levels prolong the hair's growth phase, meaning that each individual strand will grow longer and stronger before eventually falling out. Don't be surprised if you're suddenly sporting movie star hair. Between this and the boobs? Wowzers.

. . . BUT HOLD OFF ON THE HAIR DYE

If you're among the 75 percent of women who dye their hair, know that most ob-gyns and midwives recommend foregoing color until *at least* the start of the second trimester. There aren't any studies to confirm that coloring is dangerous to your pregnancy, but commercial dyes are loaded with some pretty noxious chemicals (more than five thousand of them!), many of which may be carcinogenic. (Some research suggests that professional colorists, for example, are at greater risk of developing bladder cancer.) Luckily, there are plenty of nontoxic options available if you can't go a whole nine months without touching up your roots. Henna, the same dye responsible for the temporary reddish-brown tattoos, has been used to color hair for thousands of years. Check out Morrocco Method, an all-natural, cruelty-free brand that utilizes henna and indigo. Blond mamas who want to go lighter, meanwhile, can turn to an equally old-school method: lemon juice. Dilute with some water, spritz over your hair, and dry in the sun for some natural highlights. Want blond streaks rather than all-over color? Apply the lemon juice to small sections of hair with a tooth-brush. Add some chamomile or calendula tea to lemon juice for honey tones or a darker blond color.

VISIT A PREGNANCY MASSAGE THERAPIST

A professional massage was something I always thought of as a once-in-a-blue-moon sorta thing. Something about it just seemed so *indulgent* that I had a hard time justifying having one with any regularity. Then I got pregnant. I went to a certified pregnancy massage therapist and felt uh-mazing as I left her office. Now I think of massage as an important complementary healthcare procedure. In fact, more and more midwives (and even ob-gyns!) are recommending massage therapy to relieve the unique aches and pains associated with pregnancy, not to mention increase relaxation, reduce stress, improve circulation, decrease swelling, regulate hormones, boost mood—need I go on? The great thing about certified specialists is that they have a unique understanding of prenatal physiology; they know how to position you to avoid strain or pressure on the ligaments, and can identify signs of complications like preeclampsia, one of the few circumstances in which massage isn't recommended.

SLEEP

Between the growing belly and the constant need to pee, not to mention things like restless leg syndrome, I know that getting quality shut-eye during pregnancy can seem elusive. (I even devote a whole *week* to getting your forty winks a bit later in this book.) But take it from some-one who's been there: Sleep until noon. Nap. Leisurely lie in bed reading. Whatever sleep pattern you love to indulge in, *do it.* Do it *all.* And do it often. Decorating the nursery and planning your baby shower can wait.

SEE ALL THE GOOD MOVIES

I used to love seeing all the Oscar-nominated films and then analyzing each and every one before the Academy Awards—and, yes, I was a major fan (and frequent winner) of the office Oscar pool. These days, most of the movies I see are G-rated and, frankly, not quite as gripping. So go, Mama, and eat some popcorn for me (or pack your own popcorn that doesn't taste like a salt truck exploded). Pro tip: get a seat on or near the aisle for quick and easy bathroom access.

Big fan of loud action flicks or the IMAX experience? No need to worry about the noise. Inside your uterus, floating in a sea of amniotic fluid, baby's hearing is pretty muffled (even though he will be able to hear and respond to sound by the third trimester). The only kind of noise we need to worry about as it relates to baby's future hearing is of the prolonged variety—think: eight hours a day standing on an airport tarmac.

TREAT YOURSELF TO A MANI-PEDI

The same hormones responsible for those luscious locks tend to make your nails grow faster, too. Even if getting a regular manicure-pedicure isn't your thing, consider indulging while pregnant. I found that having pretty feet gave me a much-needed self-esteem boost, even if I couldn't *see* them all that well over the mound of my growing belly. Choose a well-ventilated salon and book an appointment during a low-traffic time of day to minimize your exposure to any toxic fumes (which, aside from the obvious health implications, may be enough to trigger your extra-sensitive gag reflex). While getting your nails done is perfectly safe during pregnancy, I liked bring-ing my own nontoxic nail polish. The standard stuff your local salon stocks tends to contain chemicals like dibutyl phthalate, which has been linked to birth defects and is banned in the European Union. I'm a huge fan of Piggy Paint, which is nontoxic, hypoallergenic, cruelty-free, and completely safe to use during pregnancy (not to mention great for little girls who want their nails painted, too!). They even make a nontoxic polish remover, free of yucky stuff like formaldehyde, acetone, and BPA. Oh, you can always ditch the salon altogether and have your partner paint your piggies, too.

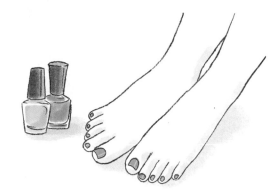

PLAYING IT SAFE WITH SELF-CARE

I'm all for pampering yourself during pregnancy, but you'll likely want to hold off on perms, relaxers, and straighteners. While there's no conclusive evidence that these processes aren't safe for baby, there's no evidence that they *are* safe during pregnancy, either. You'll also want to skip teeth bleaching or whitening kits, skin lightening or brightening creams, eyelash growth serums, and all other chemically based personal care products. Head over to mamanatural.com for some healthy, natural alternatives.

(Ridiculously Tasty) Date Oatmeal

As a nutrient, silica doesn't get much playtime, which is sort of silly when you think about it, since we literally need it to stand up straight. This important mineral helps build strong bones, as well as healthy hair, skin, and nails. And while you can boost your silica intake by eating more green beans, bananas, and brown rice, oats are one of the richest sources on the planet. My absolute favorite way to eat oats? This ridiculously tasty date oatmeal.

INGREDIENTS

2 cups organic rolled oats

5–6 cups filtered water, divided

2 scant teaspoons raw apple cider vinegar or lemon juice

3–4 coconut rolled dates

2–4 tablespoons coconut flakes

⅓ cup coconut milk

Raw honey or stevia to taste

In a large saucepan, soak the oats in 4 cups water and the vinegar for 24 hours. In the morning, drain the oats and rinse well. Add 1 to 2 more cups of water (depending on how soupy you like your oatmeal) and cook on high heat until the water comes to a boil. Reduce heat to a simmer and cook uncovered for 15 to 20 minutes. About halfway into the cook time, mince your dates and stir them into the oatmeal. Add coconut flakes and coconut milk. Finish cooking until most of the liquid has absorbed and you're left with a thick, nutty oatmeal that's still easy to dish out. Serve it up with some honey, stevia, or fresh fruit. Nuts and maple syrup make for scrumptious toppings, too. Serves 4.

GO OUT TO EAT . . . *A LOT*

I hate to break it to you, but restaurants will likely become a thing of the past, at least for a while. Think you can squeeze in a charming lunch at a café during naptime? Once you've showered (perhaps for the first time in days), gotten dressed, packed up the baby, loaded up the diaper bag, and figured out how to fold up the stroller, you'll either be too tired to go or—surprise!—baby is awake and naptime is over.

SLEEP

I really can't stress this enough. Sleep on the couch. Sleep in the car (not while you're driving, of course). Sleep on your husband's shoulder. Sleep whenever, wherever possible.

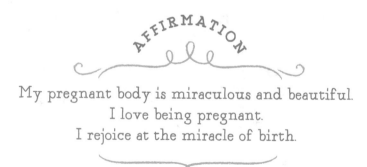

Get it while you can!

MAKE TIME FOR YOUR GIRLFRIENDS

With the arrival of a newborn, our lives start to close in around us—our entire universe is suddenly contained within the four walls of our home—and our days begin to revolve around feeding, burping, bathing, sleeping, and pooping. Trust me, it's hard to care much about the hot guy your friend is dating or even remember her birthday when the most exciting part of your Saturday is counting how many doo-doos your baby made. Socializing will become less important and our relationships can suffer. Those relationships *will* come back; many of your friends may even be in the same boat, so don't worry. Do be sure to value those old friendships, though. When baby's a little bit older, you'll be desperate to reconnect and talk about anything other than poop.

READ FOR PLEASURE

These days, reading a novel is pure luxury. Picture books or parenting books tend to fill my nightstand now. Read the bestsellers. Or the classics. Check out Oprah's Book Club or get recommendations from your friends or your local librarian.

AFFIRMATION

My pregnant body is miraculous and beautiful.
I love being pregnant.
I rejoice at the miracle of birth.

SHOULD YOU ASK FOR A PUSH PRESENT?

These days, the idea of pampering a pregnant woman has become—thankfully—pretty popular. Mamas are organizing pregnancy spa days; they're researching and planning babymoons (a trend we'll talk more about in Week 17). They're also receiving, and in some cases *asking* for, push presents.

Say what?

The "push present" is a gift mama receives from her husband or partner for having "pushed" out the baby. (It's hard work!) Though there's no real consensus on where this trend came from—Is it a conspiracy by the jewelry industry? Did Posh Spice invent this? Are modern husbands just more with-it than generations past?—one thing's for sure: push presents have exploded. According to a recent survey, 38 percent of new mamas reported receiving one (and 55 percent of pregnant women wanted one). But they've also generated a fair amount of backlash: lots of people are turned off by the implicit materialism surrounding such a sacred event. After all, isn't a brand-new, beautiful baby a nice enough present?

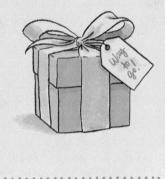

While I'm not a big gift person myself, I do like the spirit behind a push present—that is, honoring mama for a job well done. The most popular push presents are undoubtedly jewelry, and I've seen some truly charming rings and necklaces featuring baby's initials, as well as jewelry that can be added on to with the birth of each subsequent child. Push presents, however, can also be more functional and practical: some papas line up a professional housekeeper for a few weeks, for example, or contribute to baby's college fund.

FINISH UP THOSE HOME IMPROVEMENTS

The intention here is to pamper yourself, not to create an endless series of DIYs that suck your time and drain your energy. Completing some manageable projects, however, can make you feel good. So, assemble those bookshelves you purchased three years ago. Reorganize your kitchen cupboards. File your tax returns. Heck, dust the blinds! The next time you'll get around to some of this stuff your "baby" will be a kindergartner.

SLEEP

Have I mentioned this yet?

GO SHOPPING—AND *NOT* ON AMAZON.COM

Wander through a mall. Window-shop. Try on cute shoes or scarves or jackets just because you can. You don't have to buy a thing—but if you do, buy something pretty.

BLOCK OUT SOME ME TIME

It's perhaps a strange thought, but one day not long from now you will find that you miss . . . *yourself*. Or at least time alone with yourself. Solitude and privacy will seem like strange concepts you've only read about in books. And when you do have a rare, fleeting moment alone, you simply won't know what to do with yourself. Shower? Blow-dry your hair? Fill that time with someone who can speak in complete sentences?

Lock yourself in the bathroom and luxuriate in the tub. Drive around your neighborhood and sing your favorite songs at the top of your lungs. Kill two birds with one stone and see one of those Oscar-nominated movies all by yourself. Just think how much happier you'll be if you can look back on this time and say, "I took advantage" instead of "Oh, I wish I had known."

Mama, *enjoy* this phase.

mama-do list

- Make a dentist appointment, especially if you haven't been in the chair recently.

- SLEEP.

- See if there's a certified pregnancy massage therapist in your hometown. Most offer package deals, which will bring down the total cost of each rubdown. But if that's just not in the budget, set up a standing weekly date and put your partner to work. You can even make your own massage oils by adding a few drops of essential oil to your favorite lotion—plain ol' coconut oil works, too.

under the weather?

NATURAL REMEDIES FOR

cold, cough, and flu

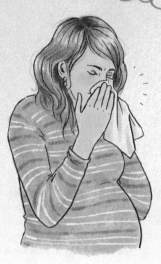

WHAT'S UP WITH *baby*?

At this point, most of baby's vital organs and major systems have formed, so the next few months are all about growth. Some of those organs, however, are on the move. Strange as it sounds, baby's intestines, for example, have spent the last few weeks not in her abdomen, where they belong, but *outside* her body, in the umbilical cord. Until now, there just wasn't enough room in her tiny tummy to accommodate all those folds of tissue. Meanwhile, the reproductive organs—ovaries for girl, testes for boy—have made their debut. It's still too early to detect baby's sex via a sonogram (for those mamas who didn't undergo cell-free DNA screening), but here's a wild thought: if you're having a girl, she's already got somewhere around two million eggs in those ovaries. Your future grandchild might even be among them. Weird, right?

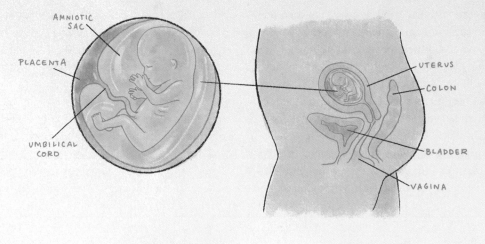

WHAT'S UP WITH *mama*?

One of the main reasons women ditch conventional or prescription prenatals is because they can lead to constipation. And let's face it, it's no fun not being able to do your daily *doo*. (Rising progesterone doesn't help matters much either, as it relaxes the stomach and intestinal muscles, triggering a slowdown in digestion.) Conventional wisdom is to drink plenty of water, exercise regularly, eat a fiber-rich diet, and switch to a natural, food-based prenatal vitamin. But while that's fine advice, sometimes we still need an extra . . . *push*. Supplementing with a little extra magnesium is one way, but I got mine in the form of two pears a day. They're high in fiber and an excellent natural laxative. You can check out my recipe for Protein Pear Pudding on page 233.

I was living in Chicago—a town famous for its brutally cold winters—when I found out that I was expecting my first child. So, when I came down with a mild case of the sniffles around Christmastime, I figured it was just the season. It wasn't until later that I realized my cold might have had less to do with the weather and more to do with the fact that I was newly (unknowingly) pregnant at the time. That's right: just like tender breasts, darkened areolas, and nausea, a mild cold may very well be a symptom of early pregnancy. Why? Because your immune system is running at less than optimal capacity (mostly so that your body doesn't reject your baby). Unfortunately, that only leaves you more susceptible to illness and infection, especially during cold and flu season. So what happens if you develop a runny nose, hacking cough, or sore throat? Is getting sick during pregnancy . . . *dangerous*?

IF *I'M* SICK, IS MY BABY SICK, TOO?

Let's start with the good news: When it comes to the common cold, the virus doesn't cross the placenta, which means that no matter how crummy you may be feeling, your baby is not and will not get "sick." (It's thought that the flu virus doesn't cross the placenta, either. Some research suggests that a few highly virulent strains—such as the avian, or bird, flu—*could*; but rest assured, that's only happened in *very* few cases.) So the real concern when you fall ill isn't about the virus itself. What you need to watch out for and be aware of is that pregnant women have a higher chance of developing illness-related complications.

Though the risk is small, we know that pregnant women with the flu, for example, are more likely to be hospitalized. For a long time, we figured that was because a suppressed immune system did a poor job of fighting off the influenza virus. New research, however—in particular, a small study from the Stanford University School of Medicine—suggests that pregnant women actually have an unusually *strong* response to the flu; they experience a kind of hyperinflammation. This may be one reason why mamas with the flu seem more susceptible to pneumonia.

The issue to really watch out for with regard to the flu is the potential for fever. Anything higher than 100.4°F is cause for concern (though you should call your healthcare provider even if you're running a very low-grade fever); some studies indicate that a high, persistent fever is linked to neural tube defects, cleft palate, congenital heart defects, autism, and premature labor.

ANTIHISTAMINES, COUGH SYRUPS, DECONGESTANTS: WHICH CAN I TAKE?

Aspirin, ibuprofen, and decongestants such as the active ingredient in products such as Sudafed (pseudoephedrine) are generally *not* considered safe to take during pregnancy. However, most doctors (and some midwives) will recommend acetaminophen (Tylenol) for fever and pain relief, Tamiflu to alleviate flu symptoms, and some over-the-counter cough and cold medicines, such as Robitussin. These are unattractive options for natural mamas who try to avoid OTCs or prescription meds whenever possible. But they may not even be all that safe to take, either.

Preliminary studies suggest that Tylenol, when taken by pregnant women for twenty-eight days or more, is linked to a higher risk of ADHD, as well as some behavioral problems and language delays. Regarding Tamiflu, there's no real evidence that antivirals are harmful, but they haven't been thoroughly tested in pregnant women. Robitussin, meanwhile—generally only recommended *after* the first

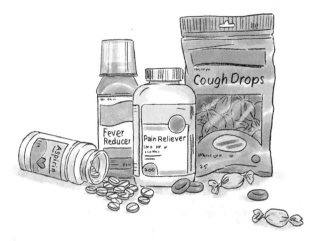

TDAP VACCINE: WHAT SAY YOU?

In addition to offering you a flu shot, your healthcare provider may recommend getting a Tdap vaccine, too. Three different diseases are addressed in the formulation—tetanus, diphtheria, and pertussis, a.k.a. whooping cough—but the priority is definitely protecting against pertussis, which can be deadly in a small percentage of infants. (Babies can't get vaccinated against whooping cough until they're two months old, so the shot is intended to "fill the gap" and protect the newborn.) The CDC, the American College of Obstetricians and Gynecologists, and the ACNM all recommend getting the Tdap shot sometime between 27 and 36 weeks.

Some natural mamas, however, aren't particularly comfortable with that recommendation, in part because vaccines can't be tested for safety on pregnant women, based on a 1976 FDA ruling. There's also some concern about the package inserts, most of which read a little something like this:

> Safety and effectiveness of this vaccine have not been established in pregnant women. Animal reproduction studies have not been conducted with this vaccine. It is not known whether this vaccine can cause fetal harm when administered to a pregnant woman or can affect reproduction capacity. This vaccine should be given to a pregnant woman only if clearly needed.

The question, of course, is: is it *clearly needed?* And that, my friend, is best determined by having a thorough discussion with your healthcare provider. If you're interested in a more natural alternative, you can also look into the homeopathic whooping cough remedy called Pertussin, which can be administered to a newborn as young as one week old. Talk to your future child's pediatrician or a naturopath for more information.

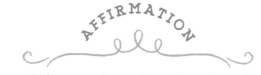
trimester—may ease some of your symptoms, but it doesn't treat, prevent, or kill the cold or flu virus. Additionally, every major health organization recommends taking medications (whether prescription or OTC) sparingly, all the more reason to give natural, drug-free remedies a try.

Two exceptions to a strict no-drugs rule? Persistent or high fever and virulent or new strains of the flu virus, since we know these can be quite dangerous if left untreated.

As a general rule, you should speak with your midwife or doctor before taking *any* medications. On the other hand, if your healthcare provider prescribes or recommends a drug you're hesitant about taking, don't just ignore the advice. Ask about appropriate dosage,

safety during pregnancy, and possible alternative therapies. Seek out a second opinion if you're still unsure, or speak with your local pharmacist. As I mentioned earlier: I took Tylenol for a few days after having a tooth pulled (I was desperate to relieve the pain), and while I worried like crazy about the consequences, it was fine.

> ### THINKING ABOUT THE FLU SHOT?
>
> Refer back to page 88 to determine if the flu vaccine is right for you.

MORE THAN JUST CHICKEN SOUP: NATURAL REMEDIES FOR COLDS AND THE FLU

Just about everybody's grandmother had the same basic prescription for treating a cold or the flu: drink plenty of fluids and get plenty of rest, sip some homemade broth or chicken soup, and up your intake of vitamin C to give the immune system a much-needed boost.

While those are all great—and important—first steps, that advice is also a little, well, *basic.*

Knock out a cold or flu quickly with the following turbocharged remedies:

RAW APPLE CIDER VINEGAR

Yes, raw apple cider vinegar (ACV) pops up once again! (This stuff is so versatile, I actually have a post featuring 101 distinct uses for it on my website.) If you're feeling under the

IS IT A COLD, THE FLU—OR SOMETHING ELSE?

The defining difference between a cold and the flu is generally the strength of the symptoms. Colds are milder; the hallmarks are sneezing and a runny nose, and rarely does a cold involve a fever. The flu, on the other hand, can hit you like a ton of bricks. Symptoms include sore throat, fever, headache, cough, vomiting, and chills, which may worsen over the first several days. But even if you're not officially sick, you might still sound like it. That's because sniffling during pregnancy is common.

Your surging hormones (it's always the hormones, isn't it?) cause swelling in the nasal passages, which can trigger the production of excess mucus—hello, runny nose. If you're congested, here's how to get some relief:

Stay Hydrated
All that blowing and sniffling and sneezing can dry out your nasal passages, so make sure you're drinking plenty of water. Sip some all-natural lemonade throughout the day, too, for a boost of vitamin C, or organic coconut water, which is high in potassium and electrolytes—add a dash of sea salt for a mineral boost and better hydration.

Try a Neti Pot
They burst onto the scene in 2007 after on-air endorsements by Oprah Winfrey and Dr. Oz, but neti pots—which look a bit like Aladdin's magic lamp—have been around for thousands of years. How do they work? Fill the pot with lukewarm filtered water, add a pinch of sea salt, place the spout inside one nostril, and pour. As the water travels through your nasal cavity (neti pots are also called "nasal irrigators" for a reason), the saline solution thins the mucus and flushes the nasal passage. And let me tell you, these things *work*. My husband used to take prescription-strength allergy medicine during hay fever season until he tried the neti pot. He's been off the drugs now for years.

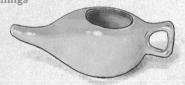

Use a Humidifier
Cold, dry air zaps moisture from your skin, but you can get some nose-soothing relief by running a warm-mist humidifier. Just make sure to change the water daily, clean the unit weekly, and replace the filter regularly, as humidifiers can breed bacteria and mold.

Try a Nasal Dilator
Another one of my husband's discoveries, nasal dilators are little silicone doohickies that fit inside your nostrils and, as the name suggests, *dilates* them. You probably won't find one at your local drugstore, but a quick search on Amazon will yield dozens of options. Michael prefers a brand called WoodyKnows, which helps him breathe at night when he's got a cold or is suffering from allergies. Bonus: they reduce snoring, too.

Supercharged Chicken Soup

Well, I had to include chicken soup in here *somewhere*! Make yours with homemade bone broth (recipe on page 89) and you'll get the added healing benefits of gelatin-based protein. Add some garlic for its cold-busting properties and Asian mushrooms (think: maitake, shiitake), which contain antiviral properties, too.

INGREDIENTS

1–2 tablespoons olive oil

2 medium onions, chopped

2 medium carrots, diced

2 celery ribs, diced

2 parsnips, diced

2 to 3 cloves garlic, crushed

1 tablespoon pastured butter

1 cup shiitake or maitake mushrooms, sliced

2–3 quarts bone broth (if you're short on broth, dilute what you have with filtered water)

1–1½ cups diced or shredded roasted or rotisserie chicken

Fresh parsley, chopped

Cayenne pepper (optional, but avoid if you're running a fever)

In a large stockpot, heat olive oil over medium heat. Add onion, carrots, celery, parsnips, garlic, and a pinch of salt and pepper to the pan. Cook until vegetables are softened (about 5 minutes). In a separate skillet, heat butter over medium heat. Add mushrooms and a pinch of salt; sauté until just brown (about 5 minutes). Add mushrooms to stockpot with vegetables. Pour in bone broth and bring to a simmer. Add chicken and parsley and simmer until heated through. Salt and pepper to taste. For a kick, add a pinch of cayenne pepper—it's a natural analgesic, or pain reliever.

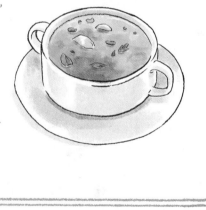

weather, mix 1 to 2 tablespoons of ACV into 8 ounces of water or tea, and drink twice a day. You can try gargling with a mixture of warm water, ACV, and salt—even more effective at soothing a sore throat than saltwater alone. ACV is also an old-school method for bringing down a fever. Add 1 cup to a lukewarm bath, or soak a washcloth in one part ACV to two parts water and place on the forehead. (Some people swear by ACV-soaked socks! Try soaking a pair in diluted ACV, wringing them out, and putting them on your feet for 10 to 15 minutes.)

AN OUNCE OF PREVENTION

Fighting the cold and flu starts *long* before you actually get sick. Reduce your chances of falling ill—as well as the likelihood that you might need prescription drug intervention—by adhering to the following guidelines:

Practice Good Hygiene.

Wash your hands often, especially before meals, and try not to touch your face. When you're at home, stick with plain ol' soap and water; I love Kiss My Face olive oil soaps. When you're out and about, a natural witch hazel or tea tree oil hand sanitizer is a good alternative when a sink isn't available. Whatever you do, steer clear of big-brand sanitizers (like the kind found in pump dispensers in public restrooms). They often contain triclosan or triclocarban, ingredients that were outlawed in soaps and hand washes by the FDA due to concerns about their safety and efficacy.

You'll also, of course, want to keep the surfaces and linens in your home sanitary. Use a nontoxic cleanser and change your sheets often. Make a point of letting in some fresh air once or twice a week, even if the temperature outside is freezing. Studies suggest that the indoor air quality in most homes is significantly worse than that outdoors.

Eat More Garlic.

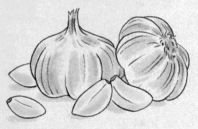

The antiviral benefits of garlic are certainly effective at treating colds, but they actually have a prophylactic (or preventive) effect, too. In fact, a study published in the medical journal *Advances in Therapy* suggests that daily consumption of an allicin-containing garlic supplement drastically lowers your chances of getting sick (study participants had 63 percent fewer colds than a placebo group), and shortens recovery time—*by 70 percent*—when you do fall ill. Aim to incorporate one clove of crushed garlic with lunch and dinner. You can toss some raw garlic into your salad dressing or pesto (check out the recipe on page 226), or try it smeared on toast with butter, avocado, or olive oil. Pro tip: wait 10 minutes after crushing the garlic before eating to allow the potent allicin to fully form.

Break a Sweat.

Aside from the obvious benefits—like maintaining a healthy weight and lowering your risk of pregnancy-related complications—regular exercise can also boost your immune system. Need proof? A study from researchers at Appalachian State University found that people who exercise at least five times a week get fewer colds than their more sedentary counterparts.

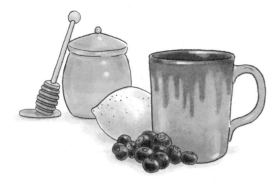

BLUEBERRY TEA WITH HONEY, LEMON, AND GINGER

Warm tea is great for relieving a sore throat and congestion, as well as soothing queasiness or an upset tummy. This version, however, packs a serious cold- and flu-fighting punch. Raw honey has antimicrobial and antibacterial properties; lemon, of course, is packed with vitamin C; ginger is a potent anti-inflammatory; while blueberries contain salicylic acid—the active ingredient in aspirin (with no side effects!).

To make a pitcher, add 8 ounces fresh or frozen blueberries and ¼ cup fresh-squeezed lemon juice to a small saucepan. Bring to a boil, simmer for about 5 minutes (stirring occasionally), then strain the mixture through a fine mesh sieve, mashing the berries to extract all the juice. Meanwhile, in a kettle or large saucepan, steep 4 bags ginger tea in 8 cups of water. Combine the tea and the blueberry mixture in a large pitcher, and sweeten with honey. Drink 1–2 cups a day. Can be served hot or cold.

COCONUT OIL PEPPERMINT BARK

Coconut oil is famous for its antiviral, antibacterial, and antifungal properties. For a sweet treat, combine 2 tablespoons raw, organic coco-nut oil with ⅛ teaspoon peppermint extract, and 1 tablespoon raw honey. Mix well, then spread the mixture thinly on a sheet of parchment paper. Pop into the freezer for 15 minutes until set. (Triple the batch if you'd like *lots* of leftovers.)

ELDERBERRY SYRUP (FOR COLDS ONLY)

Many pregnant mamas have had great success treating cough and cold symptoms with elderberry syrup (usually available in the natural section of your local supermarket or at most health food stores), but you might want to steer clear of it if you've come down with a case of the flu. Elderberry syrup is thought to be a major immune booster—potentially what you don't need if the most recent research on pregnancy and influenza is correct (meaning that pregnant women's immune systems actually *overreact* to the flu).

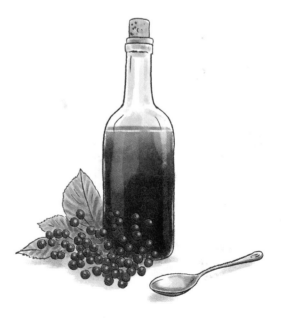

mama-do list

- If your cold is acute, you might want to consider taking a food-based vitamin C supplement (2,000 milligrams spread out over the course of the day), as well as a high-quality probiotic. Alternatively, I like mixing ½ teaspoon camu camu powder into a bowl of Greek yogurt. The camu berry is *loaded* with vitamin C— one serving has more than 1,000 percent of your daily recommended intake. Just be sure to add honey; camu camu powder is sour!

- Whether I was feeling under the weather or fit as a fiddle, I religiously took my daily dose of cod liver oil while pregnant, since it's high in immune-boosting vitamins A and D. Talk to your midwife or doctor about the dosage that's most appropriate for you.

- Your body needs significantly more fluids during pregnancy, which makes the potential for dehydration a real concern during cold and flu season. Make sure you're drinking plenty of liquids—water, coconut water, all-natural lemonade, broth—and limiting or eliminating your intake of caffeine.

baby brain
AND THE
absentminded mama

WHAT'S UP WITH *baby*?

A few months from now, baby is going to get *very* interested in the world around him. Stories—and ultrasound images—abound of babies pulling or yanking on their umbilical cord, or licking (!) the wall of the uterus. Babies have also been known to suck their thumbs—but that can start now, as early as 13 weeks. Even more interesting, some studies suggest that which thumb he chooses to suck may indicate his eventual "handedness," since the majority of babies prefer to suck their right thumb, just as the majority of grown-ups in the world are right-handed. (And, yes, babies who suck their left thumb in utero are more likely to wind up as left-handers.)

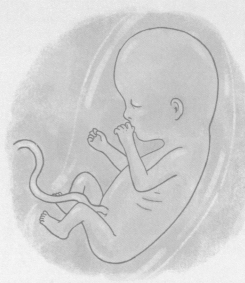

BABIES HAVE BEEN KNOWN TO SUCK THEIR THUMBS AS EARLY AS 13 WEEKS.

WHAT'S UP WITH *mama*?

Oh, happy day! This is the last week of your first trimester, Mama, and you're getting ready to enter a whole new world. One where morning sickness will likely be a thing of the past, where extreme fatigue will feel a little less, well, *extreme*, and taste and smell aversions have pretty much ceased. Your appetite is on its way back now, and you'll be able to reintroduce the foods you *used* to love but haven't been able to stomach for weeks. The second trimester is truly the sweet spot of pregnancy—in fact, it's often called the "Magic Middle." The yuck factor is gone (hopefully!), but you aren't yet so big that navigating your daily life has become awkward or uncomfortable. Prepare to feel a bit like your old self again. Yippee!

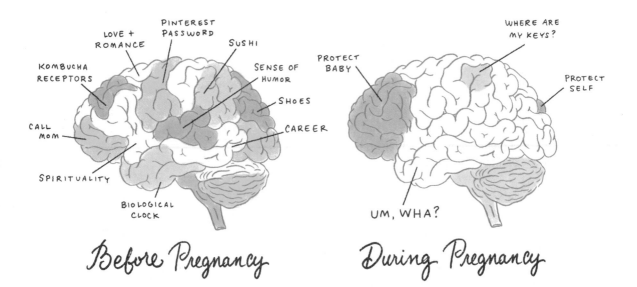

Before Pregnancy

KOMBUCHA RECEPTORS
LOVE + ROMANCE
PINTEREST PASSWORD
SUSHI
SENSE OF HUMOR
SHOES
CAREER
CALL MOM
SPIRITUALITY
BIOLOGICAL CLOCK

During Pregnancy

PROTECT BABY
WHERE ARE MY KEYS?
PROTECT SELF
UM, WHA?

I once read that each baby comes out clutching a third of his mother's brain. And in my experience, that sounds about right. Because at some point during my first pregnancy, I'd started searching around for my sunglasses when they were sitting right there on top of my head, or I'd forget to pick up half the things I had intended to buy when I went out grocery shopping. I know I'm not the only mama who's suddenly felt a bit absentminded during pregnancy, either. A slew of studies and surveys, when taken together, suggest that as many as four out of five pregnant women report lapses in memory or depressed cognitive ability. In fact, there are many terms for this phenomenon, from "pregnancy brain" to "baby brain" to "momnesia."

It's certainly true that rising hormones might affect your ability to concentrate and focus at some point in the next few weeks and months, if they haven't already (after all, it's hard to concentrate when you feel bloated, weepy, and fatigued). Lack of quality sleep, meanwhile, would make anyone feel a little bit foggy. There have been a few studies demonstrating that pregnant women may experience a *slight* dip in what's called "prospective memory" (i.e., the ability to perform an intended future action, such as remembering an appointment or taking medication at a particular time—so don't forget your prenatal vitamins!). But whereas we once thought of baby brain as an exclusively negative phenomenon, new research suggests that it's only a temporary side effect to a major neurological upgrade. Far from being a liability, it turns out that pregnancy may actually make us *smarter*.

HOW THE BRAIN CHANGES DURING PREGNANCY

Considering all the ways our bodies change when we're carrying a child—from boobs to belly to foot size—it perhaps shouldn't be surprising that pregnancy also has an effect on the brain. Twenty years ago, researchers from the Imperial College School of Medicine in London discovered that the brain actually appears to *decrease* in size—by as much as 6 percent or 7 percent—in the latter stages of pregnancy. At the time, it was thought that this shrinkage might be proof that the cognitive deficits associated with "baby brain" were real (as opposed to all in our heads).

That particular study, however, was quite small—only fourteen women's brains were scanned with MRI imaging. Much newer research, meanwhile, suggests that while the brain *may* shrink during pregnancy, in the postpartum period, certain areas of it will actually *expand*. Growth in the amygdala, for example, the area of the brain that deals with emotional reactions, helps a new mama become hypersensitive to her baby's wants and needs. (It may explain the arrival of that fierce Mama Bear protective instinct, too, since the amygdala serves as the brain's threat-processing center.) The amygdala also has a large number of receptors for oxytocin, the hormone that stimulates bonding. With each new hit of oxytocin—produced every time mama cuddles, breastfeeds, or even just stares into the face of her newborn—the amygdala may be encouraged to grow even larger; a larger amygdala, meanwhile, has even more hormone receptors. In this way, the simple act of doting on baby produces significant changes in a mama's gray matter.

And the amygdala isn't the only part of the brain that grows.

WHAT OTHER *natural mamas* SAY

emily: I definitely experienced momnesia, but now that I'm pregnant with my second child and chasing around a toddler, I'm a complete disaster. Just last week, I couldn't find my wallet anywhere. I swore I'd left it in the diaper bag. Not there. Two hours later, I rooted around in the same diaper bag, and there it was, right where I'd left it. Wow.

brandi: I'm a nurse, and I once told a patient, "I'll be right back, I'm just going to grab the wheelbarrow for you." Luckily, she realized I meant wheelchair!

hannah: I constantly felt like Dory from *Finding Nemo*.

chelsea: I left my cell phone on the hood of my car near the windshield wipers, and it flew off en route to the grocery store, smashing to smithereens. That would've been bad enough, but I managed to leave my husband's keys in the exact same spot. He looked tirelessly for them for two straight weeks. Finally, we went to get the oil changed and the mechanic asked my poor husband if he realized there was a set of car keys under the hood.

- Studies have long indicated that women are better multitaskers than men, but the gap may widen even further due to changes in the prefrontal cortex.

- Growth in the hippocampus, the region responsible for learning and memory, suggests that new mothers may actually have better recall after giving birth, not worse.

- We know that mamas are better able to recognize faces (particularly those of men) as well as better able to interpret emotions (especially emotions that are overtly negative), because they have a heightened ability to sense danger.

The changes to a new mother's brain are so rapid and so significant, in fact, that researchers have called pregnancy as important a developmental event as puberty.

Baby brain, the research indicates, doesn't leave a new mama addled; it makes her better able to cope with the demands and challenges of motherhood. And the best part? These changes don't seem to disappear or to wane. On the contrary, this enhanced cognition may very well last for a lifetime.

IF BABY BRAIN MAKES US SMARTER, WHY CAN'T I FIND MY CAR KEYS?

For decades now, pregnant women have been warned about the onset of momnesia, so it wouldn't surprise me if you've misplaced an item in your home or lost your train of thought in the middle of a conversation and figured baby brain was to blame. One theory for these bouts of absentmindedness is that your brain is busy growing, rewiring, and remodeling. In other words, your processor actually might be running a little slower during these next few months because your brain is upgrading itself to a more advanced 2.0 model.

It is also possible, however, that occasional episodes of momnesia don't have anything to do with pregnancy at all, and are caused, instead, by the mere power of suggestion.

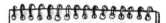

TO DO:
find keys
interview doula
apple cider vinegar
spin class
maternity bra
plan meals
recover Netflix password

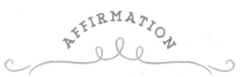

AFFIRMATION

I am grateful for every surge of nausea, every twinge of discomfort, every moment of unease. I know that these sensations are nothing compared to the joy that awaits on the other side.

DON'T FORGET TO STAY HYDRATED, MAMA!

It's important to drink plenty of fluids during pregnancy—but sometimes mama just needs something to drink other than water. (Can I get a witness?) These recipes will keep you hydrated, support digestion, ward off morning sickness, improve circulation, and satisfy your taste buds. Pick one each morning and sip throughout the day.

Citrus Cooler

1 grapefruit

1 orange

1 lime

1 lemon

1 teaspoon raw honey (optional)

1 quart filtered water

Dash of sea salt

Ice (optional)

Hand squeeze your citrus fruit and put the juices into a quart Mason jar. Mix in your honey (if using) and let it totally dissolve. Add filtered water and sea salt. Add ice if desired.

The Mama Mojito

4 limes

1 tablespoon raw honey (or 15 drops liquid stevia)

1 tablespoon raw apple cider vinegar

6 to 8 mint leaves, minced

1 quart filtered water

Ice (optional)

Juice your limes and add to a quart Mason jar. Add sweetener, apple cider vinegar, and mint leaves. Fill the jar with filtered water and mix well. Add ice if desired.

The Ginger Snap

2 lemons

1 tablespoon raw honey (or 15 drops liquid stevia)

1 tablespoon raw apple cider vinegar

1 heaping teaspoon grated fresh ginger

1 quart filtered water

Ice (optional)

Juice your lemons and add to a quart Mason jar. Add sweetener, apple cider vinegar, and ginger. Fill the jar with filtered water and mix well. Let sit for 15 minutes. Strain the ginger and add ice, if desired.

Watermelon Water

2 large slices of watermelon

Filtered water

Cut up watermelon into 1-inch cubes. Put cubes into an ice-cube tray and freeze. Once frozen, place 8 to 12 watermelon cubes in a quart Mason jar and fill with filtered water or, for a bubbly treat, sparkling water.

Red Raspberry Leaf Tea

If you talk to virtually any midwife or doula, you're practically guaranteed to hear about the miracles of red raspberry leaf, an herbal tea that's been used for thousands of years to support respiratory and digestive health and—here's where things get *really* interesting—to ease and shorten labor.

If that sounds too good to be true, there *are* some studies to back up these claims, including one published in the *Australian College of Midwives Incorporated Journal*, which suggested that women who drank the tea were less likely to need forceps or vacuum assistance or require a C-section. (Some other studies on rats, however, were less conclusive.) I put the most stock, however, in my personal experience.

Based on the advice of my midwife, I tried drinking red raspberry leaf tea during my first pregnancy, early in the first trimester. I felt some very slight uterine cramping, however, which scared me, so I quit the tea and forgot all about it. You already know how my son's birth went—twenty-seven hours of labor and a hit of Pit.

During my second pregnancy, I decided to do things differently. Starting at fourteen weeks, I made warm red raspberry leaf tea—16 ounces with a splash of coconut milk— my afternoon ritual. The week of my due date, I brewed a super-strong batch, drank it for two consecutive days, and BAM! Baby Paloma made her debut so quickly I almost didn't make it to the birth center. Call me crazy, but I am convinced the tea played a major part in making my second birth drama-free and virtually painless.

Keep in mind that most healthcare providers will recommend waiting until the second trimester—there is a slight concern (though no actual scientific evidence) that drinking the tea too early could increase your risk for miscarriage. As I mentioned, I felt some slight cramping when I tried it during my first trimester. By the second trimester, however, I was able to enjoy it (anywhere from one to two cups a day) with no problems.

Red raspberry leaf tea tastes great on its own (kind of like a weak black tea), but it *can* get a bit boring, day in, day out. So here are two easy ways to jazz it up.

For a warm, creamy treat: Steep 1 tea bag (or 1 tablespoon of loose tea) in 8 ounces of boiling water for 10 to 15 minutes. Remove the tea bag or strain and add ¼ cup coconut milk and 1 tablespoon raw honey or another natural sweetener.

For a refreshing red raspberry orange cooler: Steep 4 tea bags (or 4 tablespoons of loose tea) in a quart of boiling water, add 2 tablespoons raw honey, then put in the refrigerator. Once cooled, add a bit of fresh orange juice (about ¼ cup per serving) and garnish with an orange slice.

After all, if you're convinced that your mental acuity is going to suffer, you may become hyperaware of every memory lapse or break in your concentration. Although you've certainly misplaced your car keys before, or forgotten to mail out a holiday card, you may be much more likely now to blame that on the baby. The concept of momnesia is so well known that it may become a bit of a self-fulfilling prophecy. So do yourself a favor and don't just assume that you're suffering a cognitive decline in the event that you start to feel foggy. Instead, take some proactive steps to stay sharp, and know that baby brain is actually a *good* thing.

Get More Zzzs. Sleep deprivation has been associated with a slew of side effects that sound an awful lot like the symptoms of momnesia: problems with attention and memory, impaired judgment, slowed reaction time, and poor visuo-motor performance. In fact, operating a vehicle while drowsy can be *just* as dangerous (if not more so) than drunk driving.

Isn't it interesting that the percentage of pregnant women who suffer from sleep disorders (75) is near equal to the percentage who claim to suffer from memory problems (80)?

Get Organized. Having trouble keeping track of appointments and obligations? Well, who can blame you? You really *do* have more on your plate than you otherwise would, so make things easier on yourself. Jot down your to-dos on a giant wall calendar, carry a notepad of reminders in your jacket or purse, or start using the planner app on your iPad or smartphone.

Get Some Help. It's no secret that the busier and more distracted you are, the more likely small tasks will fall through the cracks. So, when possible, delegate some of your responsibilities. Don't be shy about asking friends, family, and your husband for help whenever you need it.

~ mama-do list ~

- We are beautifully and wonderfully made, Mama, and the changes your body (and brain!) are undergoing will only make you *better* prepared for motherhood, not worse. So cut yourself some slack, get some rest, and don't worry too much if you drive down the street with a coffee cup on the roof of your car. It happens to the best of us.

- Need a quick pick-me-up? Certain essential oils can gently stimulate the brain, particularly the limbic system, which affects mood, memories, and feelings of well-being. Some especially good ones to try: lemon oil, orange oil, spearmint oil, clove oil, and eucalyptus oil. Put a few drops into a diffuser and let run for 10 to 20 minutes.

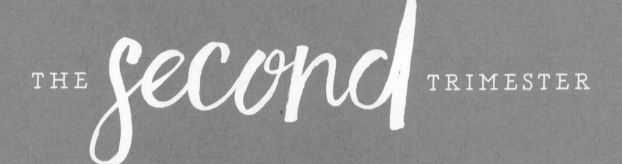

THE *second* TRIMESTER

feeling testy?

PART II

SECOND TRIMESTER CHECKUPS AND SCREENINGS

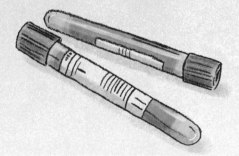

WHAT'S UP WITH *baby*?

Baby is tipping the scales at a full ounce this week! Perhaps it's all that food she's been eating? True, she doesn't technically "eat" while in utero; she consumes the byproducts of whatever you eat, after your body breaks that food down and passes along the nutrients. Starting now, however, she can discern sweet, bitter, and sour flavors in the amniotic fluid. Even more incredible, research indicates that which foods you eat during pregnancy may affect her palate later on. (Want her to love veggies? Make sure you're eating yours!) Of course, all that food has to go somewhere, so baby is hard at work producing meconium, a sticky, black or dark green tarlike substance, composed of epithelial cells, bile, mucus, and lanugo (more on that soon), that will form her first official bowel movement.

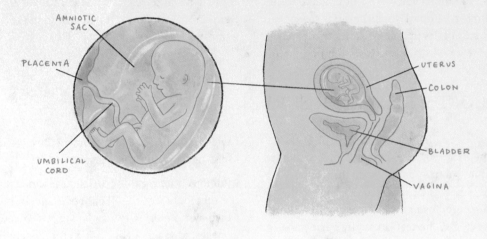

WHAT'S UP WITH *mama*?

Let me ask you a question: How *good* does it feel to be one third of the way to the big day? Congratulations, Mama! You have officially entered the second trimester. The risk of miscarriage drops significantly from here on out, and your uterus has expanded above the pelvic bone. *Voilà!* Say hello to your mini baby bump. Which makes wearing pants difficult. Ugh . . . *pants.* What on earth do you do about the pants? If your pregnancy is anything like mine were, Week 14 is like entering an ambiguous gray zone between regular clothes and maternity wear. My (misguided) solution? Wear some cheap non-maternity clothes a size or two bigger than normal. *Don't do that.* I ended up looking bigger and boxier than ever. If your clothes are snug or outright uncomfortable, you may be ready to take the leap—and we'll talk plenty more about navigating the maternity shops in Week 15. Feel free to flip ahead if you're about to pop a button!

You'd think that after all the tests you were offered back in the first trimester, we'd be just about done with the genetic screening by now, wouldn't you? I mean, sure, a doctor or midwife will continue to monitor baby's development, but didn't we *already* screen for things like Down syndrome? Turns out that when it comes to prenatal testing, your doctor or midwife was just getting started.

As you enter the second trimester, you'll be offered a whole new battery of tests, even though many of them screen for the exact same conditions you were on the lookout for months ago. In part, that's because *combining* results from the first and second trimesters tends to give your practitioner a much more accurate picture of what's going on inside your womb. This can be especially helpful if you were alerted to a potential issue with baby's health but have been on the fence about whether to proceed with more invasive procedures.

Remember that all the tests you'll be offered now can be broken into one of two types: screening tests, which determine the likelihood that baby *might* have a genetic disorder or developmental abnormality, and diagnostic tests, which are much more definitive but come with more risks to you and the baby. Here's a look at your options during the second trimester:

SECOND TRIMESTER SCREEN

Sometimes called the "quad screen" or the "sequential two," the Second Trimester Screen is actually four separate tests that, when combined, reflect the chances of having a baby with certain chromosomal abnormalities or neural tube defects. The test is usually performed between 15 and 20 weeks, and includes:

Alpha-fetoprotein (AFP): This is a blood test to determine AFP levels, a protein made by your growing baby. High levels of AFP can sometimes indicate a neural tube defect, while very low levels may indicate a chromosomal abnormality.

Beta hCG: Yup, same hormone that was present in your urine to give you a positive pregnancy test; this is a repeat of the blood test you were given during the First Trimester Screen.

Estriol: This is a blood test to determine estriol levels, a hormone (specifically, a type of estrogen) made by the baby *and* the placenta.

Levels that fall outside the "normal" range may indicate a chromosomal issue.

Inhibin A: Adding this particular blood test to the mix increases the likelihood of detecting Down syndrome, so it may be ordered if you're at risk of having a baby with a chromosomal abnormality (risk factors include advanced maternal age, a family history of chromosomal abnormalities, or a previous baby with a birth defect). If you don't have any of those risk factors, your doctor may forego this portion of the test, in which case your quad screen will be referred to as a "triple screen."

IS THIS TEST RIGHT FOR YOU?

If you did the First Trimester Screen and/or cell-free DNA screening and the results were normal, this particular test may not be a priority for you. On the other hand, all four tests in the quad screen—as you likely noticed—are blood-based (a.k.a. totally noninvasive and therefore risk-free). You should know, however, that between 3 percent and 7 percent of women will get an abnormal result. In other words, the Second Trimester Screen has an inordinately high false-positive rate. Most often, that's due to dating errors (meaning the baby is actually a few weeks older or younger than previously thought); an abnormal result could also signal the presence of twins. The Second Trimester Screen is most accurate when combined with data from the first trimester.

> As a reminder, you'll almost certainly be offered the Doppler to hear baby's heartbeat, but you can decline this if you wish. As an alternative, a fetoscope will pick up that beautiful fluttering around the time you hit 20 weeks.

AMNIOCENTESIS

This is a diagnostic test, not a screen, which means it provides *highly* accurate information about your baby's genetics and development—amnios are the most accurate of all prenatal testing, in fact—at the expense of being more invasive and thus carrying more risks. Similar to chorionic villus sampling, amnios are performed by inserting a needle into your uterus through the skin of the abdomen in order to remove a small amount (about one ounce) of amniotic fluid. Also like CVS, the insertion of the needle is guided by the use of an ultrasound. You may feel menstrual-like cramping during or after the procedure, but you should be able to resume your normal activities within a day. The risks, although rare, include injury to you or the baby, injury to the placenta, bleeding, infection, miscarriage (in less than 1 percent of cases), and preterm labor.

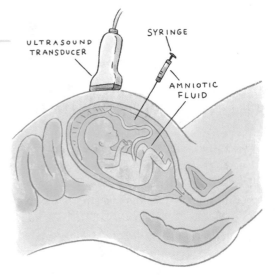

ULTRASOUND TRANSDUCER

SYRINGE

AMNIOTIC FLUID

AMNIOCENTESIS

IS THIS TEST RIGHT FOR YOU?

Amnios can technically be performed at any point during a pregnancy, but are most commonly ordered between Weeks 15 and 18, after an abnormal First and/or Second Trimester Screen. Since this is by far the most invasive of all second trimester tests, you may want to hold off until you get the results of the (less

invasive) anatomy ultrasound—we'll talk more about that in just a moment. Keep in mind, too, that virtually all women over the age of 35 are offered amnios as a matter of course, but they should by no means be considered routine. The test itself does nothing to improve baby's health or birth outcome; it's the information the test provides that may be of use. Whereas CVS cannot detect problems with the baby's brain or spinal cord, amniocentesis can detect neural tube defects (with 99 percent accuracy), as well as nearly 100 percent of all genetic

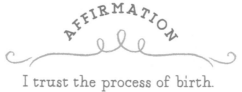
I trust the process of birth.
I know I can do this.
My baby is healthy and well.

abnormalities. For some mamas, knowing definitively that their child will have special needs has its benefits: They may be better able to plan emotionally, as well as logistically, whether that means delivering at a hospital with better resources or lining up care for the weeks and months following birth. Others believe the test will only induce stress and anxiety, and therefore choose to refrain.

ANATOMY ULTRASOUND

By the halfway point of pregnancy, it's possible to detect genetic abnormalities and congenital defects via sonogram, which is why the anatomy ultrasound—considered a standard of prenatal care and offered to virtually all pregnant women—is usually performed at 20 weeks. Your sonographer will also locate the position of the placenta to make sure it's not close to or covering the cervix (a condition called placenta previa), as well as measure amniotic fluid levels. If you didn't opt for cell-free DNA screening, you can find out baby's sex now, too. The ultrasound will be performed abdominally (using the wand on your belly), but it won't be necessary to have a full bladder. Depending on the skill of the sonographer—and how cooperative baby is feeling—the procedure usually takes about 30 minutes.

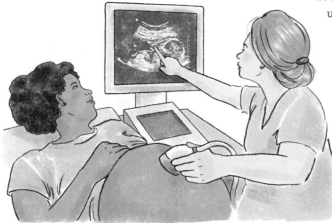

IS THIS TEST RIGHT FOR YOU?

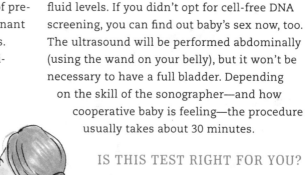

The anatomy ultrasound is not mandatory, nor does it improve maternal or fetal outcomes, statistically speaking. Just because it's routine doesn't mean you *must* have one, and some mamas won't—for religious reasons, because they want to limit baby's exposure to radiation, or because they just prefer to let nature take its course. If you're

MEASURING SMALL? COULD IT BE IUGR?

With all the fancy equipment and sophisticated blood tests at her disposal, ever wonder why your midwife or doctor uses a simple measuring tape to gauge your belly growth? She's monitoring your fundal height—that is, the distance (in cm) from your pubic bone to the top of your uterus, and it's a time-honored way to track the growth of your baby. No twenty-first-century technology required.

Don't be alarmed if you measure a little small—or a little big—on any given week, as mamas-to-be often experience fluctuations and growth spurts. Consistently or significantly measuring on the small side, however, could be an indication that your baby has something called intrauterine growth restriction (IUGR). Occurring in roughly 2 to 3 percent of pregnancies, IUGR babies are considered "small for gestational age," with an estimated weight below the 10th percentile. And while genetics can be a factor—when mama and papa are small in stature, their growing baby may be, too—IUGR can sometimes indicate a chromosomal abnormality, a problem with the placenta, or some other health issue. If your midwife or doctor suspects IUGR, he or she will order some additional testing as well as keep a close eye on the progression of your pregnancy. Intrauterine growth restriction can in some cases be severe (and can even lead to stillbirth). But the good news? The majority of these tiny babies catch up to their peers by the time they reach toddlerhood.

trying to limit the number of ultrasounds you receive but still want *one* to check baby's growth and development, however, this is the one to do. Keep in mind that there *is* a sweet spot in terms of when to undergo the procedure. Too early, and it's possible that baby's organs aren't developed enough (or visible enough) to be properly evaluated, so the test may need to be redone in a few weeks. Too late, and it becomes hard to accurately measure baby's growth.

For these reasons, my midwife recommended that I postpone the ultrasound until Week 22; you'll find that most healthcare providers have no issue with this.

Some practitioners may order a urine test at every single one of your prenatal appointments (to monitor for signs of preeclampsia, gestational diabetes, and bacteria); others may check your urine only intermittently. Either way, be prepared to pee often!

Beet Kvass

Wake up some of baby's sour taste buds (and curb a future sweet tooth) with an amazing elixir called beet kvass. I'll admit that beets are sort of like cilantro—people tend to either love 'em or hate 'em—but they're loaded with folate, iron, and betaine, as well as good bacteria and enzymes (when fermented) to support digestion. Beets are even said to cleanse the blood—and if you make the kvass, you'll look like you're *drinking* blood . . . but I digress. Here's how to whip it up:

INGREDIENTS

3 organic medium beets

2 teaspoons high-mineral sea salt

Filtered water

Wash (but don't peel) the beets, chop into 1-inch cubes, and pile into a half-gallon Mason jar. Add the sea salt, fill the jar with filtered or spring water, cover tightly with a lid, and let sit for three days in a cool, dark place. Once your kvass is done "brewing," strain and let it chill in the fridge for a few hours before drinking. Shoot for one 4-ounce serving in the morning and one at night—if the taste is overpowering, cut it with a few ounces of fresh-squeezed OJ. Recipe makes about 16 servings.

Hate beets? Other great sour foods to include this week include lacto-fermented pickles, sauerkraut, and limeade.

BASIC BLOOD WORK

Just as you underwent routine blood testing at your first prenatal appointment, you'll have another "complete blood count," or CBC test, in the second trimester, usually between 24 and 28 weeks. Your results will be compared to the baseline established by your first trimester CBC.

IS THIS TEST RIGHT FOR YOU?

Definitely. As with all blood tests, this is completely noninvasive and therefore risk-free. Your provider is watching out for signs of anemia, infection, and low thyroid function while also keeping an eye on your platelet levels (since platelets are used in clotting, a very low platelet count could lead to excessive bleed-ing during birth or Cesarean section). In other words, this is all need-to-know info.

GLUCOSE TOLERANCE TEST

Sometimes referred to as the "glucose challenge," or—more colloquially—"the diabetes test," the glucose tolerance test is a way to determine if mama has developed gestational diabetes. Sometime between Weeks 24 and 28 of your pregnancy, your healthcare provider will ask you to drink a high-sugar, pretty nasty-tasting "beverage" called Glucola. One hour later, your blood will be drawn to measure your blood sugar response. Mamas who test positive after the glucose tolerance test will be asked to take a three-hour version, which is considered diagnostic (as opposed to the one-hour screen).

It's not necessary to fast in advance of the glucose tolerance test. In fact, fasting and then drinking a sugary beverage on an empty stomach can skyrocket your blood sugar (potentially resulting in a false positive), which is why some midwives recommend that you increase your carbohydrate intake for two or three days leading up to the test, in order for your body to get used to processing the excess sugar. This may be especially helpful for women who eat a very clean, real food, low-sugar, or Paleo diet. Potential side effects of the test include feeling dizzy, jittery, or nauseous.

IS THIS TEST RIGHT FOR YOU?

While you can decline the glucose tolerance test, just as you can decline any prenatal test during your pregnancy, gestational diabetes is a condition you don't want to go unnoticed. Women with gestational diabetes are more likely to have large babies, which can be difficult to deliver vaginally (complications include shoulder dystocia, which occurs when baby gets stuck in the birth canal); they also experience higher rates of Cesarean and are more likely to develop type 2 diabetes later in life. Babies born to women with gestational diabetes, meanwhile, may have dangerously low blood sugar or problems regulating their blood sugar after birth; they're also at a higher risk of

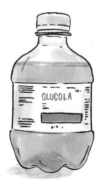
GLUCOSE DRINK

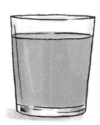
ORANGE JUICE

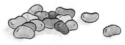
JELLY BEANS

obesity. Screening for gestational diabetes may be especially important for women who have the following risk factors:

♡ You are twenty-five years of age or older.

♡ You were overweight before becoming pregnant.

♡ You have a family history of diabetes.

♡ You are of Hispanic, African American, American Indian, Asian American, or Pacific Islander heritage.

♡ You have a previous history of abnormal glucose levels or had gestational diabetes during a previous pregnancy.

That said, I've got major issues with Glucola. For one thing, it's loaded with chemical food dyes and additives, modified food starch (which may contain gluten), brominated vegetable oil (which has been banned in Europe and Japan), and dextrose (GMO corn sugar)—exactly the type of stuff we typically try to *avoid* during pregnancy, if not *all the time.*

Luckily, there are alternatives. Midwives in particular tend to be more willing to screen for gestational diabetes using food-based tests—orange juice, dates, and all-natural jelly beans are all common stand-ins for Glucola. The makers of Glucola produce a dye-free version, which you can request. You can also inquire about "spot checking," where your health-care provider checks your blood sugar from a drop of blood drawn via a finger prick. These kinds of alternative tests have been used for years, though it's worth mentioning that from a large-scale, randomized trial standpoint, evidence that they are *as* effective as Glucola is still inconclusive.

If you're on the fence about the glucose tolerance test, you may want to consider what would happen in the event you tested positive. Treatment for gestational diabetes always includes modifying the diet and getting some exercise (in a small percentage of cases, insulin injections may be necessary, too). If you *already* eat a low-sugar, real food diet and exercise regularly, however, you likely wouldn't have to change much about your lifestyle and may be an excellent candidate for alternative testing.

If, on the other hand, you eat lots of processed foods, lead a sedentary lifestyle, and have a number of risk factors, you'll want to start focusing on improving your health *now*; don't wait for a glucose tolerance test to give you bad news.

mama-do list

- Even if you haven't been following a model pregnancy diet, it's not too late to clean up your eating habits. Remember, dining on whole, nutritious foods doesn't *just* lower your risk of complications; it affects baby's future palate, too. Studies have shown that babies who "eat" a more varied diet while in utero are more likely to be adventurous eaters when they make the switch to solid food.

- Of all your prenatal tests, the anatomy ultrasound is what you typically see depicted on TV and in the movies. Baby's big enough now to get a good view of, and you'll be able to find out the sex. So if your partner hasn't been tagging along to the midwife or doctor's office, you may want to bring him to this one. It's pretty amazing to be able to get a sneak peek inside the womb!

- Not sure if you want to move forward with the glucose tolerance test? Chat with your healthcare provider now about alternative testing options, as well as your personal risk profile. That way you'll have plenty of time to make an informed decision. Don't wait until the drink is in your hand.

dress for two

WHAT'S UP WITH *baby*?

If you could zoom in and get an up-close-and-personal view of baby in utero, you'd see that his skin is so thin that it's nearly translucent. Just under the surface, a dense network of arteries and veins is hard at work circulating blood throughout his tiny body. And *on* that skin, you'd find a soft, downy layer of hair called lanugo. This will keep him warm for the next few months, since he won't start packing on fat—responsible for those scrumptious, squishy thighs and sweet cheeks—until the final weeks of your pregnancy. By then, most of this lanugo will shed (you may remember that lanugo is one of many components that make up meconium), although some babies still have some visible at birth.

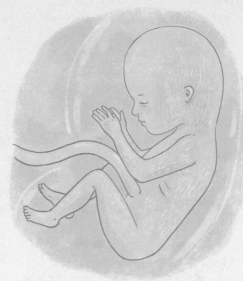

BABY'S LANUGO WILL KEEP HIM WARM FOR THE NEXT FEW MONTHS.

Speaking of hair, ever notice the circular growth pattern of hair on the back of someone's head? That's called the "parietal hair whorl" and it's forming now, too, because the thin skin of baby's scalp is being pulled and stretched to accommodate the rapid growth of his brain.

WHAT'S UP WITH *mama*?

By Week 15, most mamas have packed on about 5 pounds. Baby, however, is growing rapidly—he was about 1 ounce last week, but he's closer to 2 ounces this week—which means you'll be entering a bit of a growth spurt now, too. Though every pregnant woman will gain weight at her own pace, it's recommended that mamas-to-be add an average of a pound a week, every week, from here on out. For the first time, you may be ready to up your food intake (by about 300 calories a day, according to conventional wisdom), but remember: it's far more important to count nutrients.

At 15 weeks, I had to face reality: I could no longer button my pants. I didn't feel like I was ready for maternity clothes—I wasn't truly showing yet—but I had to do *something*, so I went out and bought the cheapest pair of pants I could find, two sizes up. Big mistake. Sure, they accommodated my bigger waistline, but they made me look bigger everywhere else, too: my thighs looked big, my butt looked big, my arms looked big. I felt fat and frumpy—a bit like a human duffel bag, in fact. I swam around in these horribly unflattering clothes for the next few weeks, until I just couldn't take it anymore.

I flung myself into the nearest maternity store and, let me tell you, what a revelation!

Lots of mamas are hesitant about making the jump to maternity wear too soon. *Am I really big enough for this yet? Can't I just tough it out in my regular wardrobe? Won't maternity clothes make me look like a whale?* Fit, however, is arguably the most important aspect of clothing even when you're not pregnant and—obvious as it seems in retrospect—maternity clothes are *made* to fit a pregnant body. They give you room where you need it (the bust and belly, mainly) without packing on bulk where you don't (arms, legs, and butt). As I stood in the dressing room, admiring my new shape, I was blown away at the difference. I actually liked the way I looked, belly and all! I felt confident for the first time in weeks. So don't make the same mistake that I did. The minute your regular clothes no longer fit, avoid drowning yourself in saggy sweatpants and head straight for maternity wear.

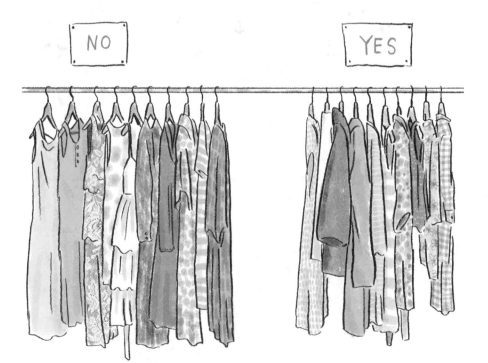

NAVIGATING THE MATERNITY DEPARTMENT

I used to think of "maternity" and "fashion" the same way I thought of "chicken nuggets" and "health food"—which is to say, two disparate concepts that just didn't mix. But maternity clothes have come a long way since the days when our mothers were pregnant. It's possible now to look not just cute and comfortable while you're carrying, but genuinely fashion-forward. That said, the maternity section can be overwhelming, especially if you're a first-timer. What should you buy? How much should you buy? How big will you be?

Start by taking inventory of the items in your closet that you may be able to continue wearing as your belly grows. Anything stretchy (fold-over yoga pants, leggings) or long and flowing (tunic tops, maxi dresses) usually makes for good maternity wear. Coats, jackets, blazers, and even some cardigans, meanwhile, can typically be worn unbuttoned or unzipped, in some cases all the way up to delivery. Next, check out a nifty little device called the Belly Band, which is a bit like a spandex belt. It'll keep your pants up even when they're unbuttoned, so you can eke out a few more weeks in your regular clothes both pre- and postpartum.

I'll be honest: I never quite cozied up to the idea of walking around with my pants essentially unzipped, but some mamas swear by it.

When you're ready to purchase some new duds, know that maternity clothes are almost always sized like regular clothing. In other words, if you're normally a medium or a size 8 you'll look for mediums or size 8s in maternity wear. Keep in mind, however, that every woman gains pregnancy weight differently. If you find that you need to go up a size or two as the months fly by, don't be surprised.

CHOOSE FABRICS WISELY

Do your best to avoid synthetic materials (polyester, rayon), as these can trap heat. It's common for pregnant women to feel warmer than usual anyway, but imagine carrying around 20 or 30 extra pounds in the middle of summer. Ugh. Anything that feels scratchy, stiff, itchy, or irritating is out, too. Instead, choose lightweight, breathable, all-natural fibers whenever possible (think: 100 percent cotton, jersey, or linen). And while no pregnant woman wants to spend time ironing—scratch that; no *person* wants to spend time ironing, *ever*—steer clear of anything labeled "wrinkle-free" or "permanent press." Items like these are chemically treated (usually with formaldehyde), so they're a no-go during pregnancy. Regardless of what you buy, wash everything before you wear it, as this can eliminate or reduce some of those toxic compounds.

PAY ATTENTION TO SHAPE

There's no need to abandon your usual style just because you're pregnant, but some shapes are universally flattering. Check out:

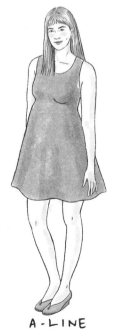

A-LINE

♡ **The A-line.** As the name suggests, A-line shirts, skirts, and dresses are narrower at the waist and flare at the hip, resembling the letter A. This versatile dress can take you from summer to fall with the addition of tights, boots, and a jacket or scarf.

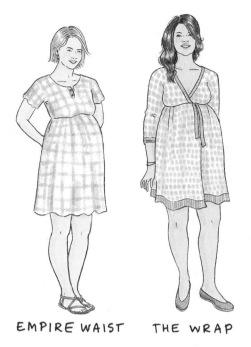

EMPIRE WAIST   THE WRAP

♡ **The Empire Waist.** Empire-waisted tops and dresses nip in tightly under the bust (soon to be the smallest part of you) and flow out. An empire waist with a scoop or V-neck will lengthen your body (so you'll look less boxy) and draw the eye away from the belly.

♡ **The Wrap.** The wrap dress—made famous in the 1970s by designer Diane von Furstenberg—is a timeless piece that never goes out of style. It's particularly useful during pregnancy since you can adjust the sash as your belly grows.

♡ **The Coat.** Many women can make it through fall and winter without the need for a true maternity coat—dressing in layers and wearing your regular coat (unbuttoned) is one option; buying a regular-size coat in a roomy style is another; trenches, pea coats, and wrap coats can more readily accommodate a growing bump.

PACE YOURSELF

On the one hand, I think it's a good idea to shop for maternity clothes early on. That way, you're less likely to get stuck buying something that's expensive or ugly (or both) just because you need *something* to wear. (By the way, lots of maternity stores stock fake baby bumps—strap one on and you can gauge how items will look as your belly grows.) On the other hand, you don't want to blow your entire clothing budget in the fourth month of pregnancy, only to realize you've outgrown everything by 32 weeks. It's virtually impossible to anticipate exactly how big you'll get, or how the weight will distribute on your body. Some women seem to gain only in the belly, while others seem to grow, well, *everywhere* (like me). But no need to purchase a whole new wardrobe. Instead, start with a few well-considered basics and buy additional items as needed. Keep in mind you can reuse these clothes in subsequent pregnancies.

WHAT TO BUY—AND WHAT NOT TO:
A CRASH COURSE IN MATERNITY BASICS

The easiest way to stretch a wardrobe? Accessories! A simple sheath dress in a neutral color can be dressed up with a cute jacket and boots, dressed down with a scarf and sandals, or made appropriate for the office with a cardigan and a chunky necklace. *Ta-da!* Three different looks, all put together with items you likely had in your closet pre-pregnancy. You'd be surprised how many looks you can throw together with just a few workhorse maternity pieces! Here's a look at what to buy—and what not to—from the maternity department:

Bras and Undies. You've probably heard it said that the vast majority of women are wearing the wrong size bra—between 60 percent and 85 percent of women, in fact, depending on which source you cite. Not surprisingly, a well-fitting bra is even more important for a mama-to-be since extra weight in your breasts means more strain on your ligaments—but it's that much more difficult to shop for.

I mean, just how big are your "girls" going to be?

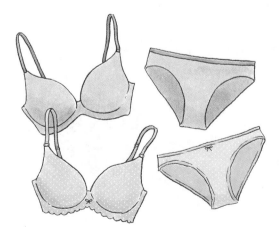

First, you'll want to know that there are two types of bras for new mamas: maternity bras and nursing bras. Maternity bras are essentially regular bras on steroids: they've got wider straps, softer cups, and way more hook-and-eye closures to account for your expanding rib cage. They also rarely have underwire since more confining bras could cause a blocked milk duct or lymph drainage issues. Nursing bras, meanwhile, have these same features, plus cups or panels that unsnap or that can be shifted to the side for easy nipple access.

Most women will need to size up at least once during their pregnancy, if not two or even three times. For this reason, it's a good idea to buy an inexpensive maternity bra, since you may not get much wear out of it. Don't, however, buy a too-big bra that you'll "grow into." It won't fit right, it'll look lumpy and bumpy under your clothes, and it won't give you the support you need. Keep in mind, too, that your breasts may expand first (as early as the first trimester), followed by expansion in your rib cage—this is when a bra with lots of hook-and-eye closures (like, *six*) or a bra extender comes in handy.

Some women opt to skip maternity bras altogether and go straight to a nursing bra, even months before they give birth. But do know that your breasts will likely continue to grow even *after* you deliver your baby. (It takes several days for your milk to come in, and several weeks for your breasts to adjust to baby's feeding schedule.) For this reason, bra-fit experts recommend getting professionally fitted for a nursing bra in the eighth month of pregnancy since this is a close approximation of what your breasts may look like four weeks postpartum.

Whether you want to jump straight to nursing bras or stick with maternity bras until the big day, make sure to purchase at least one nursing bra *before* baby arrives. Trust me, you are not going to feel like shopping for undergarments a few days after delivery, when you're exhausted, excited, and still healing.

When it comes to pregnancy panties, it's really just a matter of personal preference. You can get away with virtually any regular style, though you'll likely have to go up a size or two. However, make sure to choose breathable fabrics with a 100 percent cotton crotch. Pregnant women are more prone to vaginal infections,

NOM OF THE WEEK

Lentil Salad

Feeling hungrier now that you've hit the second trimester? Lentils are an excellent and inexpensive source of protein and fiber, which helps you feel fuller, for longer. Make an extra big batch of this lentil salad and you've got a healthy snack (or side dish) for days. Yum!

INGREDIENTS

1 pound dried green lentils (5 cups cooked)

3 medium carrots, diced

1 red pepper, chopped

½ medium onion, chopped

¼ cup fresh dill, minced

½ teaspoon sea salt

⅓ cup dried currants (optional)

Parmesan

VINAIGRETTE

4 tablespoons raw apple cider vinegar

1 tablespoons olive oil

1½ tablespoons Dijon mustard

2 cloves garlic, minced

Pinch of sea salt

Freshly ground black pepper to taste

Place your lentils in a large stockpot and cover generously with water. Add a splash of raw apple cider vinegar. Let soak overnight. In the morning, drain, rinse, and return lentils to the pot. Add enough filtered water to cover lentils by 1 inch. Cook until tender but firm (about 20 minutes). Drain and chill in the refrigerator.

In the meantime, prepare the vinaigrette by whisking the ingredients together. Once the lentils have cooled, add the chopped veggies, dill, salt, and currants, top with vinaigrette, and mix well. Serve cold with some freshly grated Parmesan. Serves 6 to 8.

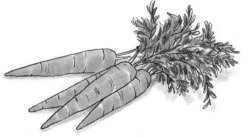

so you want a natural fabric that wicks away moisture to discourage yeast and bacterial growth. Maternity briefs are also available if you feel more comfortable and more supported by underwear that comes up over the belly.

Pajamas. You certainly don't need a matching PJ set to get you through pregnancy, but you may want to think about what you most like to sleep in. Are you an oversize T-shirt and boxers kind of gal? A fan of the satin nightgown? Whatever your preference, make sure you've got something cozy and comfortable on hand. In the eighth or ninth month, it's worth considering what you'll want to wear once baby arrives, too. A super-simple nursing nightgown or nursing tank with regular PJ bottoms can

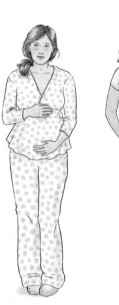

make middle-of-the-night feedings a cinch (as opposed to pulling a tight T-shirt over your head with one hand while baby's crying). Regular (i.e., non-maternity) nightgowns or sleepshirts with buttons or snaps down the front also work, and are often cheaper.

Maternity denim. If you're like most women, you will *live* in your maternity jeans so pick out a pair (or two!) that you feel great in. Don't be afraid to try on different styles, either. Even if you're not a fan of skinny jeans in your regular life, a thin, tapered leg paired with that growing belly can actually be quite flattering (in my humble fashion opinion).

Pants. How many pairs of maternity pants you'll need largely depends on your lifestyle— a stay-at-home mama, for example, may be able to skate by with mostly yoga pants and a jersey-knit dress or two, while a woman who works full-time in a corporate environment may need to invest in a decent maternity suit. Either way, plan to buy at least two pairs of maternity pants—leggings count!—in a neutral color (think: black, gray, khaki).

Tops. Shirts and blouses are an easy way to infuse some color into your pregnancy wardrobe, and it's nice to have a few different shapes and sizes for variety: a tunic, an empire blouse, an Oxford-style button down, plus a few T-shirts are all great options. But even if you plan to have more children in the future, maternity tops are the most likely to get stained or become outdated in a year or two, so shop from the sale racks and pace yourself.

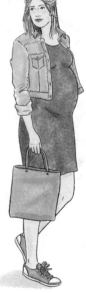

Dresses. Not everyone's a dress fan, but they're a breeze to throw on and usually *über*-comfortable. They also grow with you, can be dressed up or down, can transition from season to season, and allow for some much-needed air flow. Consider buying at least one cotton or jersey dress that can be worn again and again in different variations.

Shoes. Your belly and breasts aren't the only things growing. Relaxin, the hormone responsible for relaxing the ligaments in your pelvis in preparation for birth is also to blame for the growth in your feet. In fact, research indicates that roughly half of pregnant women will wind up with larger feet, *permanently*. (I know: the things we mamas have to go through!) So don't buy anything remotely expensive until at least a few months postpartum. Do, however, think about picking up a cheap pair of wide, comfy shoes with great arch support. Extra points for something you can slip on without lacing or buckling—by the eighth or ninth month, you may not like how it feels to bend over!

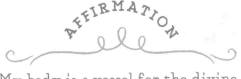

My body is a vessel for the divine.
My body is a miracle.

mama-do list

- Try experimenting with accessories this week. Google new ways to tie a scarf, or throw on some bright, bold earrings. And if you're shopping, remember that accessories don't have to accommodate the size of your growing belly, which means they'll continue to be part of your wardrobe even *after* baby is born.

- Before baby arrives, make sure you have: at least one nursing or comfort bra; comfortable loungewear that's easy to sleep and/or nurse in; and some really big, really comfortable, really cheap granny panties (you'll need room for a fairly giant maxi pad, as you'll be bleeding in the immediate days postpartum). In the meantime, try to minimize the use of your "fancy" underwear, as synthetic fibers and thong underwear can increase your risk of vaginal infection.

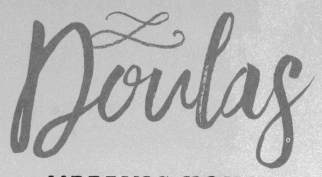

Doulas

MEETING YOUR BIRTH ANGEL

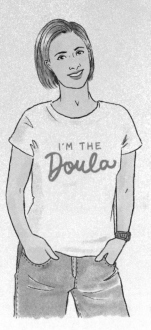

WHAT'S UP WITH *baby*?

Baby is developing lots of beautiful little details this week, including creases on the palms and her own, totally unique set of fingerprints. Something else that's developed now: her hearing. At first, most of what baby hears in utero are sounds that originate from inside your body: your heartbeat, your stomach gurgling, the whoosh of air into and out of your lungs. But soon she'll be able to pick up the sound of your voice, too. And by the time she's born, she'll be able to *recognize* it. Don't believe me? In a study by researchers at Columbia University, one-day-old newborns were given pacifiers connected to tape recorders; based on the babies' sucking pattern, the pacifiers turned on either a tape of mama speaking or the voice of a stranger. Within 10 to 20 minutes, the babies began to adjust their sucking rate, indicating a clear preference for mama's soothing tone. So don't feel weird about talking, singing, or reading directly to your stomach—baby can hear you!

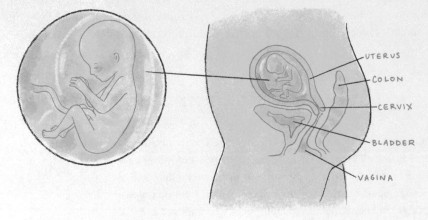

WHAT'S UP WITH *mama*?

Has anyone told you that you're "glowing" yet, Mama? It's not just a random compliment; pregnancy glow is actually a very real thing. As your blood volume increases—by as much as 50 percent, peaking around 32 weeks—more blood is diverted to the skin. Meanwhile, your surging hormones can boost oil production, giving your face a radiant, dewy flush. Although in some women, too much oil can lead to pregnancy acne, so if you look a bit like a pubescent teenager, that's normal, too. One, well, *interesting* side effect you may notice any time now (though it often peaks in the third trimester): an increase in vaginal discharge. You can thank high estrogen levels for this lovely development, but know that it happens for good reason. Vaginal discharge helps to cleanse the vagina, keeping harmful bacteria out of your body and away from your growing baby. As long as there's not a *sudden* increase in discharge, an unpleasant odor, or a yellowish or green tinge, everything down there is functioning just as it should.

Throughout history, mamas have been delivering babies with the guidance and encouragement of other women, experienced birthers trained to offer physical and emotional (if not medical) support. Today, we call these wise women *doulas*, and at my first birth I was lucky enough to have not one, but *two* of them.

Not that I planned it that way.

I went into labor on a Friday night, and the first few hours were pretty uneventful—I actually spent a fair amount of time alone in the bathroom just so my husband could get some rest before the long day ahead. Around two o'clock in the morning, contractions started to come fast and furious, and I knew it was time to phone my doula, Pam. She suggested I take a long, warm bath (which totally helped, by the way, and I was able to get some much-needed sleep). But by 8:00 a.m., when I was ready for some hands-on help, she was already headed to the hospital. You see, my doula—the queen bee of doulas—doubled as a childbirth educator, and she had a Saturday morning class to teach. So she sent over her backup doula.

Doula #2, Karen, helped me labor at home until around two o'clock and then accompanied Michael and me to the birth center. By then, Pam's class was over, and Karen could easily have gone home. She told me she was having "so much fun," however, that she didn't want to leave. Of course, *I* wasn't having much fun—I was on hour 18 of what would stretch to twenty-seven hours of labor—but I like to think that God knew I needed some extra help

DOULAS FOR HIGH-RISK PREGNANCIES?

TIPS FROM NURSE/DOULA *maura*

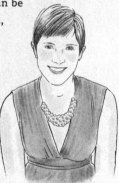

From home births to water births to scheduled Cesareans, doulas can be helpful during *all* kinds of births—really! The point of hiring a doula, after all, is to feel supported during your pregnancy, labor, and the immediate hours postpartum. All women benefit from this type of completely unbiased, nonjudgmental, totally customized care, yet they won't always receive it from other people. Your partner, for example, will be challenged by his or her own emotional response, while friends and family—no matter how loving and supportive they may be—often bring with them baggage and unsolicited advice.

For high-risk women, in particular, doulas can provide a unique kind of reassurance. Interventions can be scary, but a doula will prepare you (and your partner) for what those interventions might look like and feel like. (Know that while you may *need* a few interventions, you don't necessarily have to sign up for the whole gamut.) She can help to explain complications that may arise during the throes of labor and can assist you in developing questions to ask your primary health-care provider. She'll also provide you with support and reassurance in the event that things don't go according to plan.

that day. In fact, I can't imagine having gone through the process without these women. The word *doula* comes from the ancient Greek; roughly translated, it means a "woman's servant" or a "woman who serves." But I like to think of them as birth angels.

SO WHAT EXACTLY *IS* A DOULA?

Unlike a doctor or midwife—whose primary concern is the safe delivery of a baby—doulas are trained labor specialists who provide *non*medical care to expectant mamas. That care might come in the form of massage, to ease back pain and soothe tired muscles, or coaching, to give mama the encouragement she needs to stay centered and calm. It could mean making sure mama gets enough to eat and drink to keep up her strength, or showing mama's birth partner how best to offer support during labor. Most likely, your doula will provide a combination of *all* these services—and many more—but the scope of her practice is limited to physical, emotional, and informational support. Her entire focus is on mothering the mother.

But a doula is far more than a glorified cheerleader. In fact, doula-attended births are associated with demonstrably better outcomes.

Mountains of research, including studies published in the *Journal of Perinatal Education,* the *British Journal of Obstetrics and Gynaecology,* and by the Cochrane Review, have shown that women who receive this kind of continuous care and companionship during labor are:

♡ more likely to go into spontaneous labor,

♡ less likely to need an epidural (60 percent less likely, if you can believe that!),

♡ less likely to need vacuum extraction or forceps assistance,

♡ less likely to birth via Cesarean,

♡ less likely to have negative feelings about childbirth.

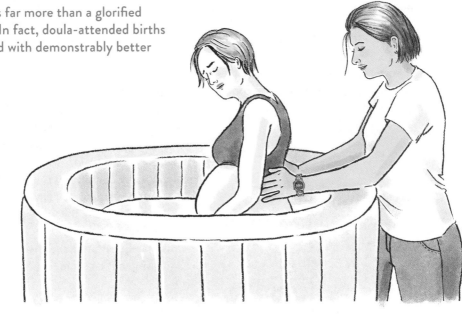

Furthermore, babies born under the care of a doula are more likely to go full-term and to have higher APGAR scores. Some studies have shown that laboring in a clinical setting—like a hospital's standard maternity ward—can undermine a mama's confidence in her ability to give birth naturally. Doulas, however, can give mama that confidence back.

Even the American College of Obstetricians and Gynecologists acknowledges that doula care is "one of the most effective tools to improve labor and delivery outcomes."

The advantages of hiring a doula, however, begin long before you ever hit the delivery room. While you can (and should) always call your midwife or doctor with medical questions, doulas are amazing resources when it comes to understanding the physiological aspects of birth. She's the perfect person to describe what you can expect *physically* on the big day, as well as help you prepare mentally and spiritually. She can also explain common procedures used by midwives and doctors, and share her experiential wisdom. When the day finally comes, your doula—unlike your midwife or doctor—will be with you right from the start; you can call her as soon as you feel that first contraction. Together, you'll decide when it's time for her to come to your home to support you during early labor. And together, you can decide when it's time to head to the hospital or birth center, or when to summon the midwife if you're planning a home birth. (Trust me: this is key. First-time mamas are notorious for showing up at the hospital *way* too early, long before they're in active labor!)

As you inch closer to delivery, your doula can suggest laboring positions that might be more effective and comfortable, and breathing and relaxation exercises to mitigate pain. Many doulas specialize in pressure point massage, counterpoint massage, and aromatherapy using essential oils, among many other (natural!) techniques. Whereas your midwife or doctor will have certain clinical tasks to complete—and other patients to attend—your doula will *always* be with you. (Case in point: my midwife was called out of the room on twelve different occasions during my labor. Apparently, it was a crazy night!) She'll also help you and your partner be better advocates, in part by encouraging you to communicate with staff about your birth plan—this is why doulas are so key when you're laboring in a high-intervention hospital! In the event that interventions *do* become necessary, a doula can support mama emotionally to ensure that she still has a positive experience despite any complications or changes to the birth plan.

Doulas are a great help after delivery, too. Many double as trained lactation consultants, so they can help you initiate a healthy breastfeeding relationship, as well as encourage mama-baby bonding after the birth. Doulas can also provide follow-up care in the coming days and weeks (we call these postpartum doulas) so you'll have someone to reach out to when you have questions about newborn care or adjusting to life as a mama.

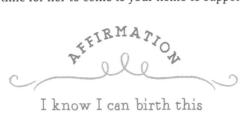

AFFIRMATION

I know I can birth this baby naturally. I trust my instincts. I trust the wisdom of my body. I believe I can, and so I will.

megan: I didn't hire a doula but ended up having one because I became high-risk when my water broke (showing meconium). My midwife sent a doula to the hospital to support me, and she is the reason I was able to endure eighteen hours of labor—and three hours of pushing—with no pain medication, no tearing, and no episiotomy!

sally: I had planned for a natural birth but was unprepared for the realities of labor. I ended up needing several interventions, including Pitocin and an epidural. Having a doula there to temper my disappointment, however, made my labor more joyful.

genevieve d.: My first birth was a long labor, and our doula gave us lots of advice and support. My second birth was so quick that the doula's main role was to drive me to the hospital! But we met a lot during the pregnancy, and her support meant so much. I'd recommend a doula to every family, but especially to first-time parents.

FINDING YOUR BIRTH ANGEL

Several different organizations provide nationally recognized certification and training for doulas, including: DONA International, Pro-Doula, toLabor, the Childbirth and Postpartum Professional Association (CAPPA), and Childbirth International (CBI). While the certification process differs slightly among these groups, all certified doulas receive childbirth and breastfeeding education, adhere to a code of ethics and standards of practice, and have attended a certain number of live births before receiving their credentials. While some doulas do have a medical background—doula Maura, for example, is an RN and a midwife-in-training—most do not. But remember, doulas do not diagnose medical conditions, prescribe or administer medications, or perform clinical procedures.

The cost of a doula usually ranges from $450 to as high as $2,500, depending on where you live and your doula's experience and unique qualifications. Many will set up a payment plan, but your insurance may cover the cost, too. Doula care is often considered preventive, since her presence can reduce your risk of interventions, including C-section.

To find a doula:

♡ Check out DoulaMatch (doulamatch.net), where you can browse through detailed profiles of doulas working in your area—a little like online dating!

♡ All five certifying organizations have a searchable database of doulas. Visit DONA International at dona.org; ProDoula at prodoula.com; toLabor at tolabor.com; Childbirth International at childbirth international.com; or check out the Childbirth and Postpartum Professional Association's Member Center at icappa.net.

♡ Ask around! Your midwife or doctor, as well as your friends and family, are (always) great resources.

NOM OF THE WEEK

Banana Almond Cake

Did you know that low levels of vitamin B_{12} and folate have been linked to hearing loss? (Seriously, what *can't* folate do?) So, this week, let's support baby's developing auditory system with some Banana Almond Cake—bananas and almonds are rich in folate, and you'll get a B_{12} boost from the cage-free eggs. This sweet cake's texture is similar to flan, and it's grain-free and gluten-free to boot!

INGREDIENTS

3 ripe bananas

½ cup creamy almond butter

¼ cup melted butter or coconut oil

3 tablespoons raw honey or organic maple syrup

1 teaspoon vanilla extract

¼ teaspoon cinnamon

¼ teaspoon nutmeg

5 cage-free eggs

⅓ cup dark chocolate chips (optional)

Preheat the oven to 300°F. Put all the ingredients into a blender or food processor. Whir on high until the mixture is smooth, like cake batter. Pour into a greased 9-inch round baking dish. Bake for 90 minutes, or until a toothpick inserted into the middle of the cake comes out clean. Let cool, slice, and top with a dollop of whipped cream.

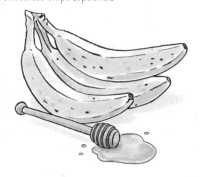

DADS AND DOULAS:
A LABOR AND DELIVERY DREAM TEAM

Papa Natural here, with just a few words about where husbands and partners fit in to all this. I'll admit that I was a little confused when Genevieve told me she wanted to hire a doula—I thought *I* would be her main support during birth! But I quickly learned that doulas don't take the place of dads. In fact, having a doula freed me up to play a more helpful and active role. I didn't have to worry if I was helping Genevieve in the "right" way, because our doula was there to model the most effective and gentle techniques. I didn't have to worry when Genevieve moaned like a wild boar (sorry, honey), because I knew from our doula's nod that this was perfectly normal. Frankly, the greatest gift was knowing that I wasn't alone. Birth is a lot to take in, and you can feel sort of helpless watching your beloved partner do all the hard work. It was comforting to share these moments with another "outsider," knowing that we'd all get through it together. Looking back, it's funny to think that I ever had doubts. I felt so much better having her in the room.

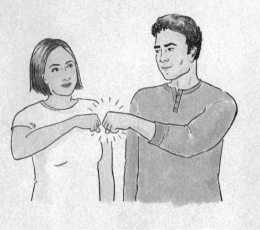

mama-do list

- Doulas may be one of the most effective tools for improving labor, but according to the American College of Obstetricians and Gynecologists, they are "underutilized." No kidding. Only 3 percent to 6 percent of mamas take advantage of this incredible resource. My advice? Make sure you're one of them! True, doula care is an investment, but I have yet to meet a woman who regrets having hired one.

- Consider bringing your partner along when you interview prospective doulas—in some ways, he or she will work more closely with your doula than *you* will.

fly me to the (baby)moon

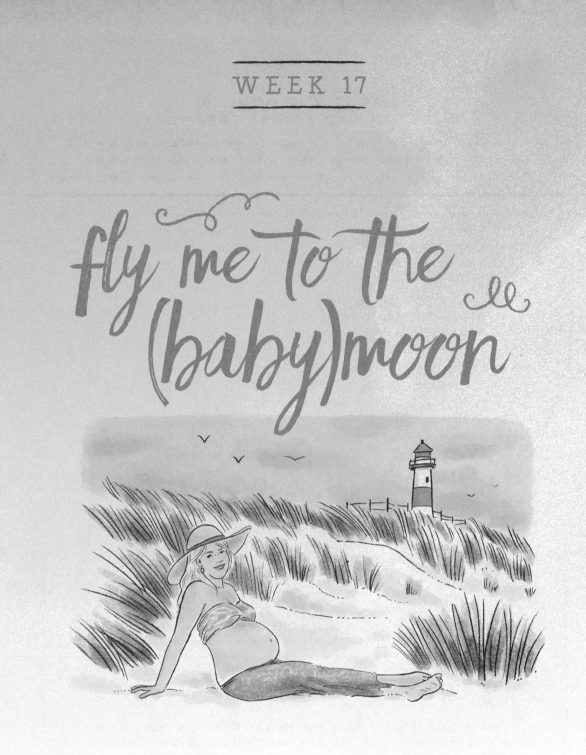

WHAT'S UP WITH *baby*?

Baby's skeleton has been pretty much all cartilage up to this point, but now it's beginning to harden into bone—around 300 bones, in fact, compared to just 206 in an adult skeleton. These bones will continue to grow and harden, fusing together in a process called ossification, until baby reaches maturity. For now, though, they're soft and malleable—the fetal skull, for example, is actually several plates that will shift and mold as he squeezes through your pelvis. (The softness also allows babies to perform those Cirque du Soleil–style moves they're known for, like sucking on their own toes.) Of course, to develop a strong, healthy skeleton, baby needs plenty of calcium—so be sure to eat plenty of dairy or other calcium-rich foods. Surprisingly, many food-based prenatals are low in this foundational nutrient.

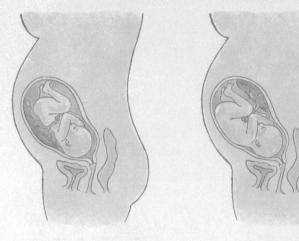

ANTERIOR
PLACENTA

POSTERIOR
PLACENTA

WHAT'S UP WITH *mama*?

Have you been feeling a fluttering in your tummy, Mama? The phenomenon is called "quickening," and while many women mistake the sensation for gas or nerves, it's really your little bambino shaking his groove thing. If you're not feeling much of anything yet, however, don't fret! Quickening might not kick in until closer to Week 20—I felt my son Griffin for the first time right around Week 18. The position of your placenta can affect when and how well you feel your baby move, too. An "anterior placenta," one positioned to the front wall as opposed to the back wall of the uterus, can cause baby's movements to be more muffled.

As best as anyone can tell, the term "baby-moon" appears to have been coined by the author and natural birth advocate Sheila Kitzinger in her 1996 book, *The Year After Childbirth*. Just as the honeymoon phase of a relationship refers to that period of head-over-heels infatuation immediately following a wedding, a babymoon (to Kitzinger, at least) was a name for the period of private bonding that occurs between parents and child in the month or so after birth. These days, however—sometime in the last four or five years, really—the definition has changed. We most readily associate baby-moons with last-hurrah-style vacations, a trip you take with your partner *before* baby arrives (when traveling does not require packing a diaper bag, car seat, foldable crib, toys, blankets, or a stroller—not to mention a baby).

I couldn't tell you what, exactly, was behind the shift, but I can tell you that Michael and I took a babymoon to sunny Puerto Rico before our son's birth—and it was amazing. Our trip was so successful, in fact (we came home reconnected, reenergized, and recharged) that I've come to think of babymoons as an important part of the preparing-for-birth process. And the second trimester is the perfect time to take one: You'll almost certainly get the all-clear to board a plane, should the trip be to a distant location. Meanwhile, you're not so big that sightseeing or snorkeling or window-shopping will zap every ounce of your energy.

But you don't have to drop tons of cash or travel to a desert island to get some much-needed R & R. You don't even have to leave town!

So pack a bag, Mama. It's time to plan a mega (or a mini) vacation.

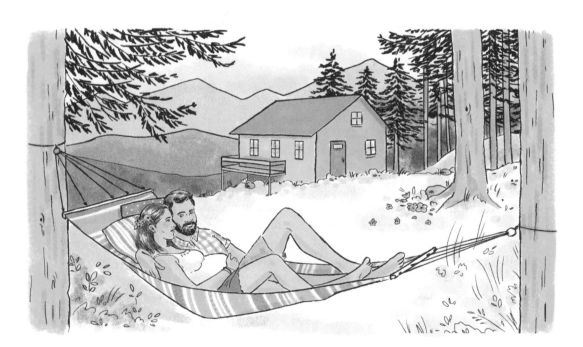

FLYING WHILE PREGNANT:
HOW LATE IS TOO LATE?

For most pregnant women, flying during the first and second trimesters is no problem. Third trimester air travel, however, gets a little more complicated. There is no explicit safety risk associated with flying—flying in and of itself doesn't trigger labor, nor will it jeopardize the health of your baby (although certain conditions, such as preeclampsia, can be exacerbated by high altitude). Rather, the concern about boarding a plane in the weeks approaching your due date is an obvious one: if you go into labor early, you'll likely be miles from home, as well as from the care of your midwife or doctor. And that's assuming you're not thirty thousand feet in the air!

Most healthcare providers will give low-risk women the go-ahead to fly right up until the 36th week, but you should probably discuss travel plans with your prenatal team—whether those plans involve hopping aboard an airliner or not—well in advance of your trip. Better yet: get a doctor's note clearing you for air travel. Some airlines *require* one for

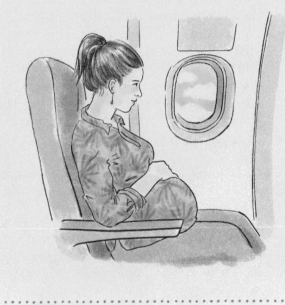

any expectant mama flying within a month or so of her due date; a few airlines restrict late–third trimester travel completely. Make sure to call ahead and double confirm their policies *before* booking your flight.

Planning a road trip (especially one late in the third trimester) instead? You'll want to follow the same guidelines as you would for air travel: get the green light from your midwife or doctor, and make sure you have his or her emergency contact information with you when you hit the road. If you're crossing state lines, you may want to jot down a list of local hospitals, too.

THE TOP 4 REASONS TO GET AWAY

There's no denying that babymoons have grown popular among the celebrity set, but this is one trend that's really *not* just for the rich and famous.

CATCH UP ON YOUR ZZZ'S

I've been preaching to you for weeks about the value of stocking up on sleep—because while parenthood is transformative and life-affirming, it is also *exhausting*. The benefit of a babymoon? Many of us get the best, most restorative sleep while on vacation. In fact, you may want to factor in "rest and relaxation" pretty heavily when planning your trip, since the last thing you want is to come home feeling like you need a vacation *from* your vacation! If that means packing your ear plugs or eye mask, do it, Mama!

REKINDLE THE ROMANCE

I'm just going to blurt it out: once you have kids, your sex life will change pretty drastically, especially during those first three months postpartum. A babymoon, however, is a great way to stock up on enough lovin' to carry you through the leaner months. Of course, romance is not just about sex, and the intimacy and alone time a babymoon affords will only strengthen your relationship. Michael and I loved being able to hang out for a whole week together.

GET CLEAR ON YOUR PARENTING GOALS

Our babymoon was a great opportunity for rest and romance, it's true, but it also gave Michael and me some time to reflect on our upcoming roles as parents. *How would we raise our child? What values did we want to instill in our son? What did we want our legacy as parents to be?* Looking back, I think the trip helped us to become more intentional about the rearing of our first child. We didn't let the pregnancy blow past us unacknowledged. Rather, we took the

---

GOING TROPICAL? EH, MAYBE NOT

It may be tempting to book an exotic getaway, but you might want to rethink that strategy. International travel can, in some cases, up your risk for food poisoning, mosquito-borne illnesses such as malaria or Zika, or encountering foreign bacteria your body hasn't met (and built up resistance to) yet. Speaking of Zika, the virus can be passed from mama to baby in utero, which can lead to birth defects like microcephaly and severe brain impairment. Visit the Centers for Disease Control and Prevention's website for a list of safe spots to travel if you're hoping to get out of the country. Since Zika can be transmitted sexually, you'll ideally want your partner to refrain from visiting infected areas, too. And if he does, the CDC recommends using condoms for the remainder of your pregnancy. We actually canceled a trip to Guatemala once I learned I was pregnant with Griffin; I can't seem to leave a Central or South American country without a case of, uh, bowel distress.

WHAT OTHER *natural mamas* SAY

mariska: We went to Berlin when I was 21 weeks pregnant, which turned out to be the perfect time to take a babymoon. I knew the baby was healthy (I'd just had my 20-week ultrasound), but I wasn't huge yet and still had plenty of energy. It was great!

samantha: My husband and I didn't take a babymoon, exactly, but we celebrated our tenth wedding anniversary during my third pregnancy by taking a "food tour" of our hometown. We tried lots of unique and delicious dishes, and it was so nice to spend some quality time together before the baby arrived.

shandy: We took one last trip before we started trying to get pregnant—I wanted to be able to fully enjoy a vacation (alcohol and all)! We went to Cancun, and it was wonderful. Now that we've had a kid, I'm even happier we went. Time as a couple is so much harder to come by now.

claudia: We didn't take a babymoon, but our doula told us to take some time out for ourselves during the last few weeks leading up to the birth, and I'm so thankful we took that advice. It was a blessing to reconnect before this little person joined our lives.

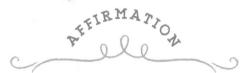

AFFIRMATION

I choose to enjoy my childbirth.
No matter how I'm feeling at any given moment,
I choose to embrace the miracle.

Cherry Chocolate Trail Mix

It can be tough to eat healthy on the go (ever try putting together a healthy meal at the airport, or—worse yet—a gas station?). Pack up some healthy trail mix, however, and you'll always have access to real food with a nice balance of fats, protein, and carbs. No matter how long your flight is delayed or how bad the traffic is, you won't have to worry about getting *hangry*.

INGREDIENTS

¾ cup raw almonds*

¾ cup raw walnuts*

½ cup dried dates

¼ cup unsweetened raisins

¼ cup unsweetened dried cherries

½ cup raw pumpkin seeds*

½ cup raw sunflower seeds*

¼ cup high-quality dark chocolate chips (check out Enjoy Life or Lily's)

Pinch of sea salt

Combine all the ingredients and store in a Mason jar or cloth baggie. Munch, munch, munch.

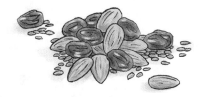

It's best to use soaked or sprouted nuts and seeds. Refer back to page 29 for more details.

time to mark the occasion, to be more present and mindful of—not to mention grateful for—the changes that were coming our way.

THE BEST REASON TO GO? BECAUSE YOU *CAN*

If you don't have children yet, you are free as a bird. Sure, you may be busy. You may even be overwhelmed or feel like you just don't have the time or the money to take an impromptu vacation. But trust me. Your life is about to change radically, and you probably won't be able to travel on a whim, just the two of you, for many, many years. So take advantage of this freedom!

If long-distance travel doesn't appeal to you or your finances don't allow for it (understandable—preparing for baby *already* requires a pretty major cash outlay!), don't forego the idea of a babymoon entirely. You can get all the benefits by choosing a place much, much closer to home. A road trip to a neighboring town, a weekend spent at a bed-and-breakfast, an afternoon at a spa (think: couples massage), or even just more regular date nights with your partner are all excellent (and cheaper!) alternatives to more extravagant trips.

Babymoons aren't just for first-time parents, either.

If you already have kids, try arranging childcare—ahem, grandparents?—even if it's just for one night. Book a hotel. Unplug. Order room service. Take a bubble bath. Sleep in.

I've yet to meet a mama who regrets having taken a little pre-baby time-out.

mama-do list

- Planning on flying? Get the all-clear from your midwife or doctor and check out airline policy *before* you book your ticket. When you're ready to purchase, select an aisle seat—it'll make frequent trips to the bathroom much, much easier.

- A little time away is just as important for couples who already have children. If you're not comfortable traveling far from home, line up a sitter and book a hotel room, even if it's just for one night.

- Single mamas can benefit from babymoons, too! If traveling alone isn't your thing, consider arranging a girls' trip or a weekend away with family or friends.

Your baby registry

CHECKLIST

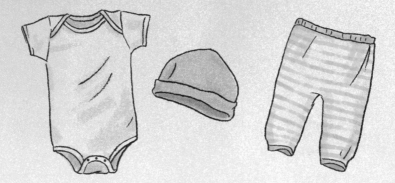

WHAT'S UP WITH *baby*?

Sure, you may have spent the bulk of the first trimester staggering around, bleary-eyed and exhausted, looking like an extra on the set of *The Walking Dead*, but sonogram images suggest that *baby* is the one yawning now. But does yawning in utero mean that she's tired? Not likely. By the second trimester, babies will begin to develop a sleeping and waking schedule, but the vast majority of time they're in a kind of deep sleep: either "active" sleep (during which she may kick and roll around) or REM sleep, characterized by the same rapid eye movement adults experience. (Some scientists even believe babies are capable of dreaming by the end of the third trimester.) It appears that a number of factors conspire to keep baby in a state of semiconscious sedation. The womb is so low in oxygen, for one thing, it's a bit like being at high altitude—researchers call the phenomenon "Mount Everest in utero." The placenta also produces a number of sleep-inducing hormones. So, why *do* babies in utero yawn? The truth is, we just don't know. There are signs, however, that fetal yawning is a hallmark of healthy development. Sweet dreams, baby!

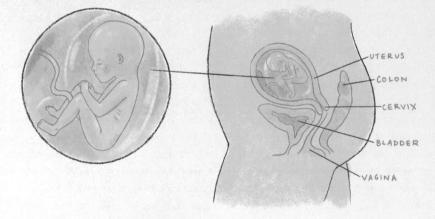

UTERUS
COLON
CERVIX
BLADDER
VAGINA

WHAT'S UP WITH *mama*?

Your pre-pregnancy uterus is usually about the size of a plum—but by Week 18, it's nearer the size of a honeydew melon. Things are getting real now, Mama! Something else that may be getting real? The pain in your back. The extra weight you're carrying around combined with changes to your posture means that aches, pains, and strains are pretty common at this stage of pregnancy. To get some relief, you might want to schedule an appointment with a Webster-certified chiropractor. Don't worry—this won't be the typical "snap, crackle, and pop" kind of adjustment. The Webster technique focuses specifically on pelvic alignment and reducing stress to the ligaments supporting your uterus, and is actually recommended by the American Pregnancy Association. Ask your midwife for a referral, or visit the International Chiropractic Pediatric Association's website (icpa4kids.org) to find a practitioner.

Ah, the baby shower. One minute you're anticipating a fun afternoon with family and friends, the next you're standing in a Babies"R"Us, armed with a barcode scanning gun, breaking into a cold sweat at the realization that it's one thing to *make* a baby and quite another to *raise* one.

Will you choose cloth diapers or disposable?

A stroller or a sling?

A crib or a co-sleeper?

Do you really need a wet-wipe warmer?

A diaper-stacker?

A mobile to hang over the crib?

And what in the *world* is a Diaper Genie?

Once I finally figured out everything I did and didn't need, I knew I had to make a registry checklist for future mamas. So this week's all about simplification, focusing on what you'll *actually use* to keep baby comfy and cared for during the first several months—and, of course, I've kept it as natural as possible.

START HERE: BIG-TICKET ITEMS

I know plenty of mamas feel queasy about registering for *über*-expensive items—I mean, isn't it tacky to "ask" your friends and family to purchase a $500 crib or changing table? But there are a few reasons it makes sense to consider it: Immediate family members, for one thing, are often inclined to spring for high-priced (read: essential) baby equipment. Friends might choose to pool their resources to purchase one major item, rather than gift you with a million bibs and teddy bears and receiving blankets. Most important, a slew of companies—including Amazon, Babies"R"Us, Target, and buybuy Baby—offer "completion discounts," which means that any unpurchased items left on your registry effectively go on sale as you get closer to your due date. So even if you wind up buying the big stuff yourself, a 10 percent or 15 percent discount off the price of a crib or stroller can add up to major bucks. (I'm especially fond of the Amazon service. It's a universal registry, which means you can add items from *any* online store, and shipping

is free for Amazon Prime members.) Let's get started.

THE CRIB

What You're Looking For: When it comes to furniture for baby's room (by the way, we'll talk more about *decorating* a natural nursery in Week 25), most cribs, changing tables, rocking chairs, and gliders are made with particleboard, press-wood, and composite materials, which means they're likely teeming with volatile organic compounds (VOCs)—a.k.a. harmful chemicals that evaporate into the air even at room temperature—as well as formaldehyde

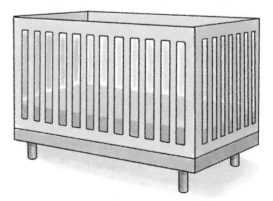

(it's in the glue). These aren't great substances for adults to be around, obviously, but they're especially troubling in a nursery, since babies are more vulnerable to the effects of noxious chemicals. Toddlers, meanwhile, have been known to chew on just about anything, including their crib rails. The safest pieces of furniture are made from solid, sustainable wood—think "solid birch" or "solid maple." If you buy an untreated, unfinished piece, you can finish it yourself with nontoxic paint or stain. Likewise, if you are co-sleeping, use a bassinet made with natural materials.

Interested in purchasing a used crib? Proceed with caution. The majority of older cribs wouldn't pass current safety regulations. Drop-side cribs, for example, can no longer be made or sold legally in the United States (though you may see them pop up at flea markets and yard sales from time to time). Check out the Consumer Product Safety Commission's updated guidelines (onsafety.cpsc.gov) before buying anything made before 2011. Portable cribs are also an option, if new furniture is out of your price range.

HOW TO FIND TOP-NOTCH BABY GEAR

Shopping for safe, eco-friendly baby gear can quickly turn into a full-time job. I mean, how *does* one choose correctly from among roughly seven thousand different types of strollers? You can narrow down your options, however, by choosing products that have been certified for meeting (or preferably exceeding) certain safety specs. Some of the organizations we gave the most credence to include:

The Greenguard Environmental Institute, which is an industry-independent organization with a focus on improving indoor air quality by reducing exposure to VOCs. The group offers two levels of certification; Greenguard Gold-certified products must meet stricter emissions standards, as they're intended for use by children in homes, schools, and daycare facilities. Look for the Greenguard Gold seal, or visit greenguard.org to find certified products in their searchable database.

The Juvenile Products Manufacturers Association (JPMA) is a national trade organization that certifies products using safety standards set by ASTM International. (Local, state, and the federal government often adopt ASTM standards, too. The legislation that outlawed drop-side cribs, for example, was inspired by ASTM recommendations.) Look for the JPMA certification seal, or visit jpma.org for a searchable database.

The Consumer Product Safety Commission is the federal agency that sets both mandatory and voluntary safety standards for manufacturers in the United States. The CPSC doesn't offer certification, but it's an excellent resource for news about product recalls and safety alerts.

What We Went With: The Oeuf Classic Crib—a splurge, no doubt, but in our opinion well worth it. Oeuf cribs are Greenguard Gold certified, meaning they're eco-friendly and certified safe for use by children and in schools. Ours is also super-low to the ground, making it extra sturdy. Bonus points for the fact that it converts to a toddler bed.

Land of Nod and Room & Board also make some reduced-toxin options. IKEA, meanwhile, offers a few nontoxic cribs for less than $200 (bless them).

For families who plan on exclusively co-sleeping—that is, sharing a bed with their newborn—a proper crib may not even be necessary. Parents who want to co-sleep but also feel *extra* secure about safety can look into a product called Snuggle Me Organic. It's a specially designed cushion that gives baby her own sleeping space within the family bed.

THE STROLLER

What You're Looking For: Plenty of natural mamas don't even have a stroller, opting instead to "wear" their babies in a wrap or a sling, but I found there were definitely occasions when I needed a set of wheels. For the first six months of Griffin's life, however, my husband and I made do with an inexpensive stroller frame that our son's car seat snapped into—buying anything fancier was just too stressful. So many options! Did we want all-terrain wheels or a city stroller? A compact, lightweight ride or one with ample storage space?

If you're planning to use a stroller right away, know that strollers for newborns *must* be (1) compatible with an infant car seat or bassinet, *or* (2) fully reclinable. Babies don't have enough head or neck strength to sit upright in a stroller meant for an older child. You can also opt for an all-in-one system, which includes a car seat, car seat base, and compatible stroller. These tend to be pricier, but they do grow with your child. Whatever you purchase, choose a stroller that's made of natural, untreated fibers. The bulk of strollers on the market are treated with flame retardants—most of which are known endocrine disruptors—as well as phthalates, BPA, and PVC. Avoid strollers with fabric that's stain resistant, waterproof, or "antibacterial," as these are treated with chemicals, too.

What We Went With: Eventually, Michael stumbled across the Bumbleride Indie, which we loved. It reclines fully, is compatible with a number of car seats, doubles as a jogging stroller, is relatively lightweight (about 20 pounds), and features all-terrain tires. The best part? Bumbleride strollers are made from eco-friendly materials including bamboo and recycled rPET (i.e., recycled water bottles). They're also PVC-, phthalate- and fire retardant–free. They're durable as all get-out, too—we're still using ours, six years later.

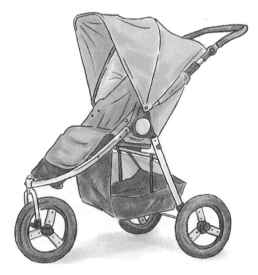

Orbit Baby and UPPAbaby make functional, eco-friendly (but still stylish) strollers, too. To save some cash, you might also consider purchasing a gently used stroller, which will have likely finished off-gassing.

THE CAR SEAT

What You're Looking For: It's gonna be a long walk home from the hospital or birth center if you don't have a car seat, so make sure you buy one—and install it—way in advance of your due date. As in, several weeks in advance, at least. Car seats are notoriously tricky for first-timers, which is perhaps why roughly 80 percent of them are installed incorrectly. And that's pretty terrifying, since proper installation is key to baby's safety.

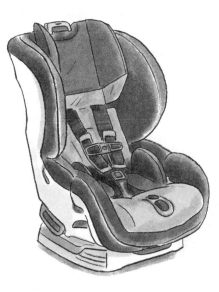

When you're ready to make the purchase, you'll be choosing from one of three types. Infant seats generally come with a carrier that connects to a base installed in the backseat—rather than strapping baby in and out of the seat itself, you'll snap the whole carrier into and out of the base (a major plus when you're transporting a sleeping baby). If you have multiple cars, you can purchase multiple bases, so you don't have to reinstall the seat every time you want to leave the house. The carrier can also be placed inside a compatible stroller or stroller frame. Infant seats should be replaced by baby's first birthday, if not sooner.

Option 2 is the convertible car seat, which starts out as a rear-facing seat and converts to a forward-facing seat (you won't make the switch until at least baby's second birthday). Pros are that convertible seats last longer—specifically, until your child outgrows the weight limit. Cons are that infants don't always fit snugly inside of convertible seats (which poses a safety issue). In fact, I know moms who had to run out and buy an infant car seat because

their convertible seat didn't pass the hospital's car seat check for proper fit.

Option 3 is to purchase an all-in-one seat, which converts from a rear-facing infant seat all the way to a booster seat. The pros and cons are the same, although all-in-one systems also tend to be bulky and expensive, and aren't always the safest choice at *every* stage of the child's life.

All car seats must meet minimum safety standards before they make it to market, and it's recommended that you have your installation job inspected. Check out seatcheck.org to find an inspector near you.

Keep in mind that car seats are the one thing you really *must* purchase new. Car seats have short lifespans—they actually come with expiration dates!—in part because the plastic they're made of can become brittle with age. Never use an old, expired, or recalled car seat.

What We Went With: Car seats are a tricky purchase for natural mamas because they're legally required to contain some kind of flame retardant. We actually (unknowingly) bought one of the most toxic seats on the market, according to a recent report from the nonprofit Ecology Center. (Boo!) Good news: UPPAbaby offers the first ever car seat that passes safety requirements *and* does not use traditional flame retardants. It's pricey, though. You can also go with Britax. They don't use halogenated flame retardants, which are some of the most harmful.

BABY CLOTHES

What You're Looking For: Lots of people will tell you not to bother registering for baby clothes, and they have a point—people *love* to pick out sweet little outfits as shower gifts, and no matter what you register for, you'll wind up with dresses and sailor suits and onesies that look like tuxedos, in sizes ranging from 0 to 3 months to whatever he's going to wear on his first day of kindergarten. Still, it's not a bad idea to choose just a few *very* basic, practical items. Aim for natural fibers and eco-friendly fabrics whenever possible, like 100 percent cotton, bamboo, and muslin. Avoid synthetic materials, as these don't breathe as well and can irritate baby's soft skin. Launder *every-thing* (in a chemical-free detergent with no fabric softener) before filling up baby's closet or dresser. And remember: newborns often fit into clothes intended for much older babies, so select items in a *wide* range of sizes.

What We Went With:

2 Stretchy Newborn Hats. Keeping a hat on a newborn is like trying to keep a bowtie on a chimpanzee; our favorites actually came from the birth center, so grab as many as you can—don't be shy! Hats help baby stay warm (newborns can't regulate their own body temperature), so they're particularly helpful when she's outdoors or if baby sleeps in a crib by herself. Just make sure they fit snugly, so they won't fall off and cover her face.

4–6 Side-Snap Shirts. Trying to get a shirt over a newborn's head isn't much easier than keeping a hat on him, but side-snap shirts are easy-on, easy-off, and great for layering. Long-sleeved shirts are better for winter babies.

4–6 Plain White Onesies. You'll no doubt receive quite a few onesies as gifts—probably with adorable sayings and slogans on them—but I used basic white onesies daily as layering shirts. They're also great for containing diaper, uh, *blowouts.*

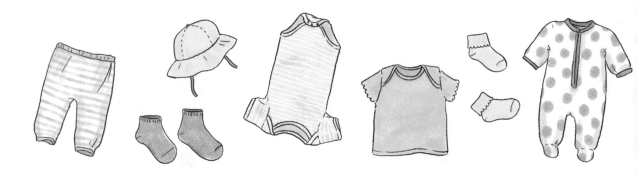

3–4 Lounge Pants. Soft, cozy pants with an elastic waistband are a must. I went with organic cotton brands including DorDor & Gor-Gor and Kushies.

4–6 Footed Onesie Pajamas. Since babies spend their first three months either napping, waking up from a nap, or being rocked back down again, you'll want lots of PJs. Get a mix of short- and long-sleeved, depending on the season. I loved the jammies from Under the Nile, which are made with eco-friendly, organic materials.

4–6 Onesie-style T-shirts. Layer these over a plain white onesie, throw on some lounge pants, and go!

4–6 Pairs of Socks. Forget about losing pairs of socks in the washer/dryer—baby socks somehow manage to get lost when they're *on the baby.* You may want to look for any brand labeled "kick-proof." Trumpette socks, made to look like little Mary Janes or sneakers, were my favorites.

BABY BEDDING

What You're Looking For: Browse through any baby goods store and you're bound to see some *elaborate* crib sets: comforters and cozy blankets and dust ruffles, all available in about a million different matchy-matchy themed sets: chickens, ducks, polka dots, bows. Here's the thing: baby can't actually sleep with *any* of that. All those adorable stuffed animals and tiny pillows are safety hazards. As for crib bumpers, there's zero evidence they do anything to prevent injury; they are, however, associated with higher rates of suffocation and sudden infant death syndrome (SIDS). All baby really needs is a mattress, a mattress cover, a fitted sheet, and maybe a swaddle or a wearable blanket. You can certainly have a beauti-

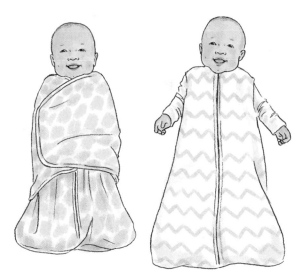

fully decorated nursery if you like, just don't put anything in or around baby's crib.

What We Went With:

Mattress. Babies need firm mattresses—anything soft or squishy could pose a suffocation risk. You'll also want one made from nontoxic materials. Babies and toddlers spend more than half their lives sleeping, yet most mattresses—just like strollers and car seats—are made with synthetic materials and treated with toxic fire retardants. We went with the Moonlight Slumber mattress, which is free of vinyl, polyethylene, PVC, lead, and phthalates. Alternatively, Naturepedic mattresses contain no flame retardants, glues, adhesives, PFCs, antibacterial treatments, or biocides, and use non-GMO fabrics and fibers. Essentia makes great organic crib mattresses, too.

2 Waterproof Mattress Liners. These are all about containing "accidents," and there will be plenty of them in the first few years. Get two, so you'll always have a clean one at the ready. I loved the organic covers from American Baby Company.

2 Fitted Sheets. Flat sheets pose a suffocation risk; stick with fitted, made from organic fibers or 100 percent cotton. Under the Nile sheets are particularly soft.

2 Sleep Sacks and 2 Swaddles. Loose blankets, quilts, and comforters all pose a suffocation risk, because infants don't have the strength to lift and turn their heads. Of course, you don't want baby to get cold at night either, which is why sleep sacks and swaddles are—at least in my opinion—a must-buy, especially if you live north of the Mason-Dixon. Newborns in particular like the sensation of being swaddled, since it's a bit like being in the womb. (I like the Summer Infant SwaddleMe Organic Adjustable Wrap, since it won't unravel; aden + anais and the Miracle Blanket Swaddle are good options, too.) Babies who are old enough to wriggle out of the swaddle or roll onto their tummies are ready to graduate to a sleep sack, which is a little like a sleeping bag that leaves baby's arms free. My favorite is the HALO organic cotton sleep slack, which is breathable and durable.

White-Noise Machine. For many mamas—including me—the white-noise machine is the go-to, numero uno, best-gift-I-ever-got, since it'll mask noises that can startle a sleeping baby (lawn mowers, doorbells, the television) while mimicking the muffled sounds he heard in the womb. We went with the Cadillac of white-noise machines, the Marpac Dohm Original Sound Conditioner. Some mamas, meanwhile, swear by the Sleep Genius Baby app, which was developed by experts in neuroscience, sleep, and sound, and features technology that's been celebrated by NASA. (Yes, *that* NASA.) Just know that noise machines and smartphones should never be placed in baby's crib or next to his head!

DIAPERS

What You're Looking For: Should you really register for diapers? In a word: *yes.* An average child will need her diaper changed anywhere from 4,000 to 8,000 times before she's ready for potty training, so it's helpful to get a leg up in this department. Of course, that means you'll have to come up with an answer to the age-old question: cloth diapers or disposable?

I'd be lying if I said I didn't approach cloth diapering with a bit of trepidation (okay, *dread*), but now I am a total convert. American parents use an estimated 27.4 billion disposable diapers every year, which end up in landfills. Factor in the petroleum-based plastic shell, the chemicals used in the production process, and 'round-the-world transportation, and the environmental footprint of disposable diapers is staggering. If that doesn't convince you to go cloth, you might want to consider the benefits to your bank account. Parents will spend roughly $2,500 on disposable diapers by the time baby is two and a half. Cloth diapers cost a fraction of that. For me, it was a no-brainer.

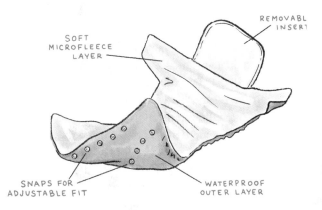

SOFT MICROFLEECE LAYER

REMOVABL INSER1

SNAPS FOR ADJUSTABLE FIT

WATERPROOF OUTER LAYER

Chia Seed Pudding

Give your baby's bones some love this week. Chia seeds have more calcium than milk, and when soaked overnight, they bloom into a glorious, gelatinous pudding. They're also an excellent yet gentle source of insoluble and soluble fiber, which will keep things, ya know, *moving*. Win-win!

INGREDIENTS

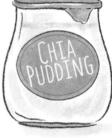

2 cups farm-fresh organic milk or fortified almond milk

⅔ cup organic chia seeds

1 teaspoon vanilla extract

½ teaspoon cinnamon

3 tablespoons organic maple syrup or raw honey, or 45 drops stevia

½ cup organic raisins (optional)

Combine all ingredients in a medium bowl, cover tightly, and refrigerate overnight. In the morning, your pudding will be set and ready for breakfast. Yum.

What We Went With:

24 Cloth Diapers. When most people think of cloth diapers, they imagine a giant handkerchief that's fastened with safety pins. (Case in point: My mom bought me safety pins as one of my shower gifts.) Cloth diapers, however, have come a long way, and there are loads of options: flats, pre-folds, all-in-ones, pockets. We went with pocket diapers from bumGenius and AppleCheeks, which come with a liner (the exterior part of the diaper) and an insert (the part you shove inside the pocket for absorbency)—24 ended up being the perfect number, since we did the laundry every three days. Wait any longer than that and you risk moldy diapers. Ew. Keep in mind there are plenty of other great brands out there; you can even purchase gently used (and sterilized!) diapers on diaperswappers.com and clothdiapertrader.com.

Diaper Pail and 2 Liners. We chose a simple hands-free pail—the kind with a pedal you step on to raise the lid—lined with a cloth laundry bag from EcoAble; wet diapers go straight into the pail. When it's time to do the wash, throw the liner in, too.

The Sprayer. Oh, if every diaper was *only* full of pee. Enter the diaper sprayer, which looks like a tiny shower head, except it attaches right to the side of your toilet. Installation is super-simple, no plumber required! Use the sprayer to blast off any fecal matter straight into the john, then toss the diaper into the pail until you're ready to launder.

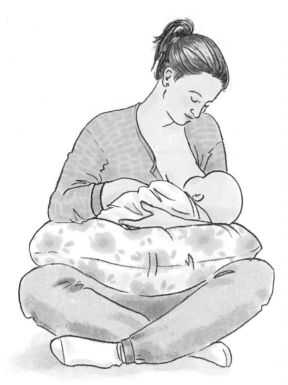

1 Package Eco-friendly Disposable Diapers. Even if you're planning to use cloth diapers, disposables are great for traveling long distances or going on vacation (unless you plan to do laundry in a hotel washroom). Disposables are also best for the first few days of baby's life, when he's still eliminating meconium. My favorite brand is Bambo Nature, but Earth's Best and Naty are pretty great, too. Whichever brand you choose, opt for a diaper that's free of dyes, phthalates, and fragrances—especially if you plan to go with disposables full-time.

1 Package Eco-friendly Baby Wipes (or reusable cloth wipes). I used disposable wipes *very judiciously*. If you go that route, be sure to buy wipes that are free of added lotions, fragrances, and unnecessary ingredients. I like WaterWipes, which are made with water and grapefruit seed extract. Earth's Best are a good option, too. Reusable cloth wipes, on the other hand, get tossed into the laundry *with* the cloth diapers.

BOTTLES, BIBS, AND BURP CLOTHS—OH, MY!

What You're Looking For: It's easy to get caught-up with adorable baby clothes and accessories, but don't forget that all the extra stuff you need to clean, bathe, and play with baby adds up!

What We Went With:

Bibs. I used mostly silicone bibs, since they're a breeze to clean and they reduce mealtime mess. (Cloth bibs, on the other hand, need to be laundered, and who needs more laundry?!) Make sure you have a few on hand by the time baby is ready for solid foods.

Burp Cloths. Spit-up may be a daily occurrence during the first few months, and unless you want to sport that telltale wet splotch on your shoulder, you'll need to use a cloth when burping. Stick with inexpensive organic cloths that are easy to wash and dry. Two to four should do, unless you've got a major spitter-upper.

Towels and Washcloths. Skip the cutesy baby robes—a nice towel or two (preferably with a hood), and 2 quality washcloths are really all you need. (Burp cloths can double as washcloths, so long as they're freshly laundered.)

YOUR *baby registry* CHECKLIST

Big-Ticket Items

- Crib, co-sleeper bassinet or pillow
- Stroller
- Car seat

Baby Clothes

- 2 Newborn hats
- 2–4 Side-snap shirts
- 4–6 Plain white onesies
- 3–4 Lounge pants
- 4–6 Footed onesie pajamas
- 2–4 Onesie-style T-shirts
- 4–6 Pairs of socks

Baby Bedding

- Crib mattress
- 2 Waterproof mattress liners
- 2 Fitted sheets
- 2 Sleep sacks
- 2 Swaddles
- White-noise machine (optional)

Cloth Diaper Setup

- 24 Cloth diapers
- Diaper pail
- 2 Diaper pail liners
- Diaper sprayer
- Eco-friendly disposable diapers
- Eco-friendly baby wipes

Bottles, Bibs, Burp Cloths, and Accessories

- 2 Silicone bibs
- 2–4 Burp cloths
- 2 Towels with hoods
- 2 Washcloths
- 1 Starter-kit glass baby bottles
- Silicone pacifiers
- Digital ear thermometer
- Bathtub
- Nursing pillow
- Infant swing
- Activity mat
- Baby carrier

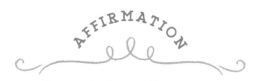

I stay active and strong.
I love being in my pregnant body.
I nourish my body, mind, and spirit each day.

Baby Soap and Lotion. Babies do not need to be bathed every day, nor do they need to be soaped from head-to-toe, as this can dry out their delicate skin and wash away good bacteria. I used a simple olive oil–based soap and only on baby's feet, hands, pits, and bum. If needed, organic virgin coconut oil makes for a great moisturizer and diaper rash cream.

Glass Baby Bottles. BPA was banned from baby bottles and sippy cups back in 2012, but new research shows that even BPA-free plastics can still leach chemicals. I like Lifefactory glass baby bottles. One of their starter kits should be enough if you're a stay-at-home mama or work part-time; get more if you work full-time outside the home.

Silicone or Natural Rubber Pacifiers. As a breastfeeding mama, I wanted to keep paci time to a minimum, but they came in handy for code-red crying spells and long car rides.

Digital Ear Thermometer. You'll want one on hand. They're less accurate than rectal thermometers, but they'll alert you to fever with less, uh, probing.

Baby Bathtub. I wasn't sure I really needed one of these, but I found it invaluable. Primo makes one that's extra-large and luxurious.

Nursing Pillow. A nursing pillow helps with the ergonomic positioning of baby during breast-feeding—and your back and arms will thank you for it, trust me. I like the Blessed Nest or the Boppy Nursing Pillow with an organic cotton cover.

Infant Swing. Greatest. Invention. Ever. When you need a little break and baby is cranky, this device will become a life-saver. I went with the Fisher-Price My Little Snugabunny, a perennial bestseller, because it was free! (We were lucky enough to get a hand-me-down.) If I were to buy new, however, I'd go with the Fisher-Price Rock 'n Play, which vibrates *and* rocks, the ultimate combo. It also encourages baby to rest at a slight incline, which be can helpful in combatting colic, indigestion, and reflux. It is also free of flame retardants.

Activity Mat. Activity mats aren't just great for entertaining infants; the stimulation and play is vital for their developing brains. We loved

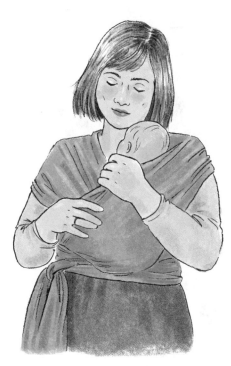

the Fisher-Price Kick & Play Piano Gym (hello, baby Mozart!).

Baby Carrier. No crunchy mama would be complete without a way to wear her baby. Wraps and carriers keep you hands-free, are great for skin-to-skin contact, and make breastfeeding a snap when you're on-the-go. For newborns, a Maya Wrap or Boba Wrap is best. When my baby hit three months, I loved my Ergobaby—good-bye, back pain!

mama-do list

- I don't know about you, but the mere thought of standing in a baby goods superstore is enough to make me feel clammy. Online registries take the leg-work—not to mention the anxiety—out of shopping.

- Want to see some cloth diapering in action? Check out mamanatural.com for more info, resources, and—yes—even videos. (Don't worry—we used a stunt baby and *unsoiled* diapers in all our demonstrations.)

- Though a car seat is something you'll likely want to purchase yourself, it's best to pick one out early since it can affect your stroller choice or vice versa. Many stores will let you test-install a seat to see how it fits in your car before making the purchase. Get your installation job checked by an inspector, and you'll have one less thing to think about when the big day comes.

catch some ZZZs

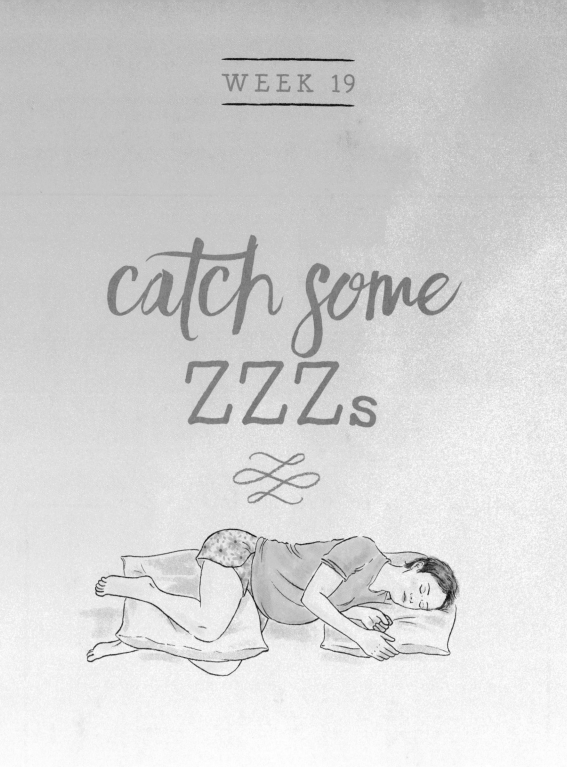

WHAT'S UP WITH *baby*?

Ever wonder why horses can walk mere hours after birth, yet it takes human babies upwards of a year? One of the reasons has to do with a process called *myelination*. Starting around Week 19, a fatty coating of insulation (called myelin) begins forming around some of the nerve fibers in baby's brain. Myelin enables the nerve fibers to transmit electrical signals quickly and efficiently. In the short term, this gives baby more control over his motor function, which is why you might feel an uptick in his movements, not to mention some much more *forceful* kicks! But the process will continue long after birth. In fact, the human brain doesn't fully mature until around age twenty-five. (No wonder teenagers and young adults are so impulsive!) And that's why human babies can't walk right away: the appropriate areas of the brain have not yet been myelinated.

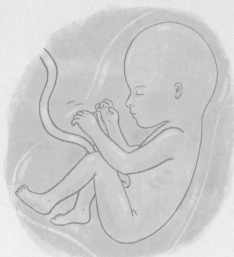

BABY'S MOVEMENTS ARE NOW FLUID AND DELIBERATE.

WHAT'S UP WITH *mama*?

Your body continues to S-T-R-E-T-C-H, and you may be *really* feeling it now. Literally. I remember once during the second trimester of my second pregnancy, I reached up into the closet and felt an intense pulling sensation in my groin area. It turned out to be "round ligament pain"—totally normal, definitely not comfortable. But what caused it? The uterus is propped up and supported by several thick ligaments, one of which is called—I bet you can guess—the round ligament. As your baby grows larger, the ligament thins and stretches, making it more susceptible to strain, especially if you make sudden movements. A dull achy feeling is common, too. Fortunately, you can ease this pain with rest, light exercise, and the use of a pregnancy support belt. You know, kind of like what weight lifters wear. Hot stuff!

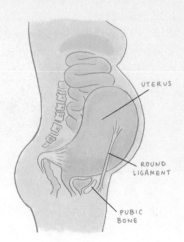

UTERUS

ROUND LIGAMENT

PUBIC BONE

The grizzly bear is definitely my spirit animal. I *love* honey. I give the best hugs. And I could sleep all. Winter. Long.

Okay, fine. Maybe my spirit animal is less "grizzly bear" and more "Winnie the Pooh." But my ability to hibernate may have been the reason I was able to sleep soundly through all nine months of my pregnancies. Most mamas aren't so lucky—the weight of the baby, the ache in your back, and the constant need to pee can make quality shut-eye elusive. In fact, a staggering 75 percent of pregnant women suffer from some sort of sleep disorder. And it's more than a mere inconvenience. Lack of sleep can hike up your blood pressure, weaken your immunity and, of course, leave you feeling fatigued, both mentally and physically. This week I've got loads of tips to help make sure you're getting your forty winks.

By the way, that thing I said before about sleeping soundly through all nine months? Don't hate me. I may have been well rested, but I snored like a linebacker and had to wear nose strips!

ASSUME THE POSITION: SAFE SLEEPING IN THE SECOND HALF OF PREGNANCY

The moment your baby bump emerges, you can pretty much rule out sleeping on your stomach. But you've likely heard that now, it's no longer safe to sleep on your back, either. What gives? Concern about lying too long in the supine position largely has to do with the vena cava—this is the largest vein in your body, and it carries blood from the lower extremities back to the heart. Too much pressure on that vein (caused, of course, by the weight of your growing bambino) can trigger nausea or dizziness in some women, not to mention restrict blood flow to the uterus. There are also concerns that sleeping on your back may increase the risk of blood clots, or lead to fetal distress.

So, out of an abundance of caution, you're left with side sleeping.

Traditionally, midwives and doctors have recommended sleeping on your left side, for many of the same reasons—the vena cava runs just to the right of the spine, so lying on your left side may allow for better circulation. (Better circulation, it's worth mentioning, can also help reduce swelling of the feet and ankles.) But let's be honest here. Sleeping on one hip night after night for twenty weeks isn't all that comfortable. And when you finally do settle into a sweet spot, you're not even conscious enough to know which side you're lying on! Some mamas can get so worked up about sleeping "correctly" that they wind up lying awake at night, wide-eyed, plagued by

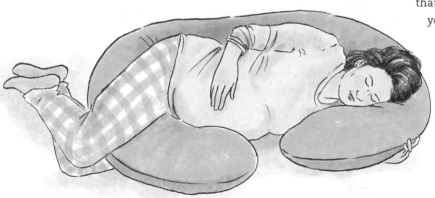

Tart Cherry Bomb

Did you know that tart cherries are one of the richest sources of melatonin on the planet? In fact, at least one small study suggests that tart cherry juice can increase sleep time by as much as *90 minutes a night*. I even tried it on my three-year-old (a notoriously early riser) to eke out some more shut-eye, and it worked! Tart cherries also help reduce inflammation, body aches, and swelling, all common pregnancy side effects. To get the most benefits, try it two ways:

In the afternoon, combine 2 tablespoons organic and unsweetened tart cherry juice concentrate, 8 to 12 ounces sparkling water, and a few drops of liquid stevia (but only if you want the sweetness). Serve over ice and enjoy.

Around 8 p.m., mix 2 tablespoons of tart cherry juice concentrate, 8 ounces of plain kefir yogurt, and liquid stevia to taste.

insomnia. And that's not doing you *or* your baby any favors.

The truth is that it's fine to sleep a little on your right side, too, just try to favor the left if you can.

Likewise, there's no need to panic if you wake up in the middle of the night and find yourself staring at the ceiling. Most mamas will instinctively shift positions if they happen to roll onto their back at some point—I know I did. As you enter your third trimester, you may even notice baby giving you a swift kick to the ribs as a not-so-gentle reminder.

If side sleeping isn't your natural position, try getting your body used to it as early as pos-

sible. If it doesn't feel comfortable, use pillows. Lots of 'em. Truly, they can save the night.

Putting a pillow between your knees, for example, will keep the hips more aligned, which can help to alleviate back pain. Hugging a pillow, meanwhile, will raise your arm, improving shoulder alignment and lessening neck strain. You might even consider springing for the mack daddy of all sleep aids: the body pillow. These days, they come in all sorts of shapes and sizes, including the "C" (which you can tuck between your knees *and* rest your head on), the "U" (sleep with your head at the bottom of the curve and the pillow will cradle you), and the "bean," which can eventually double as a nursing pillow.

BATTLING PREGNANCY INSOMNIA

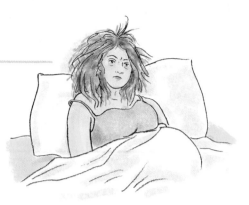

So you've got your pillows and you're doing
your best to get comfortable on your left side,
but every time you lie down it feels like there's
a German shepherd sitting on your tummy. Or
maybe you've started involuntarily kicking and
thrashing around in bed—symptoms of restless
leg syndrome (another common pregnancy

SWEET DREAMS—OR BABY-RELATED NIGHTMARES?

Are crazy dreams suddenly keeping you up at night? Are vivid memories of those dreams
haunting even your daylight hours? If so, you're not alone. (I remember dreaming that
I was on a battlefield, Rambo-style, shooting up everything in sight. What gives?) Studies show that pregnant women really *do* dream more. Well, it *seems* like they do, at least.
(In reality, pregnant women are just better able to recall those dreams upon waking.)
Most often, these nighttime imaginings have to do with the health and safety of the baby:
dreams of losing the baby, forgetting the baby, accidental death, or giving birth to an inani-
mate object are all common. In fact, research suggests that nightmares in particular may
become even more frequent in the days and weeks *after* giving birth. But what do these
dreams mean? Are they a sign that something's wrong with your pregnancy? A premoni-
tion that some awful fate will befall you or your child?

Not hardly.

While pregnancy dreams may be caused, at least in part, by wild hormonal surges,
it's more likely that all that tossing and turning, not to mention middle-of-the-night trips
to the bathroom, is interrupting your REM sleep. As for what you're dreaming about, most
experts believe this is just your subconscious working through the anxiety associated with
becoming a new mother and protecting a new life (hence my Rambo rages). In other words,
it's your brain's way of adapting to such a monumental lifestyle change.

If dark or disturbing dreams are affecting your sleep—or worse, making you afraid
to go to sleep—be extra diligent about reducing your exposure to blue light in the hours
before bedtime. Up your magnesium intake. Adopt a nighttime ritual. And don't hesitate to
speak with your midwife or doctor. While some mamas may benefit from meeting with a
therapist (your healthcare provider can refer you), sometimes just a chat with your midwife
can normalize the experience and make you feel less, well, batty.

side effect). It's a cruel irony that just when you need sleep the most—like right before you bring home a newborn—your body seems determined to keep you awake. Better sleep, however, starts *long* before it's time to turn out the lights. If you're having trouble getting enough Zs, make sure to:

Get More Exercise. It's not exactly rocket science, but you'll sleep better at night if you're physically tired. You may want to get your workouts in earlier in the day if you notice that an evening boost of adrenaline and endorphins makes it difficult to wind down. Even just some light stretching before bed can release tension in the muscles and promote relaxation. Speaking of muscles, you might ask if your partner will indulge you in a foot rub. Sure, it might not count as "exercise" (not for *you*, at least), but a foot massage can improve circulation, reduce swelling, and feels so, so good.

To Nap or Not to Nap? The short answer: it depends. Lots of mamas find that they just can't make it through the day without a quick snooze on the couch—and that's fine. If, however, you're struggling to get to sleep at night, try limiting those daytime naps to just 20 minutes. Also, don't nap in total darkness, as this can upset your wake-sleep rhythm. You might try eliminating naps altogether and moving your bedtime up by an hour or two.

Mind Your Mealtime. Since a large meal right before bed can trigger indigestion and heartburn, both of which will certainly keep you up,

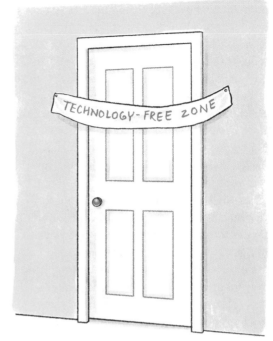

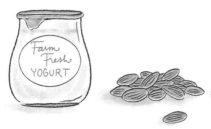

try not to eat anything after eight in the evening. (If you're ravenous by ten, a *small* serving of healthy fats—a half-cup of whole-fat yogurt or a spoonful of almond butter can be satiating.) If you're still suffering from late-night heartburn, try propping yourself up with extra pillows to limit reflux. Start drinking 1 teaspoon of raw apple cider vinegar (diluted in a few ounces of water) before each meal, as this can aid digestion. Avoid caffeinated beverages and chocolate past lunchtime, as these can keep you awake at night.

Turn Your Bedroom into a Restful Retreat. For years, sleep experts have been saying that our beds should be used for only two things, sex and sleep, and yet many of us have turned our boudoirs into veritable entertainment centers. We watch TV late into the evening, play games or surf the web on our smartphones, or drag our laptops into bed, setting up mini workstations. All those electronics, however, act as stimulants: they wake the brain up just when it should be winding down. Action movies, video games, and even work-related emails, meanwhile, can boost your stress hormones. The blue light emitted from these devices can trick our bodies into thinking it's daytime, delaying the release of the sleep-inducing hormone, melatonin. The EMF radiation may be affecting our ability to fall asleep—and stay asleep—too.

You'll sleep more soundly if you banish the electronics, turn off your Wi-Fi at night, and switch out your cell phone for a battery-operated alarm clock. You'll also want to crank up the AC or open a window. Our bodies are designed to sleep in cooler temperatures, preferably somewhere between 60 and 67 degrees. Try and make your bedroom as dark as possible; sleep masks or blackout curtains are two easy ways to keep the glare from streetlights at bay. Finally, consider purchasing a white-noise machine. These aren't just for babies; they work wonders at drowning out the rumble of a passing truck, the creaks and squeaks of the

house, or chatter coming from a nearby room. Alternatively, check out the Sleep Genius app.

Adopt a Nighttime Ritual. Keeping a consistent schedule—going to bed at the same time every night and getting up at the same time every morning—is an important part of developing healthy rest habits. But a slightly more *elaborate* bedtime ritual *really* signals to your body (and your brain!) that it's time to start sawing logs. Which is why, around eight in the evening, I don a pair of amber-tinted, $8 sunglasses I bought off Amazon. They are, admittedly, super dorky looking. (Think Bono meets construction worker or shop teacher.) They also block the blue-tinted light emitted by TV and computer screens, encouraging the body's natural melatonin production. I knock off the overheads and switch to lamp light in the evenings, too, and try to power down *all* the electronics by nine.

Of course, if you're used to being lulled to sleep by the drone of the television, the absence of all that electronic stimuli might sound less than appealing. What to do with all that free time? Try this:

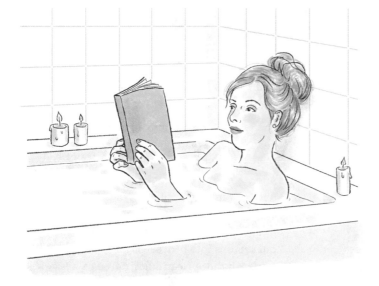

- ♡ Take a warm (not hot) bath or shower—the heat of the water will soothe tired muscles, while the rapid cool down after toweling off further signals to your body that it's time to sleep.

- ♡ Brush and floss your teeth—a gentle reminder that you're done eating.

- ♡ Drink some chamomile or lavender tea—both of these herbs calm the body in preparation for sleep.

♡ Do some very light stretching or a few low-intensity yoga poses—not enough to break a sweat, just enough to release some tension. A focus on deep breathing will further help to clear your mind.

♡ Tuck in with a good book—according to a UK-based study, reading at night is more effective at promoting sleep than listening to music, going for a walk, or having a warm cup of tea. In fact, just 6 minutes of reading reduced stress levels by a whopping 68 percent!

Try a Natural Remedy. Back in Week 7, I mentioned that a majority of Americans are likely magnesium deficient, and that boosting your stores with topical magnesium oil or a supplement can help ease the symptoms of morning sickness. But it turns out that magnesium may be a kind of cure-all for restless nights. That's

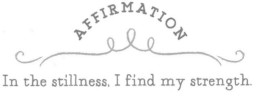

AFFIRMATION

In the stillness, I find my strength.
My job is to breathe, relax,
and work with my body.

because magnesium affects the functioning of our GABA receptors, a powerful neurotransmitter responsible for switching the brain "off" in the evening. (Incidentally, alcohol, Valium, and Xanax target the GABA receptors, too.) Talk to your doctor or midwife about supplementation.

mama-do list

○ Some mamas-to-be have more difficulty falling asleep (and staying asleep) than others, but no matter how restless or worn out you feel, resist the urge to pop a sleeping pill. There is *very* little evidence to suggest that sleep aids are safe during pregnancy, and mountains of research to suggest they may be habit-forming. They're also notorious for causing a slew of side effects.

○ "Sunglasses at Night" may be a classic song from the 1980s, but it sounds like a goofy way to improve sleep quality, doesn't it? Studies show, however, that "blue blockers" really *do* work. In fact, they may even boost your mood. I wear Uvex Skyper Safety Eyewear, which is super cheap on Amazon.

○ Round ligament or pelvic girdle pain got you feeling down? Consider picking up a maternity support belt. Though they may seem like a major fashion faux pas, they're actually surprisingly popular—probably because they work! There are loads of options out there, but you may want to check out the BellyBra, the Belly Band, or the Prenatal Cradle. Also, visit a Webster-certified chiropractor if you can.

let's get it on

WHAT'S UP WITH *baby*?

Where did the time go, Mama? You've officially reached the halfway point of your pregnancy. Wha what?! CONGRATULATIONS! It's appropriate, then, that baby is now a little more than half a foot long (around 6½ inches, crown to rump) and weighs a little more than half a pound—she's tipping the scales at 9 or 10 ounces. The midway point of pregnancy marks some other exciting milestones: For the first time, you'll likely be able to hear baby's heartbeat with a fetoscope—great news if you've been foregoing the Doppler. You may be headed in for your first and only ultrasound this week, too. If you can, however, push the anatomy scan off until Week 22—waiting a bit longer lowers the chance that you'll have to repeat the ultrasound to get a more accurate picture.

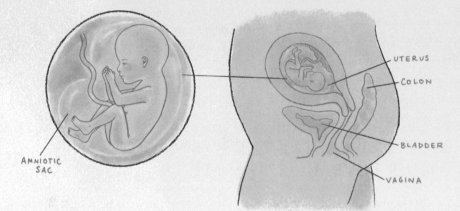

AMNIOTIC SAC

UTERUS

COLON

BLADDER

VAGINA

WHAT'S UP WITH *mama*?

Take a look at your belly button. Has your innie turned into an outie? If it hasn't yet, it probably will—the rapid expansion of the uterus causes most belly buttons to "pop" around the midpoint of pregnancy (although yours should return to its original state a few weeks or months postpartum). If you don't like the look of your outie under tight shirts, check out a product called Popper Stoppers. They're little self-stick pads that—as the name suggests—stop the navel from popping through your clothes. While we're on the subject, ever wondered why some people *have* outies? All belly buttons are essentially scars that form when the stalk of the umbilical cord dries up and falls off a few days or weeks after birth. In some cases, a small umbilical hernia or a very minor infection at the base of the cord might cause an outie, but all of them are basically just excess scar tissue.

Being pregnant is the only time in my life that I've been able to identify with a teenage boy. Because once I hit 20 weeks or so, I was suddenly insatiable. I mean, I wanted sex all. of. the. time. Feeling randy 'round the clock certainly wasn't something I'd anticipated, but after the nausea and the fatigue, here was a pregnancy side effect even my husband could get behind!

Your desire for sex will undoubtedly fluctuate over the course of your pregnancy—it's normal to feel extra interested, totally *uninterested*, or anything in between.

But many mamas do report more frequent and more satisfying romps during the second trimester.

What's behind this boost to your libido? Surging hormones, of course, are partly responsible. The increase in blood flow, meanwhile, ups sensitivity in the erogenous zones. And thanks to the movie-star hair and the major cleavage, some women actually have a better self-image when pregnant. So take full advantage, Mama, because sex during pregnancy has loads of benefits. This week we'll go over everything you need to know about getting it on.

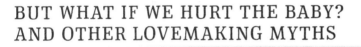

BUT WHAT IF WE HURT THE BABY? AND OTHER LOVEMAKING MYTHS

There are a few circumstances in which your midwife or doctor may advise you to abstain from intercourse (if you have placenta previa or cervical insufficiency, for example, or if you're at a high risk for preterm labor). In the vast majority of cases, though, sex during pregnancy is perfectly safe. But it doesn't help that there are so many myths floating around out there. So let's start by debunking a few of those, shall we?

MYTH #1: SEX CAN CAUSE MISCARRIAGE

Many women find that a fierce, Mama Bear–like instinct kicks in *long* before birth, so it's only natural to be worried about the safety of your growing baby. Roughly 60 percent of miscarriages, however, are the result of a chromosomal abnormality, resulting in a pregnancy that just isn't viable. Hormonal imbalance or maternal health issues, improper implantation of the egg, or certain lifestyle factors (in particular, drinking and drug use) are associated with higher rates of miscarriage, too. But none of these factors, clearly, has anything to do with intercourse.

In fact, there is *zero* evidence that sex will harm the health of your baby, assuming yours is a low-risk pregnancy.

Keep in mind that a bit of light bleeding or spotting after sex is somewhat common. Usually, this is just a side effect of the increase in your blood volume—the tiny blood vessels in your vagina and around the cervix rupture easily. If you notice a bit of blood, you should call your midwife or doctor (any bleeding, no matter how minimal, could be a symptom of a larger problem), but there's no need to panic. A small amount of spotting after sex is almost always harmless.

MYTH #2: SEX CAN SHAKE THE BABY LOOSE

Throughout pregnancy, baby is suspended in a sea of amniotic fluid. She is further protected by the amniotic sac itself and by the muscular walls of the uterus. What's more, a thick mucus plug (exactly what it sounds like, by the way) seals off the womb, protecting your baby from bacteria, pathogens and, yes, even semen. But even without all these barriers, the penis does not penetrate the cervix or the womb during sex, so it's just not possible to poke the baby, dislodge the baby, or in any way interfere with baby's development, no matter how well-endowed your partner is.

One day, your baby bump looks huge. The next, it seems to have shrunk. What gives? Baby is still pretty small (roughly the size of a banana), which means she's got plenty of room to move around down there. Depending on her position, the size and shape of your belly may change from day to day. By month six or seven, though, you'll look—and feel!—pretty big *all the time*, so enjoy this game of hide-and-seek while it lasts.

MYTH #3: BABY CAN "FEEL" PENETRATION

So, this myth is actually half-true. After all, it's certainly possible that baby might be . . . *jostled*

IS ORAL SEX SAFE?

Yes, we're going there. And yes, provided neither you nor your partner has a sexually transmitted disease, both giving and receiving oral sex during pregnancy is safe, too. However, if you were to consult any number of reputable health organizations—from the Mayo Clinic to the March of Dimes Foundation—you'd receive the same, slightly bizarre warning: oral is fine, but you should *never* let your partner blow air directly into your vagina.

I'll be honest. My first thought upon hearing this warning was: *Who is doing this? Where does such a random warning even come from?* The answer, it turns out, is from existing medical literature. See, forcing air into the vagina may cause an air embolism—basically, an air bubble that gets absorbed into the bloodstream, blocking a vein or an artery. (The risk of embolism goes up during pregnancy because the blood vessels are enlarged in order to accommodate the increase in blood volume.) And believe it or not, several large-scale studies have identified 17 or 18 fatalities from air embolism over the last century or so. It's an exceedingly rare condition, true, but one dangerous enough to merit the warning. So, no blowing air down there, okay?

FEELING YEASTY?
NATURAL REMEDIES FOR VAGINAL INFECTIONS

Sex doesn't typically cause yeast infections (a more likely culprit is rising estrogen, which can disrupt the vagina's natural pH balance), but it is possible to pass a yeast infection along to your partner—and vice versa. So, prevention is key. Keeping your genitals clean and dry, wearing cotton panties, and ditching thong underwear are all good ways to lower your risk. But if you notice any itching, burning, or discharge that's thick and white, there's likely something not quite right with your lady parts.

Before attempting to diagnose and treat a yeast infection on your own, talk to your midwife or doctor; symptoms can sometimes be confused with other issues, in particular STIs and bacterial vaginosis (another common infection) or even a UTI (more on that soon). If you get the go-ahead to try a natural remedy, you'll want to monitor your symptoms closely. The good news is that yeast infections are not dangerous for you and baby, just uncomfortable. But it's important that they be appropriately treated—it's possible to pass a yeast infection on during delivery. Vaginal yeast infections in mamas can become oral infections in infants, called thrush.

Raw Apple Cider Vinegar
To treat a yeast infection, try adding 1 cup to a warm bath and soaking for 20 minutes; it's thought that the vinegar can help rebalance the vagina's pH.

Garlic
Garlic is well known for its antifungal and antibacterial properties, and it certainly can't hurt to incorporate more fresh, raw garlic into your diet. (Pesto, anyone?) But the most effective method for treating a yeast infection is a garlic suppository. It sounds crazy, I know. But plenty of mamas and midwives actually recommend the practice. Peel one clove of garlic (gently removing the paper-like film) and slide it directly into the vagina before going to bed, then remove it in the morning.

Probiotics
The presence of good bacteria keeps yeast in check, so probiotics have long been used to restore balance to the vagina. You can incorporate more organic, whole-fat yogurt or kefir into your diet, or talk to your midwife or doctor about taking an acidophilus supplement. You'll also want to limit the amount of sugar you're eating even more than usual. Yeast feeds on sugar, and some studies suggest a relationship between high blood sugar and recurrent yeast infections.

a bit during sex. (Again, not by the penis, but by the overall rocking motion.) She may feel a slight squeeze when the uterus contracts during orgasm. And just as climax gives you a rush of adrenaline and endorphins, there's evidence to suggest that baby may feel a rush of feel-good hormones after sex, too.

It's important to point out, however, that baby doesn't *understand* any of this, nor can she see what's going on in there. (She won't even open her eyes until the third trimester, and she'd be staring at a giant wall, anyway: the cervix.)

MYTH #4: SEX CAN CAUSE PREMATURE LABOR

Sex actually may be one of the best (natural) ways to induce labor, partly because semen contains prostaglandin, a hormonelike substance that softens or "ripens" the cervix. (Synthetic forms of prostaglandin like Cervidil are sometimes used when mama is overdue and the cervix fails to efface on its own.) No amount of sex, however, will trigger cervical *dilation*. Likewise, uterine cramping that occurs during orgasm is nowhere near strong enough to expel the baby. As long as you're not at risk for preterm labor, making love will not trigger a premature birth.

SEX FOR THE WIN!

Sex during pregnancy isn't just *safe* for most mamas, it comes with a host of beneficial side effects: It's a form of exercise, for one thing, as well as a great way to relieve stress (it lowers your blood pressure, too!). Regular sex may actually lead to an easier labor and quicker

WHAT OTHER *natural mamas* SAY

stephanie: Sex in the second trimester was golden. The third trimester took some creativity—and some laughing!—for sure.

chelsea: Sex? What is that? I had zero sex drive during my first two pregnancies. I'm really hoping that changes with my third!

jennifer: As I got bigger, sex became less regular, but neither of us minded. We were just too excited to meet our little man!!

Kombucha

Can you believe we're already halfway to the big day?! If you haven't already, take a moment to relish this 20-week milestone. In fact, let's celebrate with a toast and a bit of bubbly! No, not Champagne. I'm talking about a different kind of fizzy drink: kombucha.

Made by fermenting sweetened black tea with a culture of bacteria and yeast, kombucha does contain trace amounts of alcohol, but it's generally considered safe to drink during pregnancy, if you've tried it before with no adverse reactions. Stick to small amounts: no more than 8 ounces a day, in divided doses. As for the benefits, there are plenty: kombucha is rich in polyphenols, electrolytes, enzymes, and probiotics. Some mamas swear by it to ease morning sickness (especially when it's ginger-flavored).

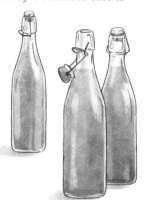

Not feeling kombucha? Try a Mama-mosa instead (equal parts fresh-squeezed orange juice and sparkling water) or a Tart Cherry Bomb (page 195). Just make sure to serve your mocktail in a wineglass—we're celebrating!

JUST FOR DADS:
HOW SEX CHANGES DURING PREGNANCY

With so much focus on the changes in mama's mind and body, it's easy to forget that husbands and partners go through a fair amount of change during a pregnancy, too. For one thing, she's not the only one whose hormones are going wild—papas experience a drop in testosterone when their partners are expecting, and that can lead to a slew of side effects. (You've heard of sympathy weight gain, right?) When it comes to sex, a plummeting libido or a sex drive that's through the roof is just as common for men as it is for women. And plenty of expectant fathers have the same fears and concerns about hurting the baby during intercourse that expectant mothers do. That's why communication during this time is so important.

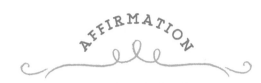

I cherish my partner. Our baby is an expression of the love and the union we share. Together, we are bringing a new life into the world.

recovery, since orgasms are like mini-workouts for the pelvic floor muscles. Getting it on may even boost your immunity. According to a study from Wilkes University in Pennsylvania, sex increases levels of an antibody called immunoglobulin A, which protects against the common cold.

That said, getting it on will get more difficult and even **comical** as your belly gets larger.

By the middle of the second trimester, for example, missionary sex is no longer comfortable for most women. The woman-on-top or "cowgirl" position can be a great alternative since it doesn't put any pressure on the stomach, but for some women it can feel a little . . . unwieldy. You'll likely need to experiment to discover positions that suit you both—you may even find that a bit of creativity in the bedroom adds a whole new level of spice to your usual routine. If you're feeling stumped, however, try these:

SPOONING

Lying side-by-side (you in front, your partner in back) keeps you off your back without having to hold up the weight of your belly. Try bending and lifting the knee of your top leg for easier, ahem, *access*—supporting that knee with a pillow can make this position even more comfortable.

EDGE OF THE BED

Scoot your rump all the way to the edge of the bed and wedge a pillow under your left side (to reduce any pressure on the vena cava). Depending on the height of the bed, your partner can stand or kneel, holding on to your legs for balance and leverage.

LOVE ON ALL FOURS (A.K.A. DOGGY-STYLE)

It may not seem like an obvious choice, but a rear-entry position precludes your partner from having to navigate around your growing baby bump. Try climbing onto the bed, resting on your elbows and knees, and supporting your stomach with a pile of pillows, or standing with both feet flat on the floor and lowering your upper body down onto the mattress.

CUDDLING FACE-TO-FACE

It's important to remember that sexual intimacy doesn't have to culminate in penetration. If intercourse is uncomfortable or you've been advised to abstain, look for other ways to satisfy one another. Lots of caressing and touching should be encouraged—and not just in the obvious places! Sensual massage, oral sex, mutual masturbation, and plain ol' skin-to-skin contact are all great ways to increase closeness and intimacy.

IS IT A YEAST INFECTION . . . OR A UTI?

TIPS FROM NURSE/DOULA *maura*

Not to be confused with yeast infections (which are caused by an overgrowth of yeast), urinary tract infections (UTIs) are caused by bacteria having worked its way into the urinary tract. Infections are most common in the bladder, but they can strike anywhere from the kidneys to the ureters (which connect the kidneys to the bladder) to the urethra (through which urine travels on its way out of the body). UTIs and yeast infections are not directly related, but they do share many of the same symptoms, including discomfort during urination. Dark or cloudy urine, a near-constant need to pee (even if you can't squeeze out more than a drop or two), abdominal pain, and low-grade fever are also hallmarks of a UTI. Chills and vomiting, meanwhile, could indicate that an infection has progressed to the kidneys.

While men can (and do) get UTIs, they're considerably more common among women, in part because our urethra is shorter and bacteria can migrate to the bladder more easily.

One thing is certain: You don't want to leave UTIs untreated. The infection can proceed to the kidneys, and in extreme cases, this can lead to permanent organ damage or even sepsis. Untreated UTIs can also trigger lower birth weight and premature labor.

Antibiotics are the most common form of treatment, and are generally considered safe for use during pregnancy. It's understandable, however, that natural mamas are hesitant about taking them.

To treat a minor infection (one that you've caught very early, that does not involve fever, vomiting, or localized pain in the abdomen, and that has not proceeded to the kidneys), you may want to ask your midwife or doctor about D-mannose. You've probably heard that cranberry juice is an effective treatment for UTIs. While that's partially true (cranberries contain a natural compound that may prevent certain types of bacteria from sticking to the walls of the bladder), the research is shaky. Studies indicate that you'd have to drink lots *and lots* of cranberry juice to get an effective dose of D-mannose (the "active ingredient" in cranberries). D-mannose supplements, however, are far more potent, and initial studies suggest that they're an effective form of both treatment and prevention. Just keep in mind that D-mannose may not be effective against *all* forms of bacteria. Regardless of how you treat the UTI, you'll also want to replenish the amount of good bacteria in your system. (Antibiotics, in particular, can sometimes kill off too much good bacteria, triggering a yeast infection.)

When it comes to preventing UTIs, make sure you're practicing excellent hygiene (always wipe front to back), staying well hydrated, urinating whenever you feel the urge (don't hold it in!), and reducing your sugar intake. You should also *always* urinate after sex—this helps flush any bacteria away from the urinary tract.

WHAT ABOUT SEX *AFTER* BABY?

In the immediate days and weeks postpartum, you likely won't be thinking much about sex at all—your primary concerns will revolve around sleep (like, the fact that you aren't getting any), learning to care for your newborn, visiting with friends or family members, and sleep (did I mention this?). Eventually, however, you'll be ready to resume being intimate with your partner. So, when *can* you expect to get frisky?

Most midwives and doctors will suggest abstaining for anywhere from four to six weeks after birth. The wait period is for obvious reasons: whether you had a vaginal or Cesarean delivery, your body needs time to recover. It takes a while for your cervix to close and your uterine lining (where the placenta was attached) to heal. The slowing and eventual end of the lochia—the bleeding and discharge that occurs in the weeks after birth—signals that this healing is nearing its end. If you didn't have any tearing and the lochia has ceased before six weeks, you may be given an early go-ahead to resume intercourse. If you did have bad tearing or an episiotomy, or if

you're still bleeding, however, you'll likely be advised to wait until your six-week postpartum appointment at minimum, to confirm that any lacerations have properly healed.

But no matter when you get the green light, keep in mind that many women aren't ready for sex right away. It's completely normal if you don't feel ready for intimacy yet. The stress and exhaustion that come with a new baby, coupled with the constant breastfeeding, can plummet your libido. Some mamas just need to feel like their body is their own for a while. Communicate with your partner about how you're feeling, and try meeting each other's needs in other ways for a few more weeks.

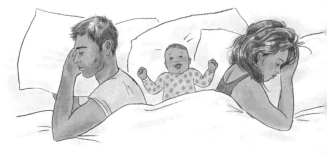

mama-do list

- Sex is a natural part of life, as well as a healthy expression of love and intimacy—so there's no reason to feel weird or guilty about wanting to tackle your partner and go to town. You won't hurt the baby and you won't "scar him for life," either. In fact, plenty of pregnant women report that orgasms seem to have a calming effect on babies in utero.

- Carve out some time to connect with your partner, even if you're not making love. Cuddling, touching, kissing, and caressing are all great ways to increase your intimacy.

get schooled

WHAT'S UP WITH *baby*?

So, it's kind of a quiet week here in utero. All of baby's major organs and systems have formed now, though they will of course continue to grow and mature. His bone marrow has begun producing blood cells (taking over that job from the liver and spleen). And while the placenta is meeting most of his nutritional needs, he's also getting a small caloric boost from the amniotic fluid. He's started to swallow it, you see, which will help with the formation of his lungs and the further development of his kidneys and digestive system. I mentioned before that baby pees directly into the amniotic sac, too—so, yes, he is essentially drinking his own urine. Gross as that sounds, however, his pee is mostly just water; the placenta (rather than his kidneys) filters out most of the waste. Whew!

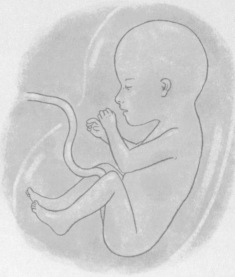

ALL OF BABY'S MAJOR ORGANS AND SYSTEMS HAVE FORMED NOW.

WHAT'S UP WITH *mama*?

Last week it was your innie turning into an outie. This week your belly has produced a new development: stripes. Okay, *one* stripe—but have you noticed a thin, dark-brown line running right up the center of your stomach? That's the *linea nigra*—Latin for "black line." It's completely normal and totally temporary; 75 percent of mamas, in fact, will experience this common pregnancy side effect. But what if I told you that you've *always* had a line there, only it's usually called the linea *alba* (white line)? Sure, you probably haven't noticed it before, but it's there—a fibrous line of cartilage separating the right and left abdominals. It's actually the same vertical line or ridge you might see running down the center of a well-defined six-pack. Hormonal surges are responsible for the color change, but the linea nigra may not be the only type of hyperpigmentation showing up on your body right about now. Little blotches of dark skin on your face (known as chloasma, melasma, or the "mask of pregnancy") are common, too. We'll talk more about skin issues, including chloasma, in Week 24.

Nine Months is an old '90s movie starring Julianne Moore (as a woman coping with an unplanned pregnancy) and Hugh Grant (the reluctant papa-to-be) that culminates in what might be the most delightfully ridiculous birth scene in all of cinema. I won't give away too much here, except to say that Robin Williams steals the show as Dr. Kosevich. This nervous Russian obstetrician confuses "epidural" with "enema" and is forced to deliver two babies simultaneously. It's outrageous and over-the-top—at one point, smelling salts are required to revive not only the dad but also the *doctor*. It's oddly charming.

It is not, however, a realistic depiction of childbirth.

Unfortunately, the bulk of what most women "know" about having babies seems to come from Hollywood, and the movies *always* feature a screaming, hysterical woman, usually in stirrups attached to a cold metal table. Don't believe me?

In *Knocked Up*, a nurse asks a mid-delivery Katherine Heigl to quiet down because her outrageous, ear-piercing, profanity-laced screams might "scare the other pregnant women."

In *The Back-up Plan*, Jennifer Lopez attends a home water birth so cringe-worthy she passes out from shock and falls in the birthing tub.

Let me tell ya, birth does not have to be like this. Birth *shouldn't* be like this—and if your doctor offers you an enema for pain relief, *run*. So, here's a better way to prepare for the big day: dust off your Trapper Keeper, sharpen your No. 2 pencils, and enroll in a natural birth course.

WHY A BIRTH COURSE?

I wouldn't blame you if taking childbirth classes seems like overkill. I mean, you're reading this book! How much information does one mama need?! Interactive classes, however, offer you experiential knowledge that you just can't get from a book, including:

♡ A deeper understanding of the physiological changes your body will go through, as well as a sense for the rhythm of labor.

♡ The ability to ask questions and talk about your fears with the instructor, as well as with other couples.

♡ The opportunity for partners to get informed and empowered, so they can better support you.

♡ The chance to bond with other natural mamas, who may become lifelong friends.

The more you understand the physiology of birth, the less fearful you'll be heading into the big day.

If you're planning a home birth, know that childbirth education courses are generally a *prerequisite* for both doctors and midwives.

One word of warning, though: if possible, sign up for a birth course that takes place *outside of the hospital*. While in-hospital classes can certainly be informative, many of them teach mama how to be a good *patient* (rather than her own advocate). They also tend to be short in duration, and few provide much education or encouragement in terms of unmedicated birth and long-term breastfeeding.

WHICH NATURAL BIRTH COURSE IS RIGHT FOR YOU?

Luckily, there are *many* natural birth courses out there, each with its own philosophy, time commitment, and fees. You'll want to find the one that best fits you—your personality, your birth goals, and your learning style. In addition to in-person classes, many methods offer online courses, home study kits, or a corresponding book on which the classes are based. Keep in mind, too, that the quality of classes can vary based on the skills of the instructor(s), so don't hesitate to shop around.

LAMAZE INTERNATIONAL

It's the oldest and best-known "natural" birth course out there: Lamaze is famous, in fact, for its style of coached breathing. Incidentally, that "hee hee, hoo hoo" breath pattern generated some controversy back in the '70s and '80s, since it apparently caused some women to hyperventilate (a big no-no in birthing). In recent years, however, Lamaze has modified and modernized its technique. Beyond breath work, classes focus on preparing expectant mamas for birth via a six-step approach to labor and delivery. Classes also provide information on the pros and cons of *all* birth choices so that parents can make informed decisions. Some women, however, have criticized the program for being too intervention-friendly.

Class duration: Roughly 12 hours of instruction, which may be divided into 6 two-hour classes or a weekend-long crash course.

Cost: Varies by location. The national average is $110.

Pros: Affordable.

Cons: Dated, possibly not enough emphasis on *natural* birth.

PFFT! I'M A SECOND-TIME MAMA—
I DON'T NEED TO TAKE A CLASS

It's common for second- (or third- or fifth-) time mamas to think they don't need a childbirth education course. They likely took one before their first birth, and more to the point, they've *already* experienced labor, so what's there to learn? A lot, actually. No two births are alike. You might not have experienced stalled labor the first time around, for example, but could during your second birth. Taking a course is also a great refresher, since it's probably been a few years since you pushed out a baby. I was pleasantly surprised to discover that more than 40 percent of the mamas enrolled in the Mama Natural Birth Course are already moms. Turns out, many of them had a challenging first birth and want to do things differently the second time around.

Coconut Chocolate Fudge

Have you been batting away chocolate cravings because you're worried it's not good for the baby? Stop! In fact, *indulge*. Researchers in Finland found that mamas who regularly ate chocolate during pregnancy had happier, livelier infants. Perhaps that's because chocolate contains phenylethylamine, which triggers the release of endorphins? Or perhaps it's just that mamas who are whacked out in chocolate bliss *perceive* their babies as being happier? Either way, you now have scientific proof that a bit of the sweet stuff is a good thing. (You're welcome, by the way.)

For an antioxidant boost, make sure you're selecting organic, fair-trade chocolate with a high cacao content (preferably over 70 percent) because you're not going to get much benefit from eating, say, a Snickers bar. Or try this delicious Coconut Fudge—it's made with antioxidant-rich dark chocolate and coconut oil, which is rich in nourishing fats. Just try not to eat the whole *pan*, as chocolate does contain caffeine. Remember, everything in moderation.

INGREDIENTS

One 14-ounce can whole-fat coconut milk

¼ cup honey

1 ½ cups dark chocolate chips (I like the ones from Enjoy Life)

2 tablespoons coconut oil

½ cup coconut flakes

In a medium-sized saucepan, empty the entire can of coconut milk. Bring to a boil, then reduce heat to medium-low. Stir in honey and mix well. Let the mixture reduce by half, stirring occasionally. (This will take about 20 to 30 minutes.) Over low heat, add the chocolate chips and coconut oil. Once completely melted, add in coconut flakes and mix well. Pour the fudge into a medium-sized baking pan, cover, and store in the fridge until completely hardened. Cut into small squares and enjoy. Makes 16 to 24 servings.

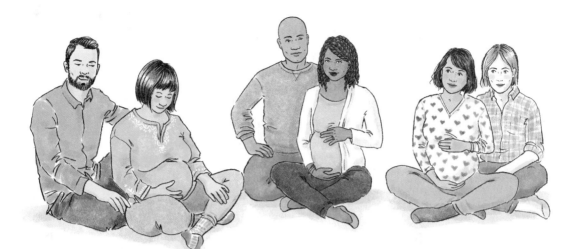

THE BRADLEY METHOD

Based on Dr. Robert A. Bradley's *Husband-Coached Childbirth* (published in 1965), Bradley birth courses focus entirely on having a nonmedicated delivery, though topics like exercise, postpartum care, and prenatal nutrition are covered, too. Speaking of nutrition, the Bradley Method supports the Brewer Diet, so prepare to hear a lot about the benefits of eating 100 grams of protein a day. Dr. Bradley also emphasized the role of the father as birth coach, rather than a doula. Some couples may appreciate this; others may find it outdated and too traditional.

Class duration: 12 two-hour classes taught over a three-month period.

Cost: $200 to $500.

Pros: Natural-minded, evidence-based.

Cons: Old-fashioned and *long*.

HYPNOBIRTHING INTERNATIONAL (A.K.A. THE MONGAN METHOD)

Instead of trying to "manage" pain, Hypno-Birthing teaches mamas how to avoid a fear-tension-pain cycle using self-hypnosis. The philosophy here is that childbirth could and even *should* be comfortable. But does it work? Maybe. A three-year study by Britain's National Institute for Health Research found that self-hypnosis made little difference in the number of women who ultimately requested pain relief during labor, but that it *did* alleviate fear of childbirth.

Class duration: Five two-and-a-half-hour classes (not including "practice" time).

Cost: $200 to $400, depending on location.

Pros: May help women alleviate fear of childbirth.

Cons: Hypnosis doesn't appeal to everyone, and has only been proven to be moderately effective.

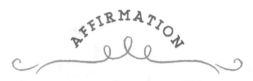
I am prepared and confident.
My baby and I work together as a team.
My body has everything it needs to birth my baby.

HYPNOBABIES

Hypno*Birthing* places an emphasis on guided relaxation and visualization. Hypno*babies*, on the other hand, focuses on hard-core "hypno-anesthesia" (which is sometimes offered in medical settings to patients who are allergic to pain meds). Classes also include general childbirth info, which is perhaps why some mamas find it to be more comprehensive. Then again, some consider Hypnobabies a little too "new age."

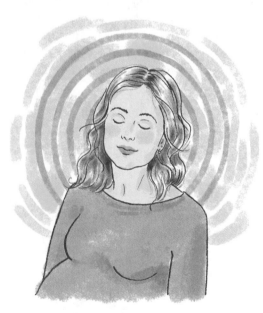

Class duration: Six weeks of three-hour classes (not including "practice" time).

Cost: $200 to $500 for in-person classes.

Pros: May be more comprehensive than Hypno-Birthing.

Cons: Again, hypnosis doesn't appeal to everyone, and has only been proven to be moderately effective.

BIRTHING FROM WITHIN

The emphasis here is that birth is a time for self-discovery, and classes are adapted to the individual needs of the woman or couple. By incorporating journaling, artwork, and other creative outlets of expression, Birthing from Within hopes to minimize emotional difficulty. This is probably the most crunchy or "hippie" of the birthing courses and is likely best for creative, free-spirited types.

Class duration: Five to six weeks of two- to three-hour classes, or a weekend intensive.

Cost: $200 to $400.

Pros: Individualized, naturally minded approach.

Cons: Available only in select markets, might be a little too "out there" for some mamas.

MAMA NATURAL BIRTH COURSE

Hosted by yours truly and doula Maura, RN, this eight-part, on-demand course is designed to educate, empower, and inspire both mamas and papas/partners to deliver naturally. (I was motivated by my own childbirth education experience to create the course. After a long day at work, I dreaded driving across town and then having to sit and listen for three hours!) Classes take you through the entire process of preparing for and experiencing childbirth. We also include modules on the first few weeks postpartum (including an entire class devoted to breastfeeding), as well as bonus segments on nutrition, natural remedies for common pregnancy complaints, and weekly practice sessions. We even have a Dudes Discuss section for dads. Mama Natural Birth Course students come together in private Facebook groups to foster a sense of community. Ten percent of proceeds are donated to nonprofits around the globe that support maternal and infant health and well-being.

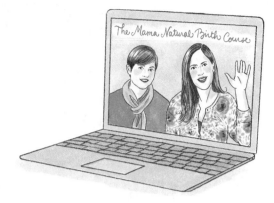

Class duration: Ten hours of content divided into 8 classes.

Cost: Starting around $275.

Pros: Online and on-demand, so you can go at your own pace, based on *your* schedule. Access to a supportive community and tons of resources. Money-back guarantee to ensure that every mama is satisfied.

Cons: Online only, which might be a drawback for some mamas.

mama-do list

- Many—though certainly not all—birth courses aim to include the partner, so make sure they're on-board. This is also a great time to consider what kind of support you'll want in the delivery room: Are you an all-hands-on-deck woman? Or a touch-me-and-I'll-kill-you kind of gal? If you're a single mama, on the other hand, you don't have to take classes alone if you don't want to. Consider asking a pregnancy pal—your mom, a close friend, or a family member—to tag along.

- True, I'm a little biased toward the Mama Natural Birth Course. But if you're deciding which childbirth education course is right for you, be sure to check out some of the videos at mamanaturalbirth.com.

high-risk pregnancies

WHAT'S UP WITH *baby*?

Each week baby's features grow cuter and cuter—and Week 22 is no exception! Her nose, lips, and eyes are more pronounced now. She's got eyelashes and eyebrows, a smattering of hair on her head and, of course, that fine coating of lanugo. But for a while yet, she'll also be pale as a ghost—there is no pigment in that hair (not even the hair on her head); it's pure white. There's no pigment in the iris, the colored part of her eye, either. Why? In utero babies don't produce a lot of melanin, the naturally occurring pigment responsible for the eventual color of our hair, eyes, and skin. So when she's born, she'll likely have light blue or steel-gray eyes, even if she's African American or Asian. Expect that to change, however. Eye color isn't really "set" until age one or two. And lots of genes contribute to eye color, so it's possible that two brown-eyed parents could have a blue- or green-eyed child. In fact, I know of a few!

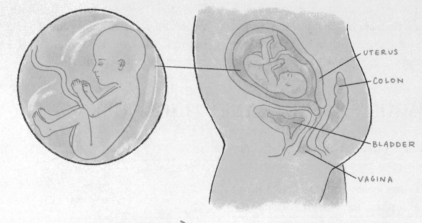

WHAT'S UP WITH *mama*?

At 22 weeks, your growing belly may soon begin to interfere with your day-to-day life, from the way you sit to the way you put on your shoes (forget fussy lace-ups!), even to the way you drive. There's no definitive cutoff for driving while pregnant, by the way—you can drive as long as you want, provided you can fit behind the wheel. Pregnant mamas, however, tend to be more tired than usual, not to mention cranked up on hormones, so be aware of how you're feeling before you back out of the driveway. And, yes, wearing a seatbelt can become increasingly cumbersome, but always wear one for the safety of you and your child. The lap belt should fit under your stomach and over your hips—not across the belly. The shoulder strap, meanwhile, should rest between your breasts and off to the side of your stomach.

As soon as my husband and I got married, lots of people—and by "people" I mean *my mother*—started hounding us about when we'd settle down and start having some kids. Of course, feeling pressure to board the baby train is common for many new brides, but in my case I figured there was a particular concern at play: my age. By the time I walked down the aisle, I was already in my thirties. (Ironic, though, that my mother was so impatient, since *she* wasn't born until her mother, my grandmother, turned forty!)

Women these days are bombarded with messages about how difficult it can be to get pregnant, or how complicated a pregnancy may be, when they are of "advanced maternal age." This term sounds positively *geriatric* even though it starts at thirty-five, which is exactly how old I was when I had Griffin. Despite eating a real food diet, having a clean bill of health, and living an active lifestyle, I was apparently so old that my pregnancy was classified as "high-risk."

It's important to point out, however, that the medical community classifies a *lot* of pregnancies this way. The label is in no way a guarantee that something will go wrong, only an indication that you *might* develop a complication. The vast majority of pregnancies—even the "risky" ones—turn out just fine. Mine did, even though I had my second baby at thirty-eight. (The horror!) High-risk mamas are more likely to receive interventions, though, so this week's all about upping your chances for a natural birth even if you fall into the high-risk category. You daredevil, you.

WHAT MAKES A PREGNANCY "HIGH-RISK"?

While not exactly a scientific term, pregnancy can be classified as high-risk because of:

Your Age. Having a baby past the age of thirty-five isn't a new phenomenon. I mentioned already that my grandmother had my mother at forty, and that wasn't even her last baby—she had one more, her seventh, two months before she turned forty-three. My paternal grandmother had her last child at forty-one. Michael's grandma had a baby at thirty-nine. And it wasn't just our families; it happened often enough that doctors had a (mildly offensive, not to mention inaccurate) name for children born to "older" women: menopause babies. Waiting longer to start a family these days, however, is much more common. The number of women having their first child between the ages of thirty-five and thirty-nine has risen steadily since 1970. Meanwhile,

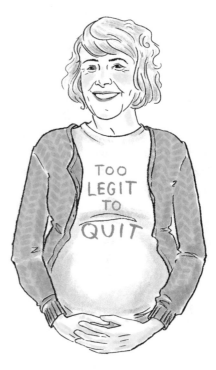

the number of women having their first baby between forty and forty-four has more than doubled since 1990. Could all of these pregnancies really be high-risk?

Eh, probably not. Turns out the idea that women over thirty-five face an uphill battle to even *get* pregnant is based on a study of French birth records from 1670 through the early 1800s. Not exactly what I'd call a recent finding. Here's a truer picture of fertility: of women trying to get pregnant, 82 percent between thirty-five and thirty-nine will conceive within a year, compared to 86 percent of women between twenty-seven and thirty-four, according to a study published in *Obstetrics & Gynecology*. Meanwhile, the chances of having a baby with Down syndrome or a spontaneous miscarriage *do* rise with age, as do the risks of preeclampsia, gestational diabetes, and protracted labor. A study from Washington University in St. Louis, however, found that women over thirty-five actually have a lower chance of having a baby with a major *congenital* defect—40 percent lower, in fact.

WHEN SHOULD YOU SEE A SPECIALIST?

There are any number of reasons a mama may want to see a specialist. A diabetic, for example, may see her midwife or ob-gyn *and* an endocrinologist. A woman with a heart condition may have a cardiologist added to her birth team. An obese woman may want to consult with a registered dietitian. It's likely that *all* of these women, however, would be transferred to a maternal-fetal medicine (MFM) specialist—also called a perinatologist— which is an ob-gyn who's had at least three additional years of training in the assessment and management of high-risk pregnancies.

Exactly how an MFM specialist will work with you varies from case to case. In some instances, you may have only one appointment with the specialist before returning to your regular doctor. (Sometimes ob-gyns and midwives order a consultation to lessen their liability or for insurance purposes.) In other situations, you'll *only* be seen by the specialist and he or she will deliver your baby. No matter what circumstances bumped you to the high-risk category, however, you always have a choice about whom you'll receive treatment from, and it is completely appropriate to "shop around" for an MFM doctor. You'll want to ask the same types of questions you had when choosing your midwife or ob-gyn, such as insurance coverage, pain management, and labor induction. A good specialist will *always* work in close concert with the members of your birth team to ensure that your care is comprehensive and that nothing "falls through the cracks." So ask how—and how often—he or she intends to collaborate with your regular doctor. Just because you've been classified as high-risk doesn't mean you should stop being your own advocate. A doula can provide a wealth of information and support, too—they're not just for low-risk mamas!

There may be other benefits to "advanced maternal age," too: older mamas tend to be better educated and more financially stable, and have a strong sense of emotional readiness for motherhood.

A study by the Boston University School of Medicine found that women who had their last child later in life (without the aid of fertility treatments) tend to live longer than women who were finished having babies by twenty-nine.

Okay, fine. That last one is probably more correlation than causation; it's not like delaying pregnancy is going to add years to your life. But as research is making increasingly clear,

the idea that older mamas-to-be are delicate flowers is largely myth. If your age is the only reason you've been elevated to "high-risk" status, you can go ahead and breathe a sigh of relief. Taken by itself, it's the least risky of all the high-risk categories.

Your Medical History. At your first prenatal checkup, your healthcare provider likely took a fairly detailed look at your medical history, and for good reason. Chronic conditions like diabetes, heart disease, obesity, epilepsy, autoimmune disorders, or high blood pressure can make a routine pregnancy innately more complicated. How *much* more complicated, of course, can only be determined on a case-by-case basis. Mamas who have diabetes, for

WHAT OTHER *natural mamas* SAY

jana: My pregnancy became high-risk at 35 weeks when I was diagnosed with polyhydramnios (excess amniotic fluid). I was referred to a doctor who recommended induction by 38 weeks due to an increased risk of cord prolapse, but I researched the risks, found a new doctor, and went on to have a natural hospital delivery at 42 weeks!

cassandra: After one of my children was born with heart disease, I had a higher-than-average risk of having another child with the same issue, so my midwife and I agreed that a hospital was the safest place for me to deliver. However, my wishes for a natural birth were respected to the fullest, and I was able to deliver with no interventions!

alexandria: I was diagnosed with gestational hypertension during each of my two pregnancies. With my first, it progressed to preeclampsia, and I risked out of the midwife suite in the hospital, which was disappointing. I felt really pleased with our choice of hospital, though. Everyone was extremely patient and seemed willing to work toward a vaginal delivery. I opted for an epidural, although there was absolutely no pressure to have one (after laboring for 14 hours, with an eventual Cesarean still a possibility, I decided the best plan was to get some pain relief and rest before seeing it through). And everything worked out just as I'd hoped, with a normal, vaginal birth!

example, may be able to mitigate some of that risk by tweaking their diet, keeping their blood sugar tightly controlled, and getting some extra exercise. In any event, your pregnancy will be monitored more closely than a low-risk mama's.

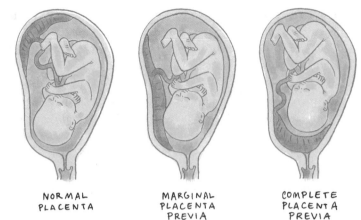

NORMAL PLACENTA

MARGINAL PLACENTA PREVIA

COMPLETE PLACENTA PREVIA

The Progression of Your Pregnancy. Older mamas, as well as mamas who are in poor health or who have a chronic medical condition, are at an increased risk for developing a pregnancy-related complication—gestational diabetes and preeclampsia are the big two, though there are certainly others. But even young mamas who started out with a clean bill of health can get bumped to the high-risk category, too. While many of these complications can be easily treated or even reversed with proper care, they all have the potential to become *very* serious, which is why close observation by your midwife or doctor is so important in these cases.

The Position of Your Placenta. During pregnancy, the placenta—that all-important organ providing nutrition to your baby—doesn't remain stationary. Early in the first trimester, it's likely positioned low in the womb, but as your uterus stretches and grows it will relo-

cate nearer the top in time for delivery. In some cases, however, the placenta does not relocate as it should and may cover part or all of the cervix. And that's a problem. Placenta previa, as the condition is called, can cause severe bleeding during labor as well as trigger early-onset labor. Depending on the severity, a Cesarean may be mandatory, which is why your sonographer will check out the placenta during your anatomy ultrasound.

Keep in mind, however, that being diagnosed with placenta previa at mid-pregnancy does *not* mean you are destined to have a C-section. In a 1990 study published in the medical journal *Lancet*, of the 250 women who were diagnosed between 16 and 20 weeks, only four actually had the condition at birth. In other words, there's a very high probability that your placenta will relocate by the third trimester. Women are typically offered a second ultrasound nearer delivery, so don't fret about this now.

The Number of Babies You Are Carrying. Although it's perhaps not surprising, the risks associated with pregnancy and childbirth go up significantly when you're carrying more than one baby at a time. Preterm labor and low birth weight are the most common concerns—

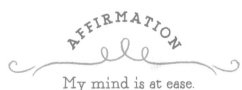

AFFIRMATION

My mind is at ease. I walk into birth with calm confidence, knowing I can handle whatever comes my way.

almost 60 percent of twins are delivered preterm, whereas 90 percent of triplets come early. Multiples pregnancies are also associated with higher rates of preeclampsia, gestational diabetes, and placental health problems. The type of multiples you're having makes quite a bit of difference, too. For example:

Monoamniotic twins—also called Mono-Mono twins—are identical twins that share the same amniotic sac and the same placenta (each baby, however, has his own umbilical cord). Of all multiples pregnancies, these are the most rare and the most risky, largely due to concerns about cord entanglement and the possibility of something called twin-to-twin transfusion syndrome (TTTS), where one baby

receives more nourishment than the other. Monoamniotic triplets or quads are possible, too, but are *extremely* rare.

Monochorionic-Diamniotic, or Mono-Di twins are identical twins that share the same placenta but each grow inside his or her own amniotic sac; TTTS is a possible concern in Mo-Di pregnancies, too.

Dichorionic diamniotic (Di-Di) twins may be either identical (two babies that came from the same egg) or fraternal (two separate eggs), but they each have their own amniotic sac and their own placenta. Di-Di twins are the least risky of all multiples pregnancies.

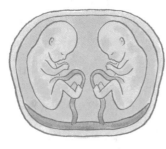

MONOAMNIOTIC
TWINS

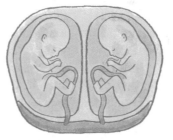

MONOCHORIONIC-DIAMNIOTIC
TWINS

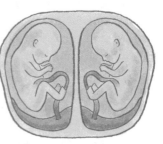

DICHORIONIC-DIAMNIOTIC
TWINS

OKAY, I'M HIGH-RISK. NOW WHAT?

Since there's no clear definition of high-risk pregnancy, circumstances (and treatment) will vary largely from mama to mama. A woman with epilepsy who's expecting Mono-Mono twins and has been diagnosed with preeclampsia, for example, would be considered higher risk than a woman with mild gestational diabetes, who may be able to treat the condition through careful monitoring of her diet. All high-risk mamas, however, can expect to be monitored more closely than low-risk women, so

expect more frequent prenatal appointments. High-risk mamas are also significantly more likely to receive interventions during birth.

In some cases, these interventions aren't just necessary; they're potentially lifesaving.

This is one of those times when we can marvel at the wonders of modern medicine—how lucky we are to live in this day and age! Sometimes, however, such interventions are not necessary. For reasons that aren't entirely

TIPS FOR HIGH-RISK MAMAS
FROM MIDWIFE *Cynthia*

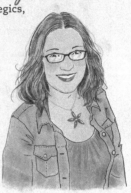

Over the years, I've attended women giving birth who are quadriplegics, cancer survivors, severe preeclamptics, women with elevated BMIs, diabetics, and users of illicit drugs, both as a labor and delivery nurse and a nurse-midwife. And what I've learned is that the definition of "high-risk" is not black and white; high-risk pregnancies fall on a *spectrum*. Some high-risk conditions are appropriately managed only by a physician—in Illinois, where I work, I'm required by law to have a collaborative agreement with a medical doctor. That agreement states, clearly and specifically, the conditions that are appropriate for midwifery management, conditions that are appropriate for co-management, and conditions that would opt a patient out of midwifery care completely. In my experience, however, the majority of patients who arrive at our office with concerns that they're "too high-risk" for midwifery care find that we're still able to participate in some aspects of their birth, whether that's attending a Cesarean delivery to facilitate skin-to-skin bonding and initiate breastfeeding, or to help the patient understand more fully the risks and benefits of (and alternatives to) birth interventions. Providing prenatal care for a high-risk mama is a team effort, but our goal as midwives is to infuse as much of our holistic philosophy into childbirth as possible.

clear, for example, the likelihood of delivering via C-section increases significantly with age, even when mama has no other risk factors and developed zero complications during pregnancy.

Your ability to have a natural birth will, of course, depend on the specific circumstances of your pregnancy, but your chances will increase dramatically based on the type of care you receive from here on out. If you've been told that you're high-risk, make sure to:

Talk with Your Midwife or Doctor. Get clear on exactly why your healthcare provider bumped you to the high-risk category and what you can expect going forward. If you've been referred to a maternal-fetal medicine specialist, ask how

your doctor expects to collaborate with him or her over the long haul. If you haven't been referred to a specialist, ask if you should consider adding another doctor to your birth team. Discuss what kind of testing might be offered from here on out, too. Very high-risk mamas may be offered a slew of ultrasounds. Ask what the sonographer would be looking for specifically during these types of scans. (For example, is baby being monitored for a possible birth defect, or are there concerns that baby may be under stress due to a pregnancy-related complication?) When it comes to amniocentesis or CVS, know that these types of tests diagnose genetic conditions and developmental abnormalities, so you may choose to opt out of this

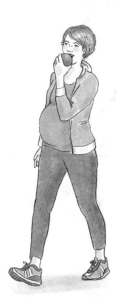

testing, even if you are high-risk. Get all the information you can so that you can make informed decisions about your health and your birth.

Pursue a Healthy Lifestyle. I can't stress this enough: the food you eat and the exercise you get (assuming you've been given the green light to work out) matters more than ever for high-risk mamas. Taking care of yourself can also *prevent* complications from appearing in the first place. You'll want to be diligent about taking your prenatal vitamins, steer clear of harmful substances (including alcohol, cigarettes, and environmental toxins), and do your best to get adequate sleep.

If you've been diagnosed with gestational diabetes, you can expect to receive a specialized meal plan and be required to monitor your blood sugar daily. You may also want to consult with a registered dietitian. Eating protein and fat with each meal, choosing whole foods, and eliminating artificially sweetened beverages

NOM OF THE WEEK

Pistachio Pesto

High-risk mamas need to pay extra attention to their health, so this week we're boosting the immune system with a dose of raw garlic. It's an important ingredient in this recipe: garlic is high in vitamin B_6, vitamin C, and manganese; it may also be helpful for high blood pressure. (Take *that*, preeclampsia!)

INGREDIENTS

5 cups organic basil

½ cup Parmigiano Reggiano cheese, grated

⅓ cup pistachios (you can substitute pine nuts or walnuts if you prefer)

2 to 3 cloves garlic

⅓ cup olive oil

Sea salt (to taste)

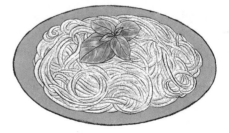

Wash and dry the basil leaves, then toss all the ingredients except the olive oil and the salt into a food processor. Pulse until blended. With the processor running, slowly drizzle in the olive oil and puree until smooth. Salt to taste, and serve over warm pasta, spaghetti squash, or zucchini "zoodles." Pesto is also delicious with eggs or spread on toast. Will keep for three to five days in the fridge, or you can freeze some in an ice cube tray. Recipe makes 4 to 6 servings.

and "juices" can also help keep your blood sugar stable.

Almost all mamas who've been diagnosed with preeclampsia, meanwhile, are advised to lower their salt intake, but speak with your doctor or midwife about the potential benefits of the Brewer Diet (see page 32). There is some (albeit conflicting and controversial) research to suggest that vitamins C and E may stave off preeclampsia, too, but stick with food-based sources, *especially* in the case of vitamin E. Excellent options (for all mamas) include sunflower seeds, almonds, spinach and dark leafy greens, avocado, butternut squash, and shellfish.

If you've developed anemia, high-quality food-based sources of iron include red meat, beef liver, and molasses (which you can use as a natural sweetener, a glaze atop roasted vegetables, or in salad dressing); vitamin C, meanwhile, can increase iron absorption from plant sources.

Identify Red Alerts. Ask your doctor or midwife to identify specific symptoms to keep an eye out for, as well as to explain what symptoms might indicate a need for emergency care. Vaginal bleeding late in the third trimester, for example, can sometimes be a sign of placenta previa or placental abruption; severe and persistent headache, extreme swelling, and vision changes can sometimes indicate preeclampsia. Other examples include pain or cramping in the abdomen, decreased fetal activity, excessive vaginal discharge, and early contractions.

Ease Your Fears. Being told that your pregnancy is high-risk is enough to make any mama feel anxious—which, ironically, can trigger its own set of problems. Likewise, it's understandable that high-risk mamas might start to dread prenatal appointments, if for no reason other than that they're terrified of receiving (more) bad news. Mama? Fight those feelings. Address the issue head-on, and chat with your healthcare provider about ways to lessen your fears. If you're in the clear to exercise, prenatal yoga or water aerobics can boost your endorphins and relieve stress. Meditation, prayer, and visualization have *proven* benefits and will help you stay positive and serene.

mama-do list

- If you're feeling anxious or worried about being classified as "high-risk," talk to your doctor about ways to improve your mental outlook. He or she may even be able to refer you to a high-risk support group in your area.

- Many mamas who have been classified as high-risk can still have a natural birth. Sometimes, however, a natural, vaginal birth just isn't possible. That can be disappointing—devastating, even—but it is nothing to feel ashamed about. We'll talk plenty more about ways to naturalize a hospital birth or even a C-section in the coming weeks.

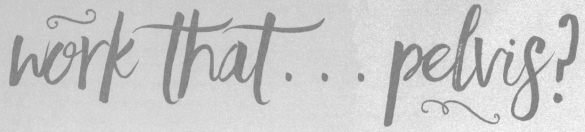

work that... pelvis?

PREPARING YOUR BODY AND BABY FOR BIRTH

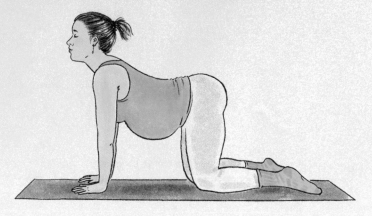

WHAT'S UP WITH *baby*?

Kicks, rolls, and punches (ouch!) will likely become more frequent as Baby Natural fights for space in your uterus. Before long, you may even see his little hands or feet poking through the skin of your belly, like something out of an alien-invasion movie. Something else he's doing in there? Walking. That is, using his feet to push off the walls of the womb. This "walking" is likely a way of preparing to breastfeed. Turns out that newborn babies—as in, babies who are only an *hour* or two old—can instinctually crawl up mama's belly, commando-style, as well as find (and latch onto) the breast all on their own. How is this possible? It's thought that

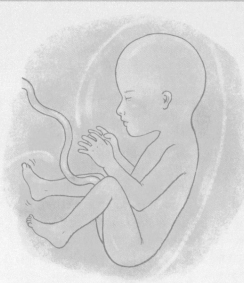

BABY NATURAL IS ON THE MOVE THIS WEEK!

infants are guided largely by smell, since the breasts and nipples smell similar to amniotic fluid. There's even a name for this breathtaking maneuver—it's called the "breast crawl," and there is some incredible footage online if you're interested in watching. Just google it!

WHAT'S UP WITH *mama*?

You've likely heard that expectant mamas shouldn't be lifting much of anything from the moment they conceive until the moment they deliver their baby. But are the warnings true? Well, yes and no. There's no evidence to suggest that lifting a heavy box or an unwieldy object is going to harm the *baby*—it's not like the stress or strain will pop your belly like a balloon!—but there's plenty of evidence to suggest that mamas-to-be are much more accident- and injury-prone than usual. Both your balance and your center of gravity have changed; meanwhile, your ligaments and tendons have relaxed (from all that—wait for it—relaxin), so the chance of tweaking something or falling down goes up during pregnancy, and there's the concern. The general consensus, then, is to reduce your "maximum lifting load" by about 25 percent—but who has any idea what her maximum lifting load is? A better idea: don't lift heavy objects if you don't have to (and that includes hefty toddlers). Luckily, when it comes to moving heavy stuff around, pregnancy is one of those magical times when partners, friends, family members—heck, even strangers!—will be more than happy to do the work for you. So let them!

When it comes to baby's positioning in utero, I was pretty much clueless during my first pregnancy. I mean, I knew that baby was supposed to come out *head first* . . . but that's about it. Then I ended up having a very long labor, which eventually stalled, in part because my son got sort of stuck underneath my pelvis. When he finally did come out, I remember just how quickly my midwife got that little newborn cap on him. His sweet little head was so cone-shaped, he looked like an alien baby!

We've all heard of breech babies, right? But did you know that there are other classifications for baby's presentation in the womb? He might be transverse, for example, meaning lying sideways in your uterus. He could be posterior, meaning facing outward looking at mama's belly (as opposed to the preferred anterior position, facing inward toward her spine). In retrospect, I know that Griffin was probably posterior and favoring my right side, which may have contributed to the problems I experienced during labor.

But is it just bad luck to have a baby who's not well positioned? Well, yes and no. You see, the trappings of modern life might contribute to the way baby situates himself in utero. After all, we:

♡ sit (usually slumped or slouched) at our desks all day,

♡ spend hours driving around in our cars, and

♡ recline in comfy loveseats and sofas at night.

These postures compress the pelvis, narrowing the passage through which baby will eventually travel on his journey to meet you. They also encourage improper alignment, which can make a natural birth not just difficult and more painful, but perhaps even impossible.

So this week we're taking a look at what you can do today to benefit your birth when the time comes.

Focusing on the proper alignment of your pelvis can encourage baby to settle (eventually) into a great position for birth. I won't pretend this topic isn't without controversy. Research on the effectiveness of prenatal exercises as they relate to baby's position in utero is largely inconclusive. But it seems logical to me (and many chiropractors, doulas, and body workers) that if your pelvis is opened, and aligned, you'll have an easier birth.

I regularly performed the following moves during my second pregnancy because I was desperate for a better delivery. You already know how that one turned out: Paloma debuted after 20 minutes of active labor. Aim

You're going about your usual routine, minding your own business, when all of a sudden it feels like you've been "zapped" or even punched in the vagina. How rude! The phenomenon is called *lightning crotch*—no joke!—and it's very real and very common. Turns out, there are quite a few nerve endings in the uterus and pelvic region, and with all the added pressure from baby, your nervous system may occasionally react by giving you a sharp shock or jab in the lower groin. (These jolts can be more frequent in mamas who've developed varicose veins in the vaginal area.) Unpleasant as this is, however, lightning crotch isn't serious, nor is it anything you need to worry about. Phew!

to incorporate the following moves into your usual workout routine:

#1: SITTING

Sure, you could argue that sitting isn't really an "exercise"—but I would have to disagree. After all, in a few months, you'll be carrying around 20-plus extra pounds in your midsection, so the way you sit can actually strengthen your core and stabilize the pelvis. The key is to resist the habit of reclining in big couches, gliders, and beds—even though kicking back in a La-Z-Boy is probably *exactly* where you'd prefer to spend the bulk of your pregnancy.

Reclining not only compresses the pelvis, it puts pressure on some major nerves and blood vessels in the back, which can cause pain during labor and deprive the baby of oxygen (not to mention leave you feeling dizzy and light-headed). Leaning backward in a chair also encourages baby to lean backward in your uterus, putting pressure on your spine. Instead, you want baby's back—the heaviest part of his little body—resting against your tummy. The best way to encourage that is to sit with your pelvis tilted slightly forward, and your hips elevated above your knees.

An exercise ball, sometimes called a birthing ball, is great for this, and an excellent substitute for a traditional office chair if you spend a lot of your day sitting in front of a computer. You'll want one firm enough and high enough that your hips stay above your knees. Another option is to sit cross-legged, which pushes your hips forward, stretches the legs, and opens up the pelvis. (I spent a lot of time sitting cross-legged with my back supported against the couch, the perfect position in which to receive a back rub!) When you really need to get comfy, try lying on your side with your upper hip leaning forward and your knee resting on a pillow. Point is, try to avoid leaning back especially as you enter your third trimester.

#2: EXERCISE

We talked a bit already about the benefits of walking for cardiovascular exercise, but putting one foot in front of the other is great for your pelvis, too. It keeps this area warm and loose, rather than locked up and tight. Try getting up and moving around every 20 or 30 minutes—

a quick bathroom break counts (which you'll do more frequently anyway once baby starts squeezing your bladder). Swimming, yoga, and stretching are excellent ways to stay limber, too.

#3: LEANING

There's an old wives' tale that a woman who spent the afternoon on her hands and knees scrubbing the floors could flip a posterior baby. Of course, I prefer using a stand-up mop, but there's a lesson here—and it doesn't require a bucket of suds or a ratty washcloth. By leaning forward—over an exercise ball, a chair,

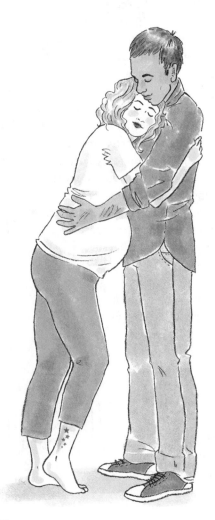

your partner, or whatever's around you—you're working with gravity to push the baby toward your belly (rather than encouraging him to fall backward and align himself with your spine).

#4: PUPPY POSE

You gotta love the name of this pose! This exercise can help encourage baby's heavy back to move toward the front of your belly (or keep your baby in an occiput anterior position). Start by getting on your hands and knees. Your knees should be in line with your hips (or wider, if needed). Walk your hands forward as your shins stay firmly planted on the ground. Press your palms into the ground while your arms stay lifted. Pull back from your shoulders for the stretch as you rest your forehead onto the floor. Keep your core engaged so that your belly doesn't drop to the floor. Stay in the pose for about 30 seconds. This position may be contraindicated for those with high blood pressure or uterine cramping so always get the okay first from your midwife or doctor.

#5: PIGEON POSE

This is an excellent position for moms struggling with lower back pain or sciatica issues. Get on your hands and knees. Slowly slide your right knee forward between your hands and straighten your left leg behind you. Rest on your right hip. For a deeper stretch, slowly bring your right foot toward your left hip and align both of your hips so that they are squared. You can lean forward and rest your arms and forehead to the floor. Stay in this pose for about 30 seconds, then switch sides.

Protein Pear Pudding

Constipation tends to come and go during pregnancy, so there's no need to be too concerned if your bowels feel a little off every now and again. But when and if you do feel, well, *stuck*, my Protein Pear Pudding is virtually guaranteed to get the party started.

INGREDIENTS

1½ cups filtered water

2 tablespoons raw honey

12 drops stevia (optional)

Cumin, cinnamon, and cloves to taste (optional)

6 ripe pears, washed and cubed (don't remove the peel!)

6 tablespoons gelatin protein powder (I like Vital Proteins)

2 tablespoons coconut oil

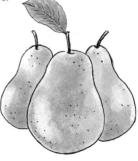

In a large saucepan combine ½ cup of water, honey, stevia, spices, and pears. Cook on medium heat for 10 to 15 minutes, or until pears are soft. Puree pears with an immersion blender or food processor. Return the mixture to the saucepan and keep warm on the lowest possible heat. In a small bowl, mix 1 cup water and gelatin, stirring quickly so the gelatin doesn't set. Pour the gelatin into the saucepan, stirring continuously until fully dissolved. Add coconut oil, allowing it to melt and blend evenly. Turn off the heat and let the mixture cool. Pour into 1-cup Mason jars and seal with a lid; place in the refrigerator for several hours until set. Pro tip: I like to leave these out for 15 minutes or so before eating, so the pudding softens a little. Makes 6 servings.

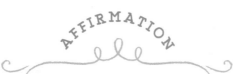

AFFIRMATION

My body was designed to do this.
I trust the process and rhythm of birth.
Each contraction brings me closer to my baby.

TRY THIS PELVIC POWER POSE!

Until fairly recently, pregnant mamas were encouraged to perform regular kegel exercises in order to strengthen the pelvic floor in preparation for birth (also to prevent urinary incontinence—so you don't pee your pants when you sneeze!). The problem with kegels, however, is that they're too targeted to *specific* pelvic floor muscles. To be more effective, you need to engage your core, your thighs, and even your glutes. And the best way to do that involves sitting and breathing.

Sounds easy enough, right?

I call this the Pelvic Power Pose. Here's how to do it:

Take a seat on your birthing ball, making sure your pelvis is higher than your knees. (If it's not, you need to inflate the ball more or get a bigger one.)

Open your legs and point your knees and feet slightly outward, for balance.

Be sure that your spine is stacked. (Not sure how to do that? Try imagining that you have a tail coming out of your tailbone. Don't sit on your imaginary tail! Instead, push your tailbone outward, so that you're sitting on the fleshy cheeks of your rump. Your shoulders should be relaxed, not thrown back or hyperextended.)

Place your hands on your belly.

Now, focus on your breath. Take slow, steady breaths through your nose. (Start by inhaling for three seconds, then exhaling for five seconds, working up to whatever feels comfortable.) As you inhale, engage your lower abdomen—your belly should expand, which pulls down the muscles of the pelvic floor. On the exhale, your pelvic floor muscles should lift and your belly should flatten (er, it should flatten a little). Pay attention to your shoulders—they should not rise or fall while you're breathing. Practice for ten minutes at a time, up to three times a day.

Want to kick things up a notch? Add in some deep squats, using a wall for support. Stand with your back against the wall. Your legs should be hip distance apart and about 2 feet in front of you. Avoid tucking your tailbone—your butt should slide up and down the wall slowly and intentionally until your knees are at a 90-degree angle. Keep your back straight, and belly engaged. Shoot for five minutes of squats, up to three times day.

#6: BUTTERFLIES

Here's another simple pose that opens your
pelvis and keeps the lower back limber. Sit
on your rump and put the soles of your feet
together. Hold your ankles, and gently pulse
your legs up and down until you feel the
stretch. For those of you who are especially
flexible, you can even have your partner add
some (gentle!) resistance for a deeper stretch.

#7: PELVIS ROCKS

Get down on all fours, with your back flat and
parallel to the floor. Then, tuck your chin to
your chest and arch your back (into a rounded
"C" shape), hold for a few minutes, and return
to a neutral position.

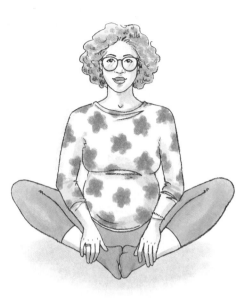

mama-do list

- Chat with your midwife or doctor and make sure you've got the okay to start
  your pelvic alignment exercises, in particular the Puppy Pose.

- Watching TV at night? Spend some time off the couch and on the floor, sitting
  cross-legged, or leaning over an exercise ball. Evening downtime is a great
  opportunity to get in some butterflies and pelvic rocks, or practice your Pelvic
  Power Pose, too.

- Wanna learn more about the "breast crawl"? Check out breastcrawl.org for
  info, pictures, and video.

love the skin you're in

WHAT'S UP WITH *baby*?

Where has the time gone, Mama? Somehow, we've reached the sixth month of your pregnancy, and baby has officially crossed the one-pound threshold. KABOOM! If you're wondering how tall she is, picture a submarine sandwich. In other words, she's about a foot long. I know, I know. It's unbelievable, right? (Remember when she was the size of a peanut?) And just think: she's got another six or seven pounds and eight more inches to go—the average weight of a newborn is 7½ pounds; the average length is 20 inches. Here's something you may be wondering: if you give birth to a longer-than-average baby, will she grow up to be a taller-than-average adult? The answer: not necessarily. While good nutrition can definitely play a role, height is mostly determined by genetics and there may be little to no correlation between her eventual height and her birth height.

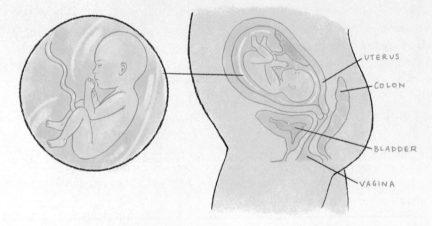

WHAT'S UP WITH *mama*?

By now, most mamas have put on somewhere around 15 pounds—roughly half the amount you can expect to gain by the time you give birth. Wait a minute. If baby is only *one* pound now, and will likely weigh between 6 and 8 pounds on D-Day, why do you have to pack on 20 or 30? Is all that extra weight . . . *fat*? Nope! By the time you deliver, only 8 of those pounds can be attributed to fat (as well as protein and nutrients), which you'll need during breastfeeding. The rest accounts for the increase in your blood volume and fluids (another 8 pounds or so), the amniotic fluid (about 2 pounds), the placenta and uterus (another 1½ to 2 pounds, each), and additional breast tissue (yet another 2 or 3 pounds). Check out the chart on page 241 to see the breakdown.

Sometimes, pregnancy definitely has its perks.

Better parking spots. Extra back massages and foot rubs. Meals delivered right to your door. Hair that grows longer and stronger. Cleavage that could make a Victoria's Secret model blush. And for many lucky women, a luminous, ethereal glow.

But for others? Not so much.

The same hormones responsible for those luscious locks and dewy complexion can *also* wreak havoc on your skin, in ways both predictable (like a night-before-prom-worthy pimple) and not (ever heard of something called PUPPS?). So this week's all about finding relief—because sometimes, pregnancy side effects are enough to make your skin crawl.

ACNE

They said you'd have a beautiful pregnancy glow—nobody said *anything* about breaking out like a teenager. Pregnancy acne, however, is almost as common as the adolescent variety. Rising levels of progesterone trigger the glands to produce more oil (a.k.a. sebum), which can clog the pores. Meanwhile, fluid retention can cause bacteria to linger in the skin, mixing with sebum and dead skin cells—and ta-da. Monster zit.

If pregnancy has you seeing spots, you'll want to take a two-pronged approach: treating the pimples from the inside out, as well as from the outside in. Here's how you can start:

TWEAKING YOUR DIET

For years, we were told that what we ate wouldn't show up on our faces. Mounting evidence, however, suggests that's just not true. For one thing, foods that are high on the glycemic index (think: refined sugars and grains) trigger a spike in insulin, which triggers your skin to produce more oil. Papa Natural is proof of this: after raiding the kids' candy bags each Halloween, his skin usually erupts in red pimples. Conventional dairy products trigger a similar insulin response; they also contain their own hormones (from the cow). Plus, research indicates that most Americans eat too many omega-6 fatty acids (which are pro-

inflammatory and worsen breakouts) and too few omega-3s (which are anti-inflammatory). You can curb your breakouts, however, by:

♡ Eating a low-sugar diet. As best you can, avoid processed foods, refined sugar (including fruit juice), and refined grains (white bread, white rice, white pasta), as all of these foods spike blood sugar.

♡ Switching to organic, cultured dairy. Cultured dairy products like whole-fat yogurt, kefir, buttermilk, and some cheeses have been fermented with probiotics, which may help reduce inflammation in the gut.

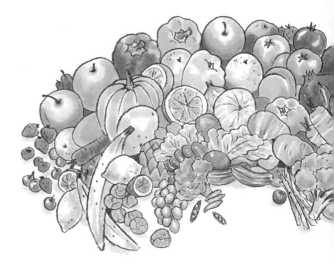

- ♡ Eating more omega-3s. Avoid seed oils (like safflower) and boost your chia seed, sardines, and salmon consumption.

- ♡ Eating more zinc. Zinc has natural anti-inflammatory and antibacterial properties, and studies have shown a link between acne and low zinc levels. Stick with dietary sources including red meat, shellfish (especially oysters), and soaked or sprouted pumpkin seeds.

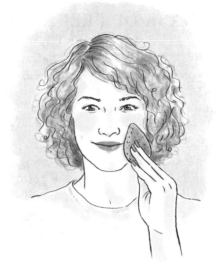

Once you've cleaned up your diet, you'll want to:

DITCH THE IRRITATING CLEANSERS

It sounds counterintuitive, but cleansing your face with oil helps *reduce* oiliness. (Ever heard the phrase "like dissolves like"?) You'll also rid the pores of dead cells, excess sebum, and other gunk while retaining your skin's natural moisture. Using overly drying cleansers, on the other hand, can aggravate acne. So for oily skin, try making an all-natural cleanser by mixing one part castor oil to one part jojoba oil. For dry skin, use castor oil and avocado oil. And for normal to combination skin, try castor oil and sunflower seed oil in equal parts. Apply liberally to the face, let it absorb for a few minutes, and then rinse with warm water (or use a washcloth for added exfoliation). *Voilà!* Clean skin that's not stripped and irritated. Raw

honey also makes an excellent cleanser, since it has natural antibacterial properties (mix one teaspoon with some warm water and massage over the face and neck). Alternatively, you might try a konjac sponge. Made from a root vegetable, these sponges gently clean and exfoliate the skin *without* the need for added soap or cleansers (really!).

For a soothing, antibacterial toner, mix one part raw apple cider vinegar with two or three parts distilled water, and swipe over your face after cleansing.

Finally, for immediate relief, dab a little tea tree oil directly onto any stubborn spots.

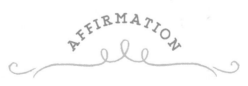

AFFIRMATION

I love and accept myself completely.
My body is amazing and working like
never before. I am so grateful today.

THE MASK OF PREGNANCY, A.K.A. CHLOASMA

Have you noticed little splotches or patches of darkened skin on your cheeks, upper lip, or forehead? Do they look kind of like ink stains or condensed freckles? Then you've likely developed chloasma (also called melasma, or more commonly the "mask of pregnancy"), which is caused by a combination of rising estrogen, progesterone, and sun exposure. Short of staying in the shade, there's not much you can do to prevent chloasma if it's already developed, but there are some steps you can take to help the splotches fade.

Lemon juice. Mix equal parts fresh-squeezed lemon juice and 3 percent hydrogen peroxide (or cucumber juice, if you prefer) and pour into a spray bottle. Spritz on your face a few times a day and let air-dry.

Turmeric milk. Some studies suggest that turmeric may prevent skin damage caused by UV radiation, as well as slow the formation of melanin, the pigment responsible for the splotches on your face. Mix up a teaspoon of turmeric powder with a bit of raw milk until it forms a paste. Apply to your spots and let sit for 10 minutes; then rinse.

Milk of magnesia. I'll be honest with you—I don't know why this stuff works, but it does. I've even used it to lighten some freckles that darkened too much in the summer sun. Before bed, apply liberally with a cotton ball to clean, dry skin. Leave it on as you sleep and wash it off in the morning.

Oatmeal honey mask. Oatmeal is a gentle exfoliator, while raw honey contains enzymes that can break down pigment. Cook up a small batch of steel-cut oats, allow to cool slightly, then mix in a bit of honey until it forms a paste. Apply to the skin, let set for 10 minutes, then rinse with cool water.

PUPPS, A.K.A. WEIRD BELLY RASH

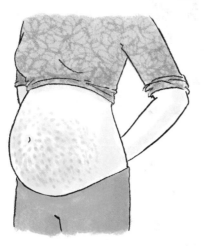

PUPPS RASH

Some mamas will get hit with an itchy, potentially painful rash on the belly known as pruritic urticarial papules and plaques of pregnancy, a.k.a. PUPPS or PUPPP.

No wonder they shortened the name, by the way—talk about a mouthful!

PUPPS starts out innocently enough: you may notice a few tiny, itchy red bumps around the navel, especially in and around the stretch marks on your abdomen. Those bumps will likely get bigger, however, morphing into large patches that can spread down the legs and buttocks and creep across the arms and chest. For some women, most of the body may be covered in the eczema-like rash by the time they hit

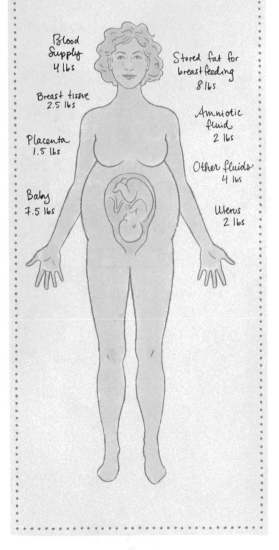

Blood Supply
4 lbs

Breast tissue
2.5 lbs

Placenta
1.5 lbs

Baby
7.5 lbs

Stored fat for breastfeeding
8 lbs

Amniotic fluid
2 lbs

Other fluids
4 lbs

Uterus
2 lbs

their due date. The good news is that PUPPS is not contagious, will not harm you or your baby, and will clear up on its own.

The bad news? We don't know exactly what causes PUPPS, and there is no known cure—other than delivering the baby, that is. The rash could be the result of stress on the skin's connective tissue due to rapid abdominal stretching. Or, it might be a sign that your liver or kidneys are overtaxed. These filtering organs are working overtime during pregnancy. PUPPS might even be an immunological issue: research indicates that fetal cells can cross the placenta and migrate to different areas of mama's body, including her skin, during pregnancy. It's possible this migration of cells can offer protective benefits from certain diseases (including Alzheimer's and breast cancer). On the other hand, it's also possible that your body might be confusing these cells with "foreign invaders," triggering a systemic immune response—hence the rash.

When it comes to treatment, conventional methods tend to focus on managing symptoms rather than addressing root causes. Topical and oral steroids are often used to relieve the itching, while antihistamines may be prescribed to treat the inflammation. It's not entirely clear how safe or effective these methods are during pregnancy, however. Better to go the all-natural route and try the following:

VEGETABLE JUICE

Although there's no clinical evidence to support the theory that vegetable juice will alleviate the PUPPS rash, lots of mamas *swear* by this method. (It's thought that the juice has a detoxifying effect on the liver.) If you're doing your own juicing, aim for a mix of fresh produce in a variety of colors: carrots, beets, ginger, fennel, apples, lemons, celery, cucumbers, and leafy greens (spinach, romaine, green leaf, and butter lettuce). If you're buying a premade or cold-pressed product, select a low-sugar, low-sodium blend and make sure the juice is pasteurized.

DANDELION ROOT AND NETTLE TEA

Not all herbs are created equal, nor are they all safe for use during pregnancy. You should always speak with your midwife or doctor before trying any herbal remedy. Dandelion root and nettles, however, have been used by midwives and herbalists to treat PUPPS for years. (It's thought that dandelion root helps nourish and detoxify the liver, while nettles are a natural antihistamine and are anti-inflammatory.) To make, steep one teabag each of dandelion root and nettles in 1 cup of boiling water for at least 10 minutes (up to one hour); enjoy hot or cold.

GRANDPA'S PINE TAR SOAP

Available online and at specialty retailers, Grandpa's Pine Tar Soap is another natural remedy that's especially popular in the blogosphere. (It's unclear exactly why this stuff works, but it can be drying, which for some reason seems to relieve the itch.) Use in your regular bath or shower, but avoid bathing in very hot water, as excessive heat can aggravate the rash and can be harmful when pregnant. Pat dry (don't rub!) and apply a soothing balm or lotion (check out my belly butter recipe below).

MAMA NATURAL'S BOOB AND BELLY BUTTER

Making my own personal care products is something I enjoy doing because I can control what goes in them! This is especially important to me during pregnancy. My recipe contains no parabens, phthalates, or artificial fragrances. Apply this soothing balm two or three times a day to the belly, breasts, and any skin irritations.

INGREDIENTS

½ cup raw cocoa butter

¼ cup raw shea butter

¼ cup extra-virgin coconut oil

1 teaspoon vitamin E oil

2 tablespoons rosehip oil

2 tablespoons sweet almond oil

20 drops geranium, lavender, and/or frankincense essential oil

In a double boiler, gently melt cocoa butter, shea butter, and coconut oil until combined. Pour into a glass container and cool to room temperature. Add in remaining ingredients and mix well. Chill in the refrigerator until butter starts to solidify (about an hour). Remove from fridge and whip with an immersion blender until the texture is similar to whipped cream. Pour into a glass container, seal tight, and store in a cool, dark place. (The lotion will further harden.) Apply to belly, breasts, and body as needed.

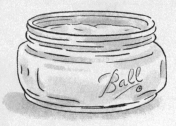

WHAT TO DO ABOUT HEMORRHOIDS

Hey, hey! It's everyone's favorite topic: hemorrhoids!

Okay, maybe not. But hemorrhoids during pregnancy are incredibly common. As your blood volume increases, more and more pressure is put on the veins in your rectum and anus, causing them to swell. In fact, that's what hemorrhoids are: swollen or inflamed veins. Another way to think about it: having hemorrhoids is a bit like having varicose veins in your bum. Yay! Constipation can also cause and exacerbate hemorrhoids due to all the, uh, *straining*. The pressure from your growing uterus can cause hemorrhoids to flare up, too. And if you thought *that* was a little TMI, here's some more info: there are actually two different types of hemorrhoids—internal and external. Internal hemorrhoids are located inside the rectum; you can't see them and often can't feel them, although they may cause some pressure, and you may notice a small amount of blood when you wipe after a bowel movement. External hemorrhoids, on the other hand, look like small pink or flesh-colored lumps or bulges on the outside of the anus (not unlike a tiny balloon). They can itch like the dickens, burn, and bleed, so they're a real pain in the . . . well, *you know*. Hemorrhoids most often appear in the third trimester or during labor (straining to push a baby out is not unlike straining to have a massive bowel movement), but they can "pop up" anytime.

So what can you do about them? First, try filling up your bathtub with two or three inches of lukewarm water, adding a half-cup of raw apple cider vinegar, and soaking for 10 to 15 minutes. This will clean the swollen area, as well as soothe irritation. Next, apply a bit of extra-virgin coconut oil directly to the hemorrhoids. (Coconut oil has antibacterial, anti-inflammatory, *and* antifungal properties, which can go a long way toward relieving pain and itching.) Finally, soak a cotton pad in a bit of organic witch hazel, freeze, and apply to the hemorrhoids for cooling relief. You also might want to invest in something called a Squatty Potty, which is sort of like a step-stool that fits around the base of your toilet. Sitting to do your doo—or worse, leaning back—pinches the intestines and puts added pressure on the rectum. Squatting, however, relaxes the muscles involved in pooping and doesn't exacerbate hemorrhoids. It's also probably closer to how we eliminated in the days before indoor plumbing came along.

Natural remedies will usually take care of hemorrhoids in a few days. However, if symptoms persist, if you're seeing more than a small amount of blood on your toilet tissue, or if you have rectal pain, call your midwife or doctor.

Healthy Gummy Men

Did you know the collagen molecule is too large to penetrate the skin when applied topically? That's why expensive collagen creams don't hold a candle to edible gelatin. I like whipping up a batch of these healthy gummy men. They're super nutritious, a snap to make, and great to eat on-the-go. Bonus: my kids *love* them.

INGREDIENTS

3 cups all-natural, chilled juice (I prefer fresh-squeezed orange juice)

½ cup grass-fed gelatin protein powder (I like the Vital Proteins brand; make sure your gelatin is *not* cold water soluble—otherwise your gummies won't set!)

¼ cup raw honey or 60 drops liquid stevia

Combine the juice and gelatin in a small saucepan, and allow the mixture to sit for a few minutes until the gelatin "blooms" or expands. Then, warm over medium-low heat until the gelatin has completely dissolved. Allow to cool slightly, then add your honey. Stir until blended and taste for sweetness. (The flavors will mellow once set, so it's okay if the mixture tastes a little too sweet at this point.) Next, transfer the mixture to a spouted measuring cup (for precision pouring), then into a silicone mold. (I use a 24-cavity mini gingerbread man mold from Wilton Silicone because I think the shapes are cute, but any design will do.) Let the gummies slightly set (takes about 10 minutes) and then transfer to the refrigerator for at least one hour, or in the freezer for 10 minutes. Eat and enjoy! Recipe makes approximately 50 mini gummy men.

STRETCH MARKS

So your belly is growing . . . and growing . . . and growing . . . and if you haven't yet, you may soon develop what I like to call "mama marks," a.k.a. stretch marks. Rapid weight gain causes the elastic fibers of the skin to snap and break, resulting in red, pink, brown, white, or gray scars. They're most likely to show up on the belly and breasts (the two areas that expand most rapidly), and they're incredibly common—roughly 90 percent of women won't escape pregnancy without a few.

Personally, I think mama marks are beautiful. You've earned them, after all—you're nurturing life in your belly! But I know that not every woman feels this way, and when it comes to swimsuit season, many mamas prefer *not* to show them off.

Too often, however, the focus is on treating stretch marks topically with creams and body butters. While lotions and potions can relieve tightness and dryness, they don't address stretch marks where they start—deep in the dermis—which is why it's important to nourish the skin internally. One way to do that? Eat more gelatin. Gelatin (from grass-fed animals) contains the amino acids glycine and proline, two fundamental building blocks of collagen and elastin, the proteins that give our skin its strength and elasticity. Bone broth is an excellent source of gelatin (you can find the recipe on page 89), as is this week's Nom of the Week.

Of course, you may still want to add a topical treatment to your daily routine, too: lotions and creams don't support the production of collagen and elastin the way that gelatin does, but they can provide relief to tight and itchy skin. Plus, there's some clinical evidence that topical vitamin E and rosehip oil in particular may be effective at reducing the appearance of stretch marks over the long term. See page 242 for my favorite balm.

mama-do list

- The best treatment for any and all pregnancy ailments? A real-food diet. Organic, nutrient-dense foods reduce heartburn, acne, and rashes, lessen the appearance of stretch marks, and keep the immune system in tip-top shape. While topical treatments can alleviate symptoms, it's always more effective to focus on whole-body health and to take care of yourself from the inside out.

- The glucose tolerance test is just around the corner—have you discussed your options with your midwife or doctor?

- Don't feel shy about talking directly to your stomach. Research indicates that by the third trimester, the fetal heartbeat actually slows down whenever mama speaks, suggesting that baby not only hears you talking but is calmed by it, too.

decorating a natural nursery

WHAT'S UP WITH *baby*?

By Week 25, baby is weighing in at 1½
pounds, and for perhaps the first time
during your pregnancy, his growth may
actually be outpacing your own. (Can I get
a hallelujah?!) Your uterus, meanwhile,
has expanded considerably: it now resem-
bles the size and shape of a soccer ball.
Something else you may be noticing: little
tiny jolts or "hops" in your belly, occurring with a surprisingly rhythmic regularity. What is that? Mama, they're hiccups
(aww!), and they're a sign that everything
is developing just as it should. Hiccups,
you see, are a reflex—they're caused by
the sudden, involuntary contraction of the
diaphragm (the muscle that separates
the chest from the abdomen). In adults,
they might be triggered by swallowing

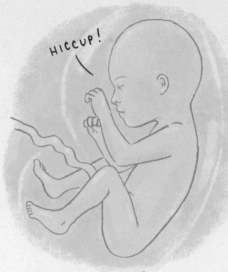

HICCUPS ARE A SIGN THAT
EVERYTHING'S A·OKAY WITH BABY.

too much air, eating too quickly, or drinking carbonated beverages. But in utero, they may be
a way of "practicing" for life outside the womb. Some researchers believe hiccupping helps
nursing mammals expel air from the stomach and is related to the suckle reflex.

WHAT'S UP WITH *mama*?

Once baby hits the 1- to 1½-pound mark, things may start to get a little, well, *tight* in that
tummy of yours. So while baby's kicks and jabs may have been noticeable before, they can
get downright uncomfortable—sometimes even a bit painful—as your pregnancy progresses.
(Just ask any mama who's been elbowed in the ribs!) If a sudden bout of tossing and turning
in utero is driving you batty, try changing positions—a slight adjustment may be enough to
coax baby into a calmer state. Still not feeling a whole lot of movement? Don't freak out, but
talk to your healthcare provider if you're concerned. Every pregnancy is different, and some
mamas don't experience "quickening"—those first noticeable flutters and twinges—until as
late as 26 weeks. Remember, too, that the position of the placenta can affect how much of
baby's movement you can feel. I had an anterior placenta during my second pregnancy, and
didn't feel my daughter consistently until around 30 weeks.

Next to navigating big box stores like Babies"R"Us, nothing gives me anxiety quite like the idea of having to decorate a baby's room. I know plenty of mamas have no problem channeling their inner Nate Berkus. I, on the other hand, just see option after option after option until I've spun myself into a vortex of panic, indecision, and fear. Clearly, it was a privilege to have this problem. But it was one I was determined to solve when it came time to set up my son's room.

Until I talked to my husband, that is. Michael's friend had just had a baby, and it was his suggestion that we not bother with a nursery *at all*. Turns out, he and his wife had invested tons of time and quite a bit of money on a room they didn't even use, as their baby ended up sleeping in the master bedroom for the first seven months.

Michael's friend had a point.

It's true that babies don't exactly *need* a Pinterest-worthy nursery.

Some especially crunchy mamas forego them entirely because a proper baby bedroom isn't exactly necessary if you're planning on co-sleeping. But even if you're a devoted follower of the "attachment parenting" movement, I still think it's a good idea for baby to have his or her own designated space if possible—for napping, playing, and daytime nursing, as well as for clothing, toy, and diaper storage. And, truth be told, I *wanted* an adorable nursery, with clouds or trains or zoo animals, but I wasn't sure where to start.

I also wanted to get the process over with as quickly as possible. I had heard nightmare stories about furniture being delayed or backordered or not being delivered in time for baby's birth, and of mamas trying to nurse on a hard-backed kitchen chair while comforting a screaming newborn—no, thank you!

So, the day I hit the six-month mark, we took the plunge. Here's everything I discovered about outfitting a nursery, and keeping it all natural.

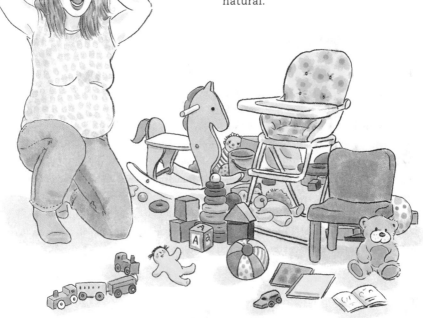

PAINT THE TOWN, ER, NURSERY RED! (OR BLUE? OR PINK? OR MAYBE YELLOW . . .)

For most mamas, the first thing they think of when they close their eyes and picture baby's future nursery is the color: pastel pinks or baby blues, or perhaps something more practical and gender neutral: like yellow.

Tell anyone your plans to paint the nursery yellow, however, and you might be met with a swift rebuke. Why? Because apparently it's a "well known" "scientifically proven" "fact" that babies cry more in yellow rooms. That's a factoid that's been floating around since at least the 1980s, and you'll find it mentioned again and again on design blogs and parenting websites across the internet. (Worth mentioning: despite a lot of references to "scientific studies," I haven't found one to back up this claim.) Here's the problem: while the psychology of color is real—we know the ways in which adults' moods can be altered and affected by color—newborns just don't see color all that well.

Infants are not actually color-blind at birth, but it's thought that they can't distinguish between colors very well until somewhere around four or five months. Newborns in particular can best discern high-contrast patterns (think: black and white stripes) and are better able to recognize bold, primary colors (as opposed to pastels). This is why so many books and toys and decorations for infants come in bright, saturated hues. It's also why, for every article warning you not to make the nursery too vibrant (your baby will cry more in a yellow room!), you'll find another suggesting that bright colors will provide necessary visual and mental stimulation.

So which is it? Busy, jazzy colors or a restful retreat? Bold patterns or soothing neutrals?

Mama? This is enough to drive any woman nuts. Babies who grow up in loving homes will get plenty of stimulation from the world around them, from toys and books and music and, most important, from you. Your kisses and cuddles, your laughter and singing, and the hours you'll spend gazing into his sweet face will provide plenty of entertainment for baby. When it comes to the nursery, the colors and decorations you pick are really for *your* benefit, not baby's. So why not think more about the *type* of paint.

Conventional paint is loaded with formaldehyde, heavy metals, and volatile organic compounds (VOCs), chemicals that "off-gas" for years after that final coat dries. In fact, the World Health Organization estimates that professional painters and decorators are as much as 40 percent more likely to develop lung cancer due to the exposure. The only consumer product that accounts for more VOCs in our atmosphere? Cars.

You might be thinking this is an easy problem to solve. After all, low- and no-VOC paint has been around for years, and stricter

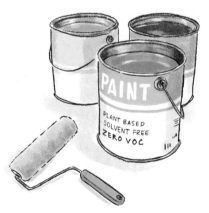

IS THE "NESTING INSTINCT" REAL?

Ask any mama, and you're bound to hear some crazy stories about the so-called nesting instinct: ironing every item of clothing in the house (T-shirts and sweatpants included), scrubbing the floors with a toothbrush, stacking and restacking—and *restacking*—onesies and blankets and diapers for hours on end . . .

But is the nesting instinct *real*, or is it all in our heads?

Although a compulsive desire to straighten and tidy in preparation for baby has been observed and documented in a wide variety of animals—including dogs, cats, rabbits, and birds—there hasn't been an enormous amount of research on the nesting instinct in humans. However, a recent study published in *Evolution and Human Behavior* confirmed what many mamas have known for years: the nesting instinct is absolutely real, and it tends to peak in the third trimester. According to the research, organizing and sorting are more common activities than cleaning, and when the nesting instinct strikes, mamas just can't seem to help themselves. Even a task that's ridiculous on its face (the study mentioned one mama who removed the knobs on her kitchen cabinets so she could disinfect the *screws*) can seem to be of the utmost importance. Sudden bursts of energy are hallmarks of nesting, too.

In fact, it's clear that nesting isn't just real, it's primal: mamas will sometimes go to extraordinary (and hilarious) lengths to get everything in order before baby arrives.

As for *why* we do this, there's almost certainly a hormonal component: oxytocin, progesterone and prolactin are all strongly associated with mama-baby bonding. There's likely a link between nesting behaviors and a fully developed protective instinct (interestingly, rats and rabbits that have their nest building interfered with often turn out to be not-so-great parents). Some researchers also believe that nesting has a survival element. For our ancient ancestors it was safer to stay close to home (away from predators) in the weeks leading up to birth, which might explain why modern mamas often turn into homebodies.

It's worth pointing out that not every mama will experience these urges so don't fret if the intense desire to bust out a label maker never kicks in. (In humans, failure to nest is *not* a reflection on the kind of mother you'll be!) But if it does, just be careful not to overexert yourself. Avoid schlepping around heavy boxes or rearranging furniture. Don't work with noxious cleansers and cleaning agents, and resist taking on overly ambitious projects (like a full-scale bathroom remodel three days before your due date). And if you do embark on some hard-core decluttering, make sure you're taking plenty of breaks to rest, rehydrate, and refuel.

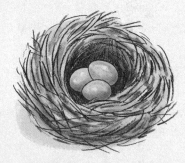

government regulations mean that VOC levels are dropping all the time. Unfortunately, not all green (as in environmentally friendly) paints are created equal. Existing regulations, for example, allow for paint with low levels of VOCs (less than 5 grams per liter) to be labeled "zero VOC." Many low-VOC paints are then tinted with high-VOC colorants. Plus, companies are not required to disclose all the chemicals they use in paint production (some ingredients may be labeled "proprietary"). This means that by the time you've applied your zero-VOC paint to the walls, it may come with a considerable toxic load.

For a safe, healthy nursery, your absolute best option is to choose a plant-based, solvent-free paint. Truly green paints use natural materials in place of petroleum solvents, biocides, and heavy metals. Some of the best brands of natural paint include ECOS Paint, Unearthed Paints, and Old Fashioned Milk Paint. Alternatively, look for a zero-VOC latex paint tinted with a zero-VOC colorant: check out Mythic Paint, Sherwin-Williams Emerald, or Benjamin Moore Natura.

Even if you choose the safest, most eco-friendly products on the market, keep in mind that it's still best to have someone *else* do the painting. Take all the usual precautions: open the windows, run a fan or a HEPA filter, and stay out of the room for at least a few days.

ARE CHANGING TABLES REALLY NECESSARY? AND OTHER PRESSING QUESTIONS ABOUT NURSERY FURNITURE

We talked about cribs (as well as crib mattresses and baby bedding) back in Week 18, if you need a refresher, but there are a few items of nursery furniture we haven't yet touched on, and we need to. I'm talking about the changing table and the rocking chair or glider.

When it comes to changing tables, the number one most-asked question mamas have is easy to guess: *Do I really have to buy one?* Plenty of women will tell you no. Changing tables often end up being the one piece of baby furniture you *won't* get much use out of unless you plan on walking back and forth to the nursery fifty times a day. Instead, you'll likely find yourself changing diapers in all corners of the house. On the other hand, some mamas find that an elevated changing station is not only more hygienic but also prevents back strain.

So what's the solution? In my opinion, your best options are to forego a traditional chang-ing table altogether, or to pick out a standard chest of drawers that can temporarily do double-duty. (Top the dresser with a nontoxic contoured changing pad, mount it securely, and *voilà*: instant changing table.) Granted,

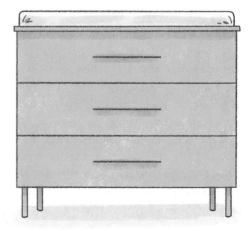

Fat Bombs!

Even before I got pregnant, I was a little like Big Ben. I'd be sitting at my desk in my stuffy old office, the clock would strike three, and 3 – 2 – 1 – out would come a giant yawn, followed by a full-body stretch. The midafternoon slump is real, Mama! And it was no less intense when I left the corporate world and started having kids. From running to prenatal appointments to chasing a toddler, pregnant mamas need energy to make it through the day.

Instead of sugar-rich treats, reach for healthy fats—they'll provide long-term energy *without the crash.* One of my favorite midafternoon pick-me-ups? I call them Fat Bombs. Funny name, I know, but they were made popular by folks following a ketogenic diet. They can be enjoyed, however, by everyone. Feel free to tinker with this recipe (add different spices or experiment with coconut oil or walnut butter). The key is to keep them fat focused.

INGREDIENTS

½ cup organic unsalted butter

½ cup raw almond butter (you can use tahini if you're nut-free)

2 tablespoons raw honey or 30 drops pure stevia

1 teaspoon cinnamon

½ teaspoon vanilla extract

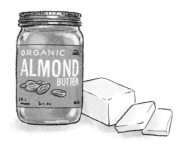

Over low heat, melt your butter and almond butter in a sauce-pan. Stir well, remove from the heat, let cool, and mix in your honey and spices. Spoon into small silicone molds (the Gummy Men molds on page 244 work great for this, too) and refrigerate for two hours. Enjoy a few each afternoon with your red raspberry leaf tea!

plenty of modern changing tables are built to grow with your child. They're designed as regular dressers that come with a removable changing tray, which makes the piece considerably more versatile. Unfortunately, the majority of new changing tables on the market are made with particleboard, press-wood, and composite materials. Just like cribs, the safest changing tables will be made from solid, sustainable materials, free of formaldehyde, VOCs, and phthalates. Secondhand furniture can easily be refinished with a nontoxic stain or paint. Meanwhile, an older piece of composite wood furniture is actually safer for baby than a new item, since it will likely have finished off-gassing.

ROCKING CHAIRS AND GLIDERS

Whereas a changing table might be an optional piece of nursery furniture, you'll be hard-pressed to find a mama who doesn't *love* her rocking chair or glider. That's because nursing and rocking a baby is practically a full-time job unto itself, so you need to be comfortable. Determining which kind to buy really comes down to personal preference. Gliders generally offer a smoother, more effortless ride (although some mamas find that gliders can trigger motion sickness). Traditional wood rockers, on the other hand, are classic and timeless, but they may begin to creak and squeak with age, and may require a cushion or back pillow to get comfy. It's worth taking a trip to your local baby goods or furniture store so you can try out a few different models. Once you've settled on the style, you may want to seek out a chair made from organic or eco-friendly materials—preferably one that's free of phthalates, formaldehyde, and flame retardants (Monte Design and Pottery Barn carry these types). Solid wood hand-me-down rockers and gliders are great options that won't break the bank.

WHAT'S THIS TOY'S STORY?
(ITS *BACK STORY*, THAT IS)

Now that you've got nontoxic paint on your walls, you'll want to make sure any toys you bring into baby's nursery are safe. Stuffed animals should be made from organic, eco-friendly fabrics, such as cotton or wool. Beware of antique and imported toys, especially those made in China, India, and Taiwan, which may contain high levels of phthalates, arsenic, or mercury or be finished with lead-based paint—eek! (A 2013 Greenpeace-IPEN study analyzed more than five hundred children's products manufactured in China and found that one third contained *at least* one toxic metal at levels considered harmful to young children!) To avoid these contaminants, stick with toys made in the United States or Northern Europe and shop from ethical stores like MightyNest and Bella Luna Toys. And remember: no need to stress out or break the bank. A few high-quality toys are plenty for a newborn, who would much prefer to gnaw on a wooden spoon.

IS CO-SLEEPING SAFE?

As much as it broke my heart, I knew that co-sleeping (well, technically bed sharing) wasn't for our family, for two main reasons. One: I am a very deep sleeper. Growing up, my family used to joke that nothing—not a thunderstorm, not a sonic boom, not an *Independence Day*-style alien invasion—could rouse me from slumber. And two: my husband is a very light sleeper. Whereas I sometimes struggle to get up in the morning, Michael struggles to stay asleep at night. Given our respective sleep baggage, we figured inviting a brand-new baby into our bed was not a particularly great way to preserve our sanity. Instead, we used a co-sleeper sidebar (i.e., a bassinet that connects to the side of the bed) for the first few months before transitioning each of our children to a crib in their own rooms.

On the other hand, I know plenty of couples who do bed share, and love it.

Certainly, sharing a bed can make middle-of-the-night nursing easier, as well as simplify the bedtime routine. Lots of families believe that co-sleeping or the "family bed" promotes better bonding and closeness. In some circles it's believed to build self-esteem and encourage independence and it's a central tenet of the "attachment parenting" movement.

It is not, however, a mainstream practice—at least not here in the States. Outside the crunchy community, co-sleeping is often met with confusion, derision, and some very stern warnings. Chief among the complaints? It's just not safe.

But is that really true?

The answer depends on how you define "co-sleeping." The term is often used interchangeably with bed sharing (a practice the American Academy of Pediatrics does *not* recommend, largely due to evidence—some would say very controversial evidence—that sharing a bed increases the risk of SIDS). But in reality, co-sleeping is more of a catch-all term; it refers not only to bed sharing but also to room sharing, a practice that's neither unsafe nor controversial. In fact, the AAP *recommends* room sharing, largely because it seems to lower the risk of SIDS.

Confused yet?

When it comes to bed sharing, specifically, it's not the practice itself that's unsafe—UNICEF and La Leche League International, for example, actually support bed sharing—but the *way* it's practiced. In other words, there is absolutely a wrong way to do it; when practiced incorrectly, sleeping alongside an infant can be exceedingly dangerous. Unfortunately, our tendency to lump together *safe* forms of co-sleeping and *unsafe* practices gives *all* forms of co-sleeping a negative connotation. This prevents many parents from talking openly about co-sleeping and bed sharing, or from seeking guidance on how to do it safely. And that's a problem. Two separate studies, both published in *JAMA Pediatrics*, suggest that as many as 50 percent of parents practice bed sharing, specifically, at least some of the time.

$\longrightarrow$

Whether you plan to bed share, room share, or put baby to sleep in a traditional nursery, I think it's important to point out that co-sleeping does not have to be an all-or-nothing prospect. Even the staunchest supporters of bed sharing may choose not to practice it *every* night. If you had a few glasses of wine, for example, it may be safer to place baby in his or her own sleeping space (another reason I think it's a good idea to have a nursery, if possible). When my babies were small, I practiced bed sharing when they—by which I mean *we*—napped. Try out different sleeping arrangements, and go with whatever works best for your family. Some parents purchase specially designed "sleepers" that fit on top of the mattress so baby has his own secure space to sleep. If you do want to practice co-sleeping, though, it's important to take note of the following guidelines:

- Babies should *always* be put to sleep on their backs, on a firm mattress with tight-fitting sheets, away from loose pillows, blankets, and stuffed animals. There should be no space between the mattress and the wall or the bedframe into which baby could roll, slip, or get stuck. Babies should not sleep between mama and papa, but rather between mama and the edge of the bed. Babies should *never* be allowed to sleep or co-sleep on sofas, recliners, or couches.

- Parents who consume or have consumed alcohol or drugs, who have taken medications that induce drowsiness, who are obese, who sleep very deeply, or who sleepwalk should consider a sidecar arrangement. Parents who smoke should likewise refrain from sharing a bed with an infant.

- Babies who are exclusively bottle-fed should sleep in a separate crib or co-sleeper sidecar. (It's thought breastfeeding makes both mama and baby more sensitive to each other's movements, and that breastfeeding, bed-sharing mamas arouse more frequently and sleep less deeply, which lowers the risk of roll-overs.)

- Babies who share a bed with their caregiver should not be swaddled.

- Babies under one year of age should not sleep next to other children.

In 2016, the American Academy of Pediatrics updated its safe sleep guidelines: new evidence suggests that sharing a room with your newborn—for *at least* the first six months, and preferably the first year—can decrease the risk of SIDS by as much as 50 percent!

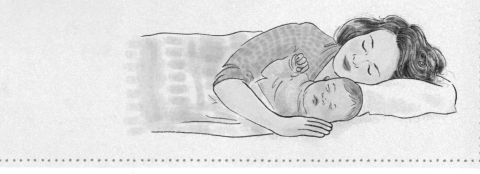

BABY-PROOFING 101

While it's true that baby won't be on the move for quite a few months, tip-over accidents are frighteningly common: falling furniture accounts for more than 25,000 injuries every year. In 2016, Ikea issued a voluntary recall of 29 million chests and dressers after the deaths of at least six children. So be sure to check the changing table as well as dressers, bookshelves, and entertainment centers throughout your home for sturdiness and stability. Keep in mind that even heavy furniture can tip when the drawers are pulled out (this shifts the center of gravity forward). Furniture or heavy electronics (like your television) that could potentially tip over need to be anchored to the wall with safety straps or L brackets. Drawer stops, which prevent children from opening drawers all the way (which they often do, in order to climb), can add increased safety. You'll also want to think twice about storing especially attractive items, such as stuffed animals or toys, on top of furniture that a child might climb.

Next, avoid hanging anything heavy on the walls above baby's crib, such as mirrors, shelving, or elaborate picture frames. Lightweight pictures should be hung at least 18 inches above the crib rail, well out of arm's reach. (Wall decals and unframed canvas prints are great alternatives to framed art, since they don't contain glass.) Crib mobiles meanwhile, should be hung *at least* 12 inches away from a newborn's face. Strings or cords should never dangle *into* the crib, and mobiles should be removed entirely as soon as baby can push himself up to his hands and knees. Be wary of mobiles with detachable parts (which could fall and present a choking hazard), as well as old or antique mobiles, which may not pass current safety inspections. I preferred to hang my mobile over the glider because it gave baby something to look at while nursing. You could also hang one over the diaper station to distract baby while wiping his tush.

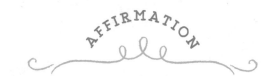

AFFIRMATION

I embrace the profound gift of motherhood.
I am blessed by the awesome opportunity to raise
a kind and compassionate citizen of the world.

DECORATIONS AND TOYS

It's tempting to buy every toy and stuffed animal and baby book and rattle you can get your hands on, especially if you're a first-time mama. But a fully stocked toy box is a waste of time, money, *and* space—after all, kids get bored quickly, and it's a well-known fact that small children are often more enamored with the box a toy was packaged in than with the toy itself! Another important factor to consider: the clutter. The more knick-knacks and playthings you stuff in the nursery, the more likely you are to step on or trip over something in the middle of the night. (Stubbed toes hurt!!) If you get a toy store's worth of goodies at your baby shower, consider packing most of them away for now. Rotate the toys periodically, and you'll extend the life of each item by years.

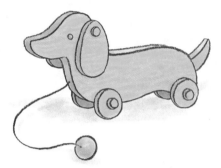

mama-do list

- There may be loads of adorable blankets and toys and stuffed animals to choose from, but babies don't need a whole lot of *stuff*—nor do they have a particularly discerning eye when it comes to interior design. So when creating a nursery, remember to KISS—Keep It Simple, Sweetie. Have fun with it, make it functional, but don't sweat the small stuff.

- True milk paint is some of the most environmentally friendly, nontoxic stuff on the market, but it doesn't provide much in the way of color consistency—milk paint is known for its ability to give furniture a mottled, "old world" look. Do a Google image or Pinterest search for "milk paint," and you'll find loads of charmingly distressed pieces and DIY tutorials. Who knows? You might be inspired to go in a whole different design direction.

- For more tips about safe co-sleeping and bed sharing, check out the Mother-Baby Behavioral Sleep Laboratory at the University of Notre Dame (cosleeping .nd.edu).

VBAC

THE ODDS
ARE WITH YOU

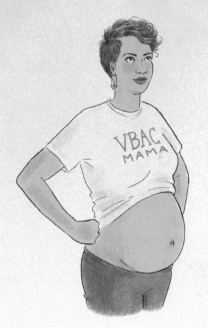

WHAT'S UP WITH *baby*?

Ever looked at a diagram of the human lungs? Inside each one is a dense network of airways (called bronchioles) that look like an insanely intricate set of tree branches. At the end of each branch is a cluster of air sacs (called alveoli), which look like bunches of grapes. Each time we breathe, air passes through the bronchioles, inflating the alveoli; it's from these mini pockets of air that our blood takes up oxygen. But while in utero, baby's lungs are filled with amniotic fluid. This causes the alveoli to stick together, making it difficult to inflate at the moment of birth. And that's why Week 26 is such a vital stage of baby's development. Right now, her lungs are transitioning from the "canalicular" to the "saccular" phase, and have started to produce a soap-like substance called surfactant. Just as dish soap breaks water's surface tension (add a dollop of dish soap and a perfectly round droplet of water will flatten out), soapy surfactant breaks the surface tension of the fluid in the alveoli—this allows baby's lungs to drain and fill with air; it also prevents the air sacs from collapsing each time she exhales. All this is preparation to make those gigantic but oh-so-sweet cries.

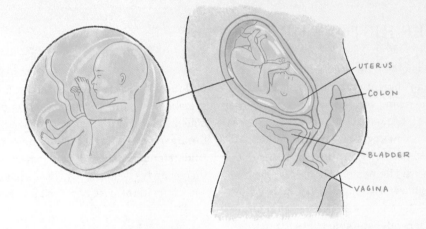

UTERUS

COLON

BLADDER

VAGINA

WHAT'S UP WITH *mama*?

Speaking of, well, *airways*, here's something you might be noticing now: gas. That's right. The slowdown in your digestion means there's more time for gas to build up in the gut, and there are only two ways for that gas to escape: burps or toots. And as baby gets bigger and bigger, the organs of your digestive system will only get more compressed. Plus, the relaxing of your muscles triggered by progesterone makes you less able to . . . *clench*. The result? Bombs away! Don't worry, Mama. Flatulence is common during pregnancy, embarrassing as it may be. However, if a case of the farts has you feeling flustered, try eliminating carbonated drinks and fried foods from your diet, since they can cause GI distress. A digestive enzyme taken with meals may help, too. And if all else fails, you can always blame it on the baby.

It used to be standard medical thinking: "Once a Cesarean, always a Cesarean." In other words, once a mama had delivered a child via C-section, she could never again experience vaginal birth. These days, however, more and more women are trying for a VBAC—vaginal birth after Cesarean (pronounced "vee-back"). And, statistically speaking, the odds are definitely in their favor.

Between 60 percent and 80 percent of women who delivered their first baby via Cesarean and try for a VBAC will be successful.

Some midwifery practices (and some especially natural-minded OBs) have VBAC success rates north of 90 percent. Even the American College of Obstetricians and Gynecologists recommends the practice for certain kinds of low-risk women. But this is not the message of hope you'll receive when talking to *most* ob-gyns. In fact, many physicians will try to talk you out of it—and that's assuming the hospital you're planning to birth at doesn't have a VBAC ban. What gives?

A BRIEF HISTORY OF THE VBAC

Though it might come as a surprise, Cesarean section is an ancient procedure. The first successful American C-section was performed way back in the late 1700s, but there are references to the surgery in Egyptian, Greek, and Roman folklore and mythology, as well as in ancient Chinese texts. The name itself, Cesarean, was thought to have originated with Julius Caesar's birth in the 1st century BC—although that's a matter of some debate, since Caesar's mother apparently survived long enough to see her son to adulthood. Because that's the thing about old-school C-sections: they weren't just dangerous; they were deadly. In fact, they were performed *only* to save the life of the baby when the mother was sure to die during childbirth. (*Grim.*)

What was once a fairly gruesome operation, however, changed dramatically thanks to the miracle of modern medicine. The development of local (as opposed to general) anesthesia,

the discovery of antibiotics to treat infection, and the advancement of surgical techniques (notably, switching to a transverse or side-to-side incision, rather than a vertical cut) made Cesareans exceedingly safe for most women. Understandably, then, doctors began to rely increasingly on this newly safe form of delivery, especially in the case of breech babies and as a

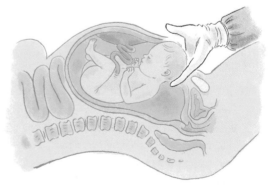

CESAREAN DELIVERY

way of avoiding forceps assistance (which at the time carried a high rate of injury to both mama and baby).

Meanwhile, the growing popularity of continuous electronic fetal monitoring and labor aids like Pitocin pushed a climbing Cesarean rate even higher. What had once been relatively rare—only 5 percent of births in 1970 ended in C-section—had suddenly become increasingly, disturbingly common. By 1980, the rates had jumped to 16 percent. By the late 1980s, nearly a quarter of all births were surgical. When you factor in that any woman who'd had a C-section was doomed to have another—remember: Once a Cesarean, always a Cesarean—surgical births were poised to skyrocket.

And that triggered a bit of a public health crisis. VBACs—fairly common in Europe, but virtually unheard of in the States until the 1950s—were suddenly back on the menu. Several large-scale studies confirmed their relative safety. And by the mid-1990s, the American College of Obstetricians and Gynecologists' official position was that a trial of labor after

WHAT OTHER *natural mamas* SAY

ashley: After my C-section, I wanted to prove to myself that I could birth my child, and that my body wasn't broken. My VBAC was beautiful and healing—an incredible success!

vanessa: The morning after my VBAC, I told my husband that I felt like I'd been hit by a Mack truck—but I also felt like I could throw a Mack truck. I went into it with the confidence that my body could do this, and no one could change my mind. The whole experience was extremely empowering.

hanna: I was all about the VBAC until my daughter's heart rate dropped and I had no choice but to opt for another C-section. I'm a very active person, but the recovery took much longer than I expected.

kelly: With my second birth I knew I wanted a VBAC. I went to 42 weeks and everyone was getting nervous. But through faith, prayer, and preparedness, my daughter was born easily and gently. It was the most amazing birth!

kimberly: There were doubts and concerns from the people around me, but my husband and I pressed forward! We read and read and researched and researched, and the loving guidance of a great midwife helped us feel like we could do it. I've now had three VBACs, and it was blissful being able to do it the natural way.

Cesarean (TOLAC) was appropriate for most women. Thus, the number of VBACs began to rise dramatically, while the number of Cesareans began to fall.

That might have been the end of our story. But guess what happened next?

VBACs began to be treated an awful lot like regular births. More and more women attempting VBACs were induced, even though the research clearly showed that induction increased the risk of eventual complication. Also troubling? The College reported that some insurance companies were attempting to make TOLACs *mandatory*, rather than determined on a case-by-case basis after a discussion between patient and doctor. (Why? Because vaginal birth is cheaper than Cesarean.)

Not surprisingly, doctors began to see an uptick in the rates of injury and, in some cases, even fetal death after VBACs gone wrong. (They were also served with quite a few lawsuits.) By 1999, the College had reversed course; new guidelines stated that both a physician and an anesthesiologist should be on call during all TOLACs "just in case." Malpractice insurance rates went through the roof. Today, despite support for the TOLAC from the American College of Nurse-Midwives *and* the College of Obstetricians and Gynecologists (which softened their guidelines again in 2010), almost half of American hospitals enforce practice-wide VBAC bans. Vaginal birth after Cesarean is often considered to be risky, dangerous, and definitely controversial. And the C-section rate? At 33 percent, it's the highest it's ever been.

ABOUT THOSE RISKS . . .

So, what exactly is "risky" about VBACs?

Far and away, the number-one concern as it relates to VBAC is the potential for uterine rupture—that is, a separation or tear of the uterus at the site of the previous incision (a.k.a. the scar). Though extremely rare, uterine rupture is actually possible during *any* birth—whether you've had a C-section before or not. "Uterine rupture" is also something of an umbrella term, encompassing several different types of complications. In the most serious of circumstances—a "catastrophic rupture"—the uterus tears open at the site of the scar, the amniotic sac ruptures, and the baby is pushed into the abdominal cavity. As the name suggests, a catastrophic rupture is a very big deal. It requires immediate surgical intervention and, in 6 percent of cases, results in fetal death.

The other type of rupture—what's known as an incomplete rupture—is far less serious, in that the scar only thins or stretches, but the uterus and the amniotic sac stay fully intact.

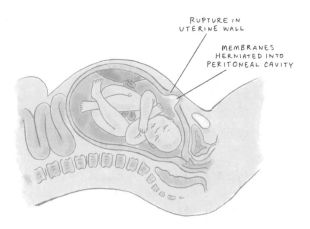

RUPTURE IN
UTERINE WALL

MEMBRANES
HERNIATED INTO
PERITONEAL CAVITY

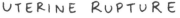

UTERINE RUPTURE

MORE ABOUT VBACS

FROM MIDWIFE *cynthia*

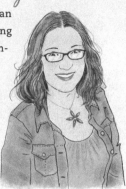

Trial of labor after Cesarean (TOLAC) and vaginal birth after Cesarean (VBAC) is a service that I'm proud to offer. One of the most frustrating things from my perspective as a midwife, however, is meeting potential clients whose previous providers did not support their attempt at a vaginal birth. Both the American College of Obstetricians and Gynecologists and the American College of Nurse-Midwives have position statements supporting TOLAC and VBAC, and when attended by skilled providers in a hospital setting with a readily available operating room and anesthesia team, a TOLAC should be a no-brainer.

What concerns me is that more and more women who live in rural or remote areas or in places where the "Once a C-section, always a C-section" dictum constitutes official policy are seeking to VBAC *outside* of the hospital—home birth after Cesarean (HBAC) is a rising trend in the United States. While I do support home birth for low-risk women, I do not personally support home birth in situations where there are true and documented medical risks for mother and baby.

If VBAC is not an option in your community, ask your provider *why* it's not! Is it because the hospital in question isn't equipped with in-house anesthesia? Is it because of the provider's fear or risk of perceived liability? Demand to know your options, and don't hesitate to get referrals for providers that are willing and able to offer VBAC.

In addition to the potential for uterine rupture, there are some concerns about the risks associated with placenta accreta, a condition in which the blood vessels of the placenta attach too deeply within the wall of the uterus. Placenta accreta is not *caused* by VBAC—the condition itself develops long before birth. It is, however, a very serious, potentially life-threatening emergency. The failure of the placenta to detach from the uterus can trigger a massive hemorrhage. The placenta must then be surgically removed, sometimes via emergency hysterectomy. Placenta accreta has a high (7 percent) maternal death rate.

Blueberry Ginger Smoothie

Support baby's growing lungs this week with a blast of antioxidants. These amazing agents are excellent for supporting bronchial and capillary health and provide loads of other benefits, too. Foods that are especially high in antioxidants include goji berries, raspberries, dark chocolate, turmeric, and garlic but this refreshing smoothie utilizes berries, grapes, and ginger. The protein powder, meanwhile, adds staying power.

INGREDIENTS

1 cup frozen organic blueberries

1 cup frozen organic red grapes

1½ cups unsweetened coconut water

1 teaspoon freshly grated ginger

1 tablespoon raw honey

2 scoops protein powder (optional)

Toss everything in a blender (add some ice if necessary) and blend away. To keep your blood sugar steady, drink alongside eggs in the morning or with a handful of nuts as an afternoon snack. Recipe makes 2 servings.

GIVEN THE RISKS, WHY WOULD *ANYONE* EVER EVEN ATTEMPT A VBAC?

I'll admit that just writing about uterine rupture and placenta accreta is pretty scary, and it's understandable that women would be fearful of the risks associated with VBAC. I mean, why *would* anyone attempt this? And—more to the point—why would any medical association recommend it?

The answer is actually pretty simple: the risks associated with VBAC are *lower* than the risks associated with repeat Cesarean.

I'll give you just a minute to let that sink in.

See, among women who have had one previous C-section and have a low transverse scar (that is, a side-to-side or "bikini" incision), the risk of uterine rupture during a VBAC is less than 1 percent. According to some studies, it can be as low as 0.2 percent, or 1 in 500. This means that depending on which statistics you cite, the risk of uterine rupture is comparable to—or even less than—the risk of miscarriage during amniocentesis (a procedure, it's worth pointing out, that doctors recommend with surprising regularity).

In the case of placenta accreta, it's not VBAC that ups your risk—it's *Cesareans*. In fact, the chance of developing accreta increases with each subsequent surgery you have (as does your risk of infection, bleeding or hemorrhage, bladder or bowel injury, and troublesome scar tissue known as adhesions). The risk of accreta after just two C-sections is *greater* than the risk of uterine rupture during a non-induced, planned VBAC.

Isn't it interesting that your healthcare provider may counsel you on the risks of VBAC, but might not say anything about the risks of repeat abdominal surgery?

Assuming you're a good candidate for VBAC, there are tons of benefits to going the vaginal route: fewer complications, a shorter hospital stay, a faster recovery. You'll get a boost from the hormones associated with labor, in particular oxytocin, which helps relieve pain, promote mama-baby bonding, and shrink the uterus following birth. Baby reaps benefits from vaginal delivery, too: traveling through the birth canal, for example, forces amniotic fluid out of baby's lungs, lowering her future risk of developing allergies and asthma. It also exposes her to a plethora of good bacteria, which may lower her risk of developing inflammatory illnesses later in life, such as Crohn's disease.

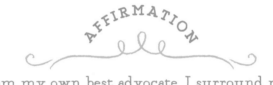

AFFIRMATION

I am my own best advocate. I surround myself with supportive people. I make perfect decisions for myself and my baby.

ARE YOU A GOOD CANDIDATE FOR VBAC?

While the majority of women who've had a Cesarean—more than 90 percent, according to the American Pregnancy Association—are candidates, VBAC is definitely not for everyone. You'll want to discuss the pros and cons and the specifics of your pregnancy with your healthcare provider. But generally speaking, women who have no major medical problems, who've experienced no previous uterine ruptures, and whose baby is in the head-down position can expect a good outcome. (Women who've experienced a previous vaginal birth have especially high VBAC success rates.) Additionally, mamas hoping for a VBAC will have a greater chance of success if they meet the following criteria:

♡ Your pregnancy is low-risk, and you've gained an appropriate amount of weight. Women who are overweight or obese or who have gained more than 40 pounds during pregnancy are less likely to VBAC successfully.

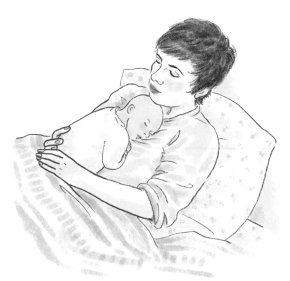

♡ You've had no more than two previous C-sections.

♡ You had a low transverse incision during your previous C-section. Women with vertical or T-shaped scars are generally not good candidates for VBAC, since these types of incisions are more likely to rupture.

♡ Your previous C-section was the result of an isolated incident (for example, a breech presentation) that has not recurred during your current pregnancy.

♡ Your placenta is not covering your C-section scar (which ups your risk of placenta accreta).

♡ Your baby is not more than one week over-due.

PREPARING FOR A VBAC

Want to increase your chances for a successful vaginal birth? Then you'll need to:

♡ Collect your medical records. It's the only way to be certain about the type of scar you have—it's actually possible to have a side-to-side scar on the *outside*, but a vertical incision on the *inside*. You'll also be able to tell exactly what factors contributed to your previous C-section.

♡ Find a VBAC-friendly provider. Even if your doctor is pro-VBAC, the hospital where he or she delivers may not be. Find out the official policy on VBAC at the location where you plan to give birth, and keep in mind that partnering with a midwife may significantly improve your odds. If you don't feel comfortable with your provider, switch!

♡ Hire a qualified doula. Her encouragement and experience will likely prove invaluable

during your birth. Doulas can also help to calm and empower nervous partners.

♡ Write a birth plan. The truth is that every birth is unique and unpredictable—but writing down your preferences will help get you prepared for whatever surprises or complications might come your way. We'll talk more about birth plans next week.

♡ Get your mind right. Just as you committed to a natural pregnancy and childbirth, it's important to commit to a TOLAC—it's just too easy to be swayed or discouraged if you don't go in with a positive, determined outlook. Seek help from VBAC support groups, listen to birth affirmations, read empowering birth stories (we have thousands at mama natural.com), and visualize yourself having a successful vaginal delivery. If your spouse or partner is resistant to the idea, consider making an appointment with your midwife so you can both talk through any concerns.

♡ Take care of yourself. The most important things you can do to increase your odds for a successful VBAC are to eat a healthy diet, exercise regularly, and get adequate rest. Making your health a priority lowers your risk for complications that might bump you into the high-risk category. It also reduces the chance that you'll need interventions during delivery—all things that can make or break a VBAC.

♡ Rock your pelvic poses. A balanced and aligned pelvis will not only help you feel better during pregnancy but could result in an easier birth. Be sure you're doing your pelvic exercises daily (see Week 23) and consider regular care from a Webster-certified chiropractor. Don't forget the Pelvic Power Pose on page 234, which helps strengthen your pelvic floor while you practice deep breathing, both essentials to unmedicated, vaginal births.

mama-do list

○ The International Cesarean Awareness Network (ICAN) is a phenomenal resource for C-section mamas who need support or are seeking a VBAC. Local chapters offer weekly or monthly meetings, and the ICAN website (ican-online.org) is loaded with valuable information. Check them out!

○ VBAC may still be an option even if you don't meet all the criteria on pages 265–266. For example, induction during a VBAC is not a total no-go, it just needs to be approached with quite a bit of caution. Chat with your provider about the specifics of your pregnancy and don't hesitate to seek out a second opinion.

○ Have you been to the dentist yet, Mama? No? Well, it's not too late to slip in for a routine cleaning. Remember, rising hormones associated with pregnancy can cause swollen gums and plaque build-up, and may contribute to cavities, whereas tooth decay has been linked to premature labor.

should you really write a birth plan?

WHAT'S UP WITH *baby*?

Anyone who's ever witnessed a live birth—whether in person or via "reality" baby shows or YouTube videos—knows that newborns don't come out of the womb looking pristinely clean and perfectly pink. But did you know that their slippery, slimy appearance isn't just caused by blood and bodily fluids? Many babies emerge from the womb sporting a waxy, creamy coating that smells like breast milk and looks like feta. It's called *vernix caseosa* (which, believe it or not, is Latin for "cheese varnish"). And at 27 Weeks, your baby has started to produce it. Why? Vernix is a bit like waterproofing, in that it prevents babies from getting pruny after floating in amniotic fluid for nine long months. It protects him

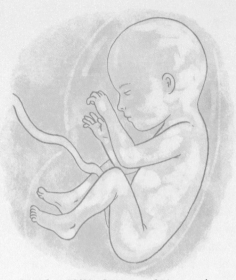

AT 27 WEEKS, BABY IS BEGINNING TO PRODUCE VERNIX.

from bacteria and pathogens, both inside *and* outside the womb (vernix has immune proteins similar to those found in breast milk). It likewise protects him from meconium exposure, and is quite possibly the world's best moisturizer. But vernix is also—if we're being honest here—a little bit gross looking, which is why so many nurses will rush to towel it off right away. Mama? Don't let them do this. Aside from myriad health benefits, studies show that delaying baby's first bath—preferably for at least 24 hours—significantly improves breastfeeding. Even the World Health Organization recommends leaving the vernix alone. Don't wash away this amazing gift from nature. Rub it in.

WHAT'S UP WITH *mama*?

During my first pregnancy, a dear friend of mine issued me a warning: don't wait to tackle big projects like decorating the nursery, she said, because you'll be too big and too tired to do much of anything once you hit 34 weeks. It's certainly true that every pregnancy is different, and that every mama is different. Some women feel wretched from the first month to the last, while others stay surprisingly active right up until their water breaks. But one thing is for certain: as you head into the third trimester, things are going to start changing—and fast! So if you haven't yet signed up for a childbirth education class, thought about having a baby shower, or started making decisions about where baby will eat, sleep, and poop, now's the time.

Here's a secret most doctors and nurses won't tell you: Nobody cares a whit about your birth plan.

Sorry. I know that sounds harsh, but it's nonetheless true—birth plans have become a bit of a joke in quite a few labor-and-delivery nurses' stations. A very popular refrain in maternity wards across the country is: "The more detailed the birth plan, the more likely the C-section." In fact, you can even find a number of parody birth plans floating around on the web. (One of the funniest, published in the literary journal *McSweeney's*, lists the obnoxious, over-the-top demands of fictional parents-to-be Jeff and Jamie: "When the crown of the head appears, please turn down the music as Jeff will be reading aloud from *Be Here Now* by Ram Dass.")

So, where's all this birth plan backlash coming from?

Birth plans—completely nonexistent before the 1980s—came about as a way to facilitate communication between expectant parents and their healthcare providers. They were also supposed to prevent making important medical decisions in the heat of labor. Simply put, they are written documents that include your preferences regarding birth. This includes everything from pain medication to the use of routine interventions, and some even include notes on the music you'd like to listen to or the type of lighting you'd prefer. Sounds innocuous enough, right? Somewhere along the way, however, birth plans took on a distinctly "us versus them" kind of tone. Rather than a list of *preferences*, they became a set of *demands*. Rather than evolving documents, they became increasingly rigid and inflexible. Hospital staffers began to perceive women who wrote elaborate, multipage instruction manuals to be controlling, ill informed, and high maintenance.

The great irony, of course, is that the fear that their wishes won't be respected in the delivery room is the very reason many women write rigid birth plans in the first place.

Here's the thing: birth plans *are* helpful and they *are* important, especially if you're seeking a natural, unmedicated childbirth. The process of writing one is a great way to educate yourself about the options you'll have during labor and delivery. It also gives you a chance to think about how you might like to handle a complication. But there is a helpful way—and a not-so-helpful way—to go about writing one.

UNDERSTANDING WHAT A BIRTH PLAN IS— AND WHAT IT'S NOT

Consult virtually any baby book or parenting website, and many will tell you that a birth plan is like a guide or a roadmap to realizing your specific vision of an ideal childbirth. But while that's partially true, it's definitely not the whole story—in fact, even the term "birth plan" is a bit misleading. Because as anyone with experience will tell you, the one thing you can reliably plan on is that every birth is unique and unpredictable. A document you wrote weeks or even months in advance, then, will likely need some minor (if not major) adjustments come D-Day. Once those contractions kick in, for example, you may realize that you really *do* want that epidural. Or you might discover that you really *do* need that C-section. That's why a good plan shouldn't just describe your best-case scenario; it should also include your preferences in case things *don't* go according to plan.

Keep in mind that you may not be ready to begin writing your birth plan for several more weeks—and that's okay. Because before you start putting pen to paper, there are a few things you'll need to figure out:

Know Your Priorities. In the last few years, a slew of downloadable, fill-in-the-blank style birth plans have popped up all over the internet. While these can be handy thought starters, many of them are pages and pages long, and/or contain outdated, no-longer-relevant medical info. (Enemas and pubic hair shaving, for example, are no longer routine at most hospitals, yet you'll find those things listed on virtually all predesigned birth plans.) Even more troubling? Internet-generated birth plans rarely come with a set of instructions, so first-time parents often just start checking off boxes willy-nilly or include things on their plan merely because they "sound" good.

For instance, you may decide that you'd like to labor in whatever positions feel most comfortable—on a birthing ball, on your hands and knees, etc. But if you state that you'd *also* prefer continuous electronic fetal monitoring, you'll likely be confined to a bed and won't be able to move freely. These two preferences, then, are fundamentally incompatible. Or you might specify that you don't want a "saline lock" or a "hep-lock" under any circumstances, but if you opt for an epidural, you *must* have one. The point is, you need to understand everything you include on a birth plan and get really honest about what you want. Don't write down anything just because you feel like you *should*. Birth plans are very personal and highly individualized. They should reflect your views and nobody else's.

Know Your Options. Your ideal birthing experience might involve a whirlpool tub and a roomful of candles, but know that if you're planning to deliver in an ultraconservative hospital—where women in active labor are denied food, strapped to a fetal monitor, and forced to lie on their backs—you can forget all of that. (In fact, you'd be hard-pressed to find *any* hospital that would green-light candles—major fire hazard!)

This is why it's so important to get clear on your hospital or birth center's policies *long* before the day of delivery.

Likewise, you'll want to talk through your birth plan with your healthcare provider well before you go into labor. And if at some point you realize that your plans and your chosen practitioner are just not compatible, you might even consider changing providers.

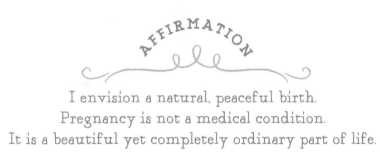

AFFIRMATION

I envision a natural, peaceful birth.
Pregnancy is not a medical condition.
It is a beautiful yet completely ordinary part of life.

A BIRTH PLAN REALITY CHECK

FROM NURSE/DOULA *maura*

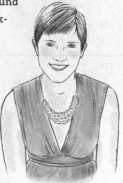

I've attended more than one hundred fifty births, and I have *never* found a birth plan to be helpful in the delivery room. That may sound shocking, but the truth is that no birth plan, no matter how meticulously written, can protect you from a difficult birth or unexpected complications on the big day.

So, does that mean you shouldn't bother writing one? No way! I have seen some amazing things come from a birth plan, although the benefits often kick in well before baby's birthday. One client in particular comes to mind. This mama was *prepared*: she enrolled in a natural childbirth education course, read all the books about birth and breastfeeding, hired a doula, and scoured the internet for evidence-based information. She and her husband were clear and confident about how they wanted things to proceed. But when they brought their birth plan along on their 36-week checkup, their healthcare provider scoffed at their wishes.

My client had planned to use intermittent monitoring with a Doppler—turns out that hospital policy dictated the use of continuous electronic fetal monitoring.

My client wanted to avoid receiving IV fluids during labor—her provider insisted that IV fluids were nonnegotiable.

My client had hoped that her water might break on its own—her provider told her it was standard practice to break the bag of waters upon admittance.

What did this woman do? She took her birth plan and *ran*. With only a few weeks left before delivery, she switched to a midwifery practice and ended up having exactly the birth she had wanted. The best part? Every aspect of her birth plan was followed so closely that she didn't even have to take it out during labor.

Just because a birth plan isn't (usually) much help when you're already in the thick of contractions doesn't mean that writing one can't be useful. A birth plan is a wonderful educational tool for you and your partner. It might even provide the last-minute reality check you need. Hopefully, you've been discussing your preferences with your midwife or doctor all along, but presenting a birth plan will help you determine if your wishes and your healthcare provider's standards of practice are truly compatible.

Know That Life Happens. I'd known long before I got pregnant that I wanted a vaginal birth, but I also knew there was always a chance of having a C-section. That's why my first birth plan included my preferences in the event that I ended up in the OR. (My highest priorities? Immediate skin-to-skin contact and immediate breastfeeding, if at all possible.) Nobody *wants* to think about all the things that could go wrong during delivery, of course, but you also don't want to be making important decisions in between contractions (for obvious reasons!). Check out the Gentle Cesarean chapter (Week 38) for ways to naturalize a surgical birth, if one proves necessary. Imagine all the possibilities now, and you'll feel more secure about your choices on baby's birthday.

Think About What Happens *After* **Birth, Too.** Mamas-to-be (and papas!) have lots of decisions to make relating to labor and delivery, but the decision making doesn't stop once you stop pushing. On the contrary, it's just getting started. Will you breastfeed or bottle-feed? Will you circumcise your son (and if so, when)? Will you be saving or donating baby's cord blood? While every birth plan is different, the following is a list of topics you'll want to start thinking about. (And don't worry if you don't know all these terms. We'll address them throughout the remainder of this book.)

DURING LABOR

Electronic Fetal Monitoring (EFM). Continuous or intermittent?

Freedom of Movement. Would you like to be up and walking around during labor? Permitted the use of a birthing ball, bar, or stool? Would you like to choose the position in which you deliver?

Eating and Drinking. Would you like the option to snack during labor? Administered IV fluids? Would you prefer to avoid getting a routine IV?

Pain Medication. Would you like pain medications to be made available only upon request? Would you like to be notified as soon as you're eligible for an epidural?

Induction and Labor Augmentation. Would you prefer to avoid the use of Pitocin, if possible? Have your bag of waters artificially broken or allowed to rupture naturally?

Photos and Video. Do you plan to hire a photographer or videographer?

Method of Delivery. Are you planning a vaginal, Cesarean, VBAC, or water birth?

AFTER DELIVERY

Mama-Baby Bonding. Is immediate skin-to-skin contact important to you? Would you like to delay routine newborn exams other than the APGAR?

Breastfeeding. Would you like to initiate breastfeeding ASAP? Would you like to meet with a lactation consultant? Would you like to avoid pacifiers, formula, artificial nipples, and supplementation?

Umbilical cord. Would you like to delay clamping of the umbilical cord? Do you plan to bank or donate the cord blood?

Placenta. Do you intend to save the placenta?

Routine Newborn Exams. Would you like to delay or decline any of the following routine newborn exams: heel prick, eye ointment, vitamin K shot, hepatitis B?

Newborn Bathing. Would you like to specify that baby's first bath be delayed? Performed only by you or your partner?

Circumcision. Yes or no?

IF BIRTHING VIA C-SECTION (WHETHER PLANNED OR UNEXPECTED)

Visitors. If possible, would you like your partner and/or doula present during the surgery?

Surgical Drape. If possible, would you prefer a clear surgical drape or a mirror to watch baby being delivered? Alternatively, would you prefer the drape to be lowered—or baby lifted—so you can catch a glimpse as soon as possible?

Style of Incision and Suturing. Would you prefer a low transverse incision? Single- or double-layer uterine suturing?

Vaginal Swab. Would you like a vaginal swab collected and wiped on baby's skin following delivery?

Mama-Baby Bonding. Would you like EKG or monitoring devices placed in areas that won't infringe on your ability to bond with your baby? Would you like immediate skin-to-skin contact? In the event that you cannot be conscious (i.e., you need general anesthesia), would you prefer that your partner be allowed

to hold baby skin-to-skin immediately after birth, barring any medical complications?

Breastfeeding. If possible, would you like to initiate breastfeeding immediately (while still in the operating room)?

NOM OF THE WEEK

Sauerkraut

As baby comes down the birth canal (covered in cheesy vernix), he'll pick up beneficial bacteria, which will help him establish a healthy microbiome. So this week, let's give your inner ecosystem a boost. The easiest (and cheapest) way to support gut health is to eat fermented foods, which are rich in lactic acid–producing bacteria. Unfortunately, most "fermented" foods on the market today aren't fermented *naturally*, so they don't offer much in the way of beneficial probiotics. Thankfully, you can make your own. I love this simple recipe for classic sauerkraut.

INGREDIENTS

1 small head organic green cabbage
1 tablespoon fine-grain Celtic sea salt
1 tablespoon caraway seeds
Filtered water

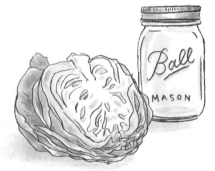

Finely chop the cabbage, wash and allow to dry for an hour or so, then place into a large glass bowl. Add salt and caraway seeds, and with clean hands, mix well. Let marinate for 10 to 15 minutes. Next, use your hands or a potato masher to smash the cabbage, releasing as much liquid as possible—this will serve as your brine. (If you're having trouble producing much liquid, add up to ¼ cup filtered water.) Pound and mix until you've got about ½ cup of liquid in your bowl. Transport the contents into a wide-mouthed half-gallon Mason jar. The brine should cover the cabbage as it protects it from mold. Leave at least an inch of space at the top of the jar for expansion. Cover loosely with a plastic lid or cloth, and let sit at room temperature for at least three days. Taste with a clean fork (no double-dipping) until the sourness is to your liking. The cabbage should be soft and have a zippy tang. Serve as a condiment with eggs, whole grains, burgers, or anything else that strikes your fancy. Recipe makes about thirty servings, and it should keep for about a month in the fridge.

MY NATURAL BIRTH PLAN

DURING LABOR

NO PAIN MEDICATION   FREE MOVEMENT   NATURAL WATER RUPTURE   INTERMITTENT MONITORING   LIGHTS DIM

WATER BIRTH   NO EPISIOTOMY   LIMITED CERVICAL EXAMS

AFTER DELIVERY

IMMEDIATE SKIN-TO-SKIN   DELAYED CORD CLAMPING   SAVE PLACENTA   PARTNER TO CUT CORD   BREASTFEEDING ASAP

NO VITAMIN K   NO HEPATITIS B   NO EYE OINTMENT   NO BATH FOR BABY   DELAY EXAMS FOR BONDING

PUTTING IT ALL TOGETHER: THE VISUAL ONE-PAGER

So, you've researched all your options, you've thought about the best- *and* worst-case scenarios, and now you're ready to put it all together. But how best to do that? Sure, you could just write all your preferences down or type them up in a bullet-point list. But—let's be honest here—who wants to read through all of that? A long list of instructions, especially one that spans several pages, is tedious for the reader. On the day of delivery, busy nurses and doctors just don't have time to flip through pages and pages of information. What's a mama to do?

Enter the one-page, visual birth plan—check out the sample opposite. It's simple, respectful, and clear; it provides information at a glance; and it's perfect for getting your birth wishes across without any resistance.

When you're ready, you can find a printable, customizable version of this birth plan—featuring these and many more icons—at mamanatural.com. (I know, I warned you about birth plans you can download from the internet. But this one has no blanks to fill out and contains no outdated medical info. You decide what's on it and what's not, so it will be uniquely yours!) Then, once you've created your plan, make sure to review it closely with your healthcare provider. You'll also want to share it with anyone who might be in the delivery room with you, including family members and your doula.

mama-do list

- Keep your birth plan short and sweet. Feeling compelled to write a birth plan from a defensive posture or write one that's several pages long may be a sign that you haven't chosen the right provider or birth location. If that's the case, think about making a switch. It's not too late!

- Once your midwife or doctor signs off on your birth plan, it should be added to your medical chart. However, don't forget to bring along several copies on the big day, in case there's a nurse shift-change. Pro tip: attach some mints or chocolates as a thank you treat—kindness goes a long way. Share it with the attendants when you check in at the hospital or birth center, and make sure everyone caring for you is on the same page.

- Complications can render parts of your birth plan irrelevant, so be prepared to be a little flexible on D-Day. Remember: your and baby's health is everyone's number one priority.

THE *third* TRIMESTER

feeling testy?

PART III

THIRD TRIMESTER
CHECKUPS AND SCREENINGS

WHAT'S UP WITH *baby*?

Yippee! We have officially entered the third—which is to say, *final*—trimester. Baby Natural is continuing to grow like a weed. She weighs a little more than 2 pounds now, and measures somewhere around 15 to 16 inches. But growing isn't the only thing she's doing this week: She's also started batting those pretty eyelashes at you, the little flirt. That's right. For the first time, she's opening her eyes, taking a look around the womb, and blinking. True, she can't actually *see* much of anything yet (it's not only dark in there, but her eyesight is quite poor). Sometime around Week 33, however, her pupils will begin to constrict and dilate, which means she may be able to make out some basic shapes—her hand in front of her face, perhaps, or the curve of the umbilical cord.

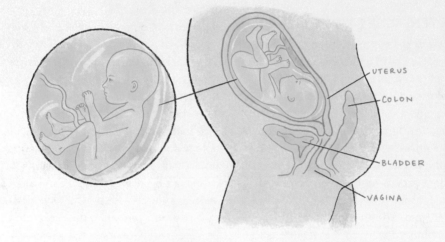

UTERUS

COLON

BLADDER

VAGINA

WHAT'S UP WITH *mama*?

Hey, Mama? Is it *hot* in here . . . or is it just me? Like, *Death Valley hot.* You might even be feeling positively menopausal—which is weird, considering the fact that you're pregnant. What's up with all the hot flashes? Turns out that feeling like a sweaty mess is another common pregnancy side effect, caused by—what else?—your surging hormones. In fact, your core temperature can actually rise by as much as a whole degree during pregnancy. Wearing natural fibers may help (since synthetic materials can trap heat), as can dressing in layers. You may also want to avoid caffeine, as hot flashes seem to be triggered by anxiety, stress, and blood sugar spikes. Reduce the temptation to forego your regular workouts—some studies suggest that working up a sweat can actually *prevent* hot flashes. Finally, let your partner know that the pregnant person in the relationship gets control of the thermostat. I'm pretty sure it's the law.

Given all the strain on your body—and your brain!—during the third trimester, it's a gift that you'll have considerably fewer decisions to make when it comes to prenatal testing from here on out. In fact, you likely won't even be offered many of the following tests unless your pregnancy has been designated high-risk or you go past your due date. Here's a quick rundown of the most common exams performed during the final three months.

THIRD TRIMESTER ULTRASOUND(S)

Nothin' special about the way ultrasounds are performed at this stage—however, you may notice significantly *less* of your baby on the screen, now that she's gotten so big!

IS THIS TEST RIGHT FOR YOU?

Assuming you're healthy, low-risk, and haven't had any problems with the pregnancy, there's rarely need for an ultrasound in the third trimester. They aren't routine, and if you have a more holistic healthcare provider, you likely won't even be offered one. In some cases, however, a late ultrasound *could* give you the all clear to proceed with a vaginal birth. For example, placenta previa—most often diagnosed during an anatomy ultrasound at the halfway point of pregnancy—is a condition that, given time, will almost always correct itself. (As the uterus continues to grow and stretch, a low-lying placenta often repositions itself higher in the womb, away from the cervix.) Confirming that your placenta has indeed relocated via an ultrasound may save you the need for an otherwise unnecessary C-section.

If, however, your doctor just wants to confirm that your baby hasn't gotten "too big," you might choose to decline additional screening. Ob-gyns often prefer to deliver "macrosomic" babies (a.k.a. big babies, weighing more than 8 pounds, 13 ounces) via Cesarean, even though it's not medically necessary to do so. The American College of Obstetricians and Gynecologists does not recommend a planned Cesarean due to size unless baby is *at least* 11 pounds, or 9 pounds 4 ounces if mama has gestational diabetes; and even then, Cesarean is only an option. Further complicating matters? Ultrasound estimates of baby's weight can be off by as much as a pound or two, so the estimate you receive may not even be accurate.

Make sure you understand exactly why your provider wants to order an ultrasound. And remember that you can always negotiate how detailed the procedure will be. If your doctor or midwife just wants to double-check that baby is head down, for example, she may be able to take a quick peek herself, rather than sending you out for a lengthier screening.

NON-STRESS TEST

A non-stress test, or NST, is a way of confirming baby's well-being in utero by monitoring his heart rate over a twenty- to thirty-minute period. To do that, two monitors will be strapped to your belly, one that detects contractions (the frequency of them, not the strength), and another that detects baby's heartbeat. This is actually the same setup you'll experience if you choose to undergo continuous electronic fetal monitoring once you're

Crunchy Kale Chips

Now that baby's winking and blinking, let's support the health of her developing peepers with a hefty dose of lutein and zeaxanthin. Say what? Okay, in *human speak*, these carotenoids are considered some of the most important vitamins for maintaining good eye health. In fact, quite a few studies suggest that they can protect against cataracts and age-related eye diseases, including macular degeneration. Kale—often called the king of green leafy veggies—is loaded with lutein and zeaxanthin (not to mention folate, iron, potassium, and vitamins A, C, and K). And for those who love to crunch and munch, these easy-to-make kale chips are an awesome alternative to, well, just about every other chip on the market.

INGREDIENTS

2 pounds curly kale (curly kale makes for a milder, crispier chip than lacinato or dinosaur)

1 tablespoon olive oil

Salt and pepper to taste

Optional toppings:

¼ cup grated Parmesan

¼ cup nutritional yeast flakes

Red pepper flakes

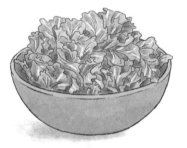

Preheat the oven to 275°F. Remove kale stems, wash and dry leaves well, then chop into small, bite-sized pieces. Place the pieces in a large bowl with all remaining ingredients. Massage the oil and spices into the leaves. Arrange the chips in a single layer on two cookie sheets lined with parchment paper. Bake for 20 to 30 minutes, or until chips are slightly crispy. Let cool and enjoy. Store any leftovers in an airtight container.

in labor. Together, the monitors will create a "tracing," a.k.a. a paper printout (which looks a bit like the results of a mini lie-detector test, if you ask me). This allows your midwife or doctor to see the heart rate pattern, as well as determine how well baby's heart rate responds to contractions—assuming you're having any.

What your healthcare provider *wants* to see is a lot of variability in the heart rate, which indicates that baby is doing well and is in good health. Decelerations, or decreases in the heart rate, on the other hand, suggest that baby is perhaps not doing so well, and delivery—whether by induction or C-section—may

SHOULD I BANK MY BABY'S CORD BLOOD?

In the last decade or so, preserving, or "banking," the blood from a newborn's umbilical cord has become a surprisingly common practice among new parents. But . . . *why?* And—more to the point—should *you* do it?

Cord blood is loaded with stem cells, which are capable of growing into specialized cells throughout the human body (think: brain cells, blood cells, nerve cells, etc.). It's this ability to morph into virtually any type of healthy tissue that makes them ideal for treating a wide array of blood-based disorders, certain cancers, and immune deficiencies. In fact, cord blood transplants have already been used to treat more than seventy different diseases, and stem cell therapy is an exploding field of medical research. Which is exactly why so many people are scrambling to save it: on the off chance that your child developed a life-threatening illness, his or her cord blood might provide the cure.

Banking baby's cord blood, however, doesn't come cheap. It's also not without controversy. For one thing, there are a slew of private cord blood banks in the United States, but the industry is loosely regulated, so they're not all equally reputable. (A 2014 investigative report in the *Wall Street Journal* unearthed instances of contaminated or degraded samples, dirty storage conditions, and banks going out of business.) The odds are also extremely low that you'll ever use it. Diseases that might be treatable with cord blood are themselves rare. Certain genetic conditions are not treatable with cord blood at all (because the blood itself would contain the same defect). It's also possible there wouldn't be *enough* blood, since only a few ounces of blood are extracted from the cord, which may contain an adequate number of cells for a transplant. As for how much it costs, you're looking at anywhere from $1,000 to $2,000 up front (for collection and registration), and an addition $100 to $200 a year for storage. For these reasons and more, the American Academy of Pediatrics and the American College of Obstetricians and Gynecologists actually discourage private cord blood banking when used as "biological insurance"—in other words, "just in case." Better, more appropriate candidates for private storage are those with a family history of disease that might require a stem cell transplant (say, a sibling or relative with leukemia), or ethnic minorities, who might have a harder time finding a match from a public bank.

Yes, match. You see, private banking is not your only option. There are also a number of public banks to which you could *donate* your child's cord blood (which is free), but there's no guarantee you'd have access to that blood should you need it. However, choosing to forego private banking doesn't mean your child would have no hope for a transplant if he needed one, provided he could find a matching donor. In contrast to private banking, most major medical associations are advocates of public storage.

If you're interested in cord blood donation, check out the National Marrow Donor Program (bethematch.org), where you'll find a list of hospitals across the country that collect cord blood. If your hospital participates, you can contact the public bank with which

$\longrightarrow$

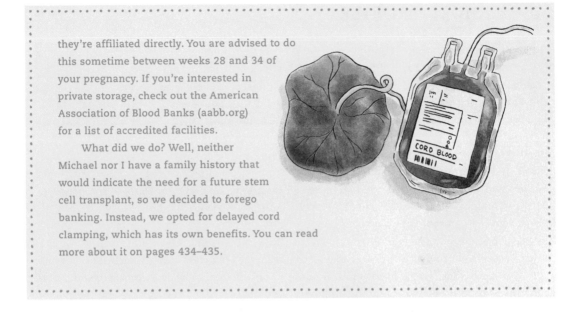

they're affiliated directly. You are advised to do this sometime between weeks 28 and 34 of your pregnancy. If you're interested in private storage, check out the American Association of Blood Banks (aabb.org) for a list of accredited facilities.

What did we do? Well, neither Michael nor I have a family history that would indicate the need for a future stem cell transplant, so we decided to forego banking. Instead, we opted for delayed cord clamping, which has its own benefits. You can read more about it on pages 434–435.

be a good option. Based on the results of the test, your baby will be classified as "reactive" or "nonreactive." A nonreactive result might indicate the need for additional testing, in particular the biophysical profile (more on that in a bit).

IS THIS TEST RIGHT FOR YOU?

For women who are low-risk, the most common reason to undergo a non-stress test is because you've gone past your due date. In fact, many providers will recommend repeat NSTs—as often as one or two times a week—once you hit 40 or 41 weeks. Some mamas, however, may start undergoing NSTs a bit earlier if they have gestational diabetes or pre-eclampsia, are over the age of thirty-five, or if an abnormality was detected via ultrasound.

Because active babies tend to have more variability and accelerations in their heart rate—which is what we *want* to see—it's a good idea to eat and drink a little something just prior to the procedure to perk her up a bit. It will take longer to get an accurate reading if baby is sleeping.

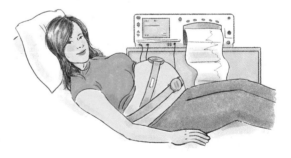

NON-STRESS TEST

BIOPHYSICAL PROFILE

A biophysical profile, or BPP, actually consists of two separate tests: (1) a non-stress test—the exact same version described on the previous pages, after which your baby will be given a "reactive" or "nonreactive" classification—and (2) an ultrasound. During the ultrasound portion, baby's movements, breathing, and muscle tone, as well as the amniotic fluid level, will be assessed and scored, for a total possible score of 10. Anything between 8 and 10 suggests that baby is doing well; a score of 6 or below, however, may indicate some level of fetal distress. In these cases, your midwife or doctor may order a follow-up BPP within twenty-four hours or may want to induce you, depending on how far along you are in the pregnancy.

IS THIS TEST RIGHT FOR YOU?

Like the NST, biophysical profiles are most commonly ordered for low-risk women when they've gone past their due date. Mamas who are expecting multiples, who've had a previous stillbirth, who have medical issues or who are expecting a baby with a genetic or congenital abnormality may be asked to submit to a biophysical profile, too. You'll want to eat and drink a little something just prior to the procedure—again, just like a regular NST. You'll also want to drink plenty of water in the twenty-four hours leading up to the test, because dehydration can lower the level of amniotic fluid in the womb. Low fluid levels can be a reason to induce labor. If the level of amniotic fluid is the only low score on the test, however, you may consider asking to repeat the procedure within twenty-four hours after hydrating adequately (i.e., drinking at least two liters of fluid). By doing so, you could avoid induction.

GROUP B STREP

Group B Strep (GBS) is a type of bacteria that exists naturally (and harmlessly) in about 25 percent of women but can (in rare cases) cause infection and serious complications if it spreads to the baby. That's why all pregnant women in the United States are tested—via a vaginal and anal swab—prior to birth, usually between 35 and 37 weeks. (Occasionally, GBS is detected during a routine urine test, in which case mama will be categorized as a "heavy colonizer" and considered to be GBS-positive for the remainder of her pregnancy.) GBS-positive mamas are typically treated with antibiotics during labor.

IS THIS TEST RIGHT FOR YOU?

We'll go over Group B Strep testing in detail in Week 35.

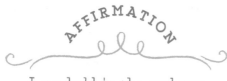

AFFIRMATION

I am held in the embrace of my Creator, just as I hold my baby in my womb. I am loved.

BASIC BLOOD WORK

Lab work at this stage (usually ordered sometime between weeks 26 and 30) isn't generally as comprehensive. In fact, third trimester blood work is often performed around the same time as the glucose screen, so you might actually undergo these tests nearer the end of the second trimester. In addition to another "complete blood count," you'll have something called a rapid plasma reagin (RPR), which screens for syphilis, and the GC/CT, which checks for gonorrhea and chlamydia. Both the RPR and the GC/CT are repeats, by the way; you were screened for all three STIs way back in the first trimester.

IS THIS TEST RIGHT FOR YOU?

Yup! As with all blood tests, this is completely noninvasive and therefore risk-free. Some women do choose to decline the RPR and GC/CT if they've already tested negative at some point during the pregnancy. Keep in mind, however, that all three STIs (syphilis, gonorrhea, and chlamydia) are caused by bacterial infections, and all three can infect baby either before or during delivery. Women under the age of twenty-five or who in engage in "high-risk" sexual activity are particularly encouraged to retest in the third trimester. If you're planning to decline erythromycin, an antibiotic eye ointment given to almost all babies within twenty-four hours of birth (we'll talk plenty more about this soon; for now just know that erythromycin prevents STI-related eye infections in newborns), you also may want to move forward with this screening. After all, it certainly can't hurt.

mama-do list

- Now that you're in the third trimester, you want to start monitoring your baby's movements in utero. Pick a time of day when your baby is active, like mid-morning or right before dinner. Get still and start counting all of your baby's kicks, rolls, jabs, and wiggles. Do so until you feel ten distinct movements. Repeat this daily, preferably at the same time. If you notice changes in your baby's movement pattern, call your midwife or doctor right away. By doing this important daily practice, you could potentially save your baby's life. Go to countthekicks.org to learn more.

- Have a chat with your partner this week about the pros and cons of cord blood banking. If you're planning to go the private storage route—which may be an appropriate choice for you if you have a family history of certain diseases—you'll want to start doing your research. Cord blood banks suggest making contact before 34 weeks.

- Make sure you're staying adequately hydrated, *especially* in the event your healthcare provider orders a biophysical profile. Too little hydration can lead to low amniotic fluid, which ups your chance for induction. Bottoms up!

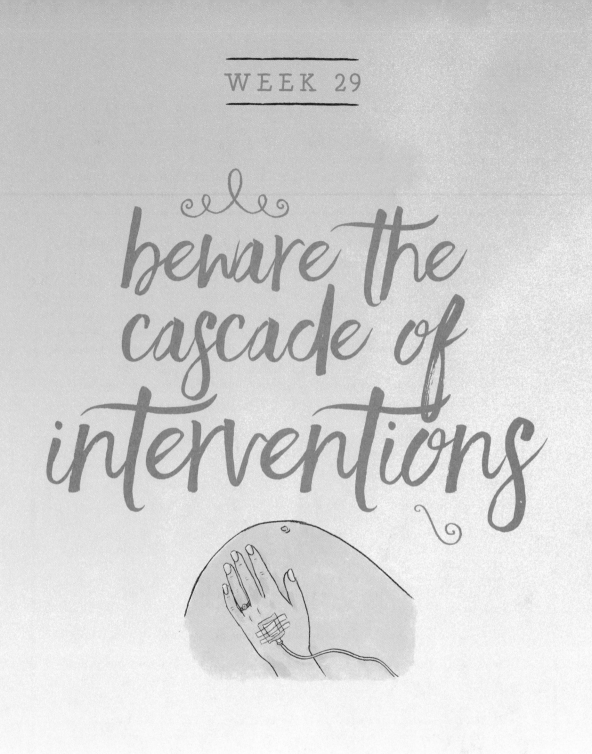

beware the cascade of interventions

WHAT'S UP WITH *baby*?

Welp, this week your little peach is approaching 3 whole pounds in weight and 17 inches in length, Mama. Come to think of it, that makes him less like a peach—and more like a large butternut squash. As for your uterus? Your healthcare provider has been diligently measuring its *fundal height*—that is, the distance from your pubic bone to the top of the womb—at each of your prenatal appointments. And as of a few weeks ago, the measurement started to correspond with the progression of your pregnancy. In other words, at 29 weeks, the fundal height should be around 29 centimeters. (By 36 to 38 weeks, your uterus will be sitting right up under the sternum, a.k.a. the breastbone. Hello heartburn!)

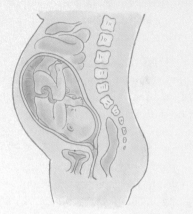 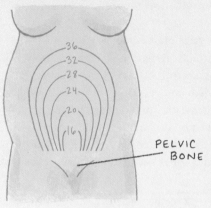

PELVIC BONE

WHAT'S UP WITH *mama*?

Blood volume isn't the only thing that increases during pregnancy, Mama. You're carrying around a lot of extra fluid now, too. While this fluid helps your body and joints to expand in preparation for delivery, it can sometimes lead to edema. That's the technical term for swelling, which most often occurs in the hands, legs, feet, and cankles—you know, the place where you *used* to have ankles. Here's the thing: a certain amount of swelling during pregnancy is normal. Pressure on the vena cava slows the circulatory system, causing blood and fluid to pool in your lower extremities. Relaxin, meanwhile, causes the bones in your feet to spread, which is why you may suddenly be sporting Hobbit feet. (If you have *sudden* swelling, or swelling that doesn't seem to improve overnight, call your midwife or doctor, as this can sometimes be a sign of preeclampsia.) As for how to relieve it? Going for a walk first thing in the morning and elevating your feet at night may help. Sleeping on your left side exclusively can improve circulation too. Gentle skin brushing, starting at the feet and working up to the heart, can also promote healthy blood flow. And whenever possible, avoid sitting or standing for long periods of time.

Some midwives and doulas believe that the minute you step into a hospital and put on that gown, you've had your first official birth intervention.

Does that sound a bit overdramatic? I mean, the hospital gown *does* have a purpose. For one thing, it keeps your regular clothes from getting stained with blood, bodily fluids, or poop (both your baby's and your *own*). In the event of an emergency, that easy-access gown helps your birth team do their thing. And furthermore, it's just a hospital gown! What possible difference could it make whether you agree to wear one or not?

For plenty of mamas, not a lick. Some women actually prefer the gown to their own clothes (and certainly, having one less item to launder when you get home isn't a bad thing). But the significance of the gown, I think, is this: It's the first domino to fall. It's the first action many mamas perform without giving it a second thought. They just put it on because

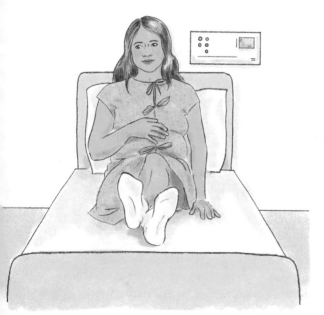

they're "supposed" to, or because they're expected to, or because putting on the gown is just part of giving birth these days. Right?

The problem, however, is that many women submit to far more than a uniform—like, a whole host of "routine" procedures and protocols because they believe they're "supposed to," without questioning one bit. They don't realize that each seemingly innocuous intervention may lead to another and another and another.

Before you know it, the few minor interventions you accepted—just to "move things along"—have derailed your plans for a natural childbirth.

This is the Cascade of Interventions we've spent so much time talking about, a symptom of the medical management approach to labor and delivery, and arguably one of the main reasons the United States has such a high C-section rate.

I know what you're thinking. Isn't the health and safety of my baby more important than going *au naturel*? Of course, it is. It's also true that some women will *need* a few—or perhaps many—interventions. I needed a "hit of Pit" when labor stalled during my first birth, and it may have saved me from an eventual forceps delivery or vacuum extraction. Not all interventions are bad. Not all interventions should be avoided (on the contrary, some can be lifesaving). But not all interventions are *necessary*—even though they may seem as harmless as that hospital gown.

That's why it's important to understand the ways in which one *elective* intervention might lead to a slew of interventions you *don't* want.

For most mamas—especially those laboring in a hospital—the Cascade of Interventions usually goes something like this:

INTERVENTION #1: THE ROUTINE IV

Shortly after putting on the hospital gown, you'll likely be hooked up to an IV, whether you need one right away or not. Why? There are a few reasons. Since the majority of women laboring in hospitals are denied food and drink, dehydration is a real concern, and an IV allows mama to get any fluids she needs dripped straight into her veins. (Wait a minute. Wouldn't it be easier to let her drink some water or juice? Of course, it would! However, concerns about the potential danger of aspiration—in the unlikely event that you're put under general anesthesia—linger, despite the fact that the American Society of Anesthesiologists has called the practice of restricting food and drink both unnecessary and unwarranted.) An all-ready-in-place IV also makes it easier to administer medications, from antibiotics to labor-inducing drugs like Pitocin. And, truth be told, having an IV in place can certainly be helpful in an emergency: no need to fiddle with getting a line in place.

But there are some disadvantages associated with a routine IV, too.

In the event that you're receiving fluids or drugs, you'll be tethered to an IV pole, which limits mobility. If your labor turns out to be a long one (think: twenty hours or more) it's actually possible to receive too much fluid; large amounts of fluid have been linked to edema (a.k.a. swelling in the extremities), as well as engorgement of the breasts, which can affect breastfeeding. And believe it or not, IV tubing and bags are riddled with phthalates. While there aren't any studies that focus on the effects of IV-related phthalate exposure during labor, several studies *have* indicated a higher rate of ADHD among critically ill children who spend significant time in the ICU or NICU. One type of phthalate in particular,

DEHP, has been permanently banned from toys and care products intended for use by children under the age of twelve due to its potential toxicity, yet it's still present in medical tubing.

To be clear, you should never refuse IV therapy when it's medically necessary just because you're concerned about potential phthalate exposure. But doesn't it make sense to *avoid* exposure when IVs *aren't* necessary?

Potential Alternatives: If you're laboring at a birth center, you likely won't be offered a "routine" IV at all. Most birth centers support a woman's right to eat and drink as she pleases. If, however, you're laboring at a hospital and don't want a routine IV, just say so. (Better yet, discuss this with your doctor or midwife well in advance, and add "no routine IV" to your birth plan.) Keep in mind that in certain circumstances, you *must* have one: if you opt for an epidural, for example. Know, too, that many ob-gyns will insist that you have one "just in case."

Rather than strapping mama to an IV pole straight out of the gate, some nurses will instead offer you a "saline lock" or a "heparin lock." In both cases, a flexible catheter (a.k.a. a thin, hollow tube) with be threaded into a vein in your hand; at the end of the tube is a small chamber that's then filled (or "locked") with saline or heparin (a blood thinner) to prevent clotting. Saline and hep locks give hospital staff access to an open vein should an emergency arise, but you won't be tethered to an IV pole in the meantime. You can decline a saline or hep lock, but if hospital policy dictates that you must have an IV, these are your best options.

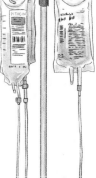

INTERVENTION #2:
CONTINUOUS ELECTRONIC FETAL MONITORING

I've been saying it for pages and pages now: continuous electronic fetal monitoring restricts your movement during labor and is associated with higher rates of eventual C-section. But *why?*

During labor, your baby's heart rate will fluctuate in response to the pattern of your contractions. When the uterine muscles clamp down and clench together, for example, blood flow to the baby is temporarily restricted. Decreased blood flow, in turn, temporarily restricts the amount of oxygen making its way to your baby, which lowers baby's heart rate. When your contraction ends and the uterine muscles relax, however, blood flow returns to normal, oxygen levels increase, and the fetal heart rate rises. This is a normal, natural, safe phenomenon. Minor fluctuations occur during every woman's labor. Occasionally, however, blood flow is restricted too much or for too long. In that case, the fetal heart rate will drop significantly, which can be a sign of fetal distress. If baby's heart rate cannot or will not return to normal, any number of interventions might become necessary to ensure his safe delivery, all the way up to and including emergency C-section.

With me so far? Okay, because here's where things get a little more complicated:

Back in the 1940s and '50s, it was thought that fetal hypoxia—that is, lack of oxygen to the baby while in utero—was the primary cause of stillbirth, mental retardation, cerebral palsy, and other types of neurological damage in newborns. And in those days, a relatively high number of babies were born with these types of issues. (Not surprisingly, these babies were disproportionately born to high-risk women.) But the only way to monitor the fetal heartbeat was with a fetoscope (a stethoscope-like instrument pressed to mama's belly) via a technique called auscultation.

You can imagine, then, why electronic fetal monitoring (EFM)— first introduced in the late 1950s—was almost immediately considered to be a superior technique. I mean, here was a fancy *machine* (presumably more accurate and more sensitive than the human ear), that could provide a steady, constant stream of important information! Even though EFM was originally intended for high-risk pregnancies

only, its use exploded. By the mid-1970s, EFM had become a standard of care during labor. And today, it's near universal. Continuous electronic fetal monitoring is the most common birth intervention, used in more than 85 percent of American births.

As EFM became ubiquitous, however, research into the actual benefits of the practice began to produce some unexpected results. Turns out, for example, that a baby must be deprived of oxygen for a longer period than previously thought before problems develop. When it comes to cerebral palsy, fetal hypoxia is rarely the cause (intrauterine infection is more frequently to blame). Further complicating matters, the heart-rate patterns printed by the electronic monitor must be *interpreted*. In other words, there is no super-precise definition for what exactly constitutes "fetal distress." What one doctor considers nonreassuring may differ widely from another doctor's interpretation. And that's one of the reasons EFM is associated with "false alarms" or high

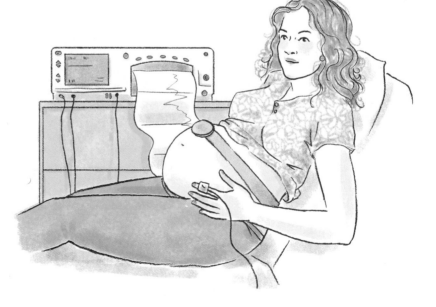

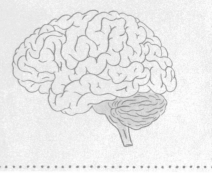
false-positive rates. According to the American College of Obstetricians and Gynecologists, the false-positive rate for predicting cerebral palsy via EFM is *greater than 99 percent*.

This means that babies who aren't really in distress are more likely to be ushered into the world via C-section (unnecessarily). Furthermore, research has shown that EFM does not improve infant mortality rates, is not associated with higher APGAR scores, does not lessen admissions to the NICU, nor does it lessen instances of low-oxygen-related brain damage. Put another way: Electronic fetal monitoring does not improve fetal outcomes when used by low-risk women. And if all that weren't

enough, submitting to continuous monitoring can require mama to labor flat on her back, stuck in a bed, which not only compresses the pelvis but also constricts some of her major blood vessels, which—ironically—can deprive the baby of oxygen. Yeesh.

Potential Alternatives: If you're low-risk and your labor is progressing normally, you can request "intermittent auscultation"—that is, intermittent fetal heart rate monitoring via handheld Doppler—instead of EFM. Understand that intermittent auscultation is different than "intermittent EFM," which would require you to strap up to the electronic monitor for 10 to 15 minutes every hour. Understand, too, that your ability to request intermittent auscultation will depend on hospital policy; some ob-gyns will insist on continuous electronic monitoring. And, of course, some mamas might prefer continuous monitoring, for various reasons. If that's the case, you can inquire about telemetry—a.k.a. wireless monitoring. It's not available everywhere and it won't improve the risk of false-positives, but it will improve mobility during labor.

INTERVENTION #3: LABOR AUGMENTATION

During unmedicated, spontaneous labor, your body will at some point begin to produce oxytocin, one of the hormones that triggers contractions. (Although it's worth pointing out: Oxytocin has a lot of other functions, too. It's commonly referred to as the "cuddle hormone" or the "love hormone" because it facilitates mama-baby bonding after birth. It's also secreted when people snuggle, hug, or bond socially.) But unlike some other hormones involved in babymaking—which might be produced primarily in the ovaries and/or the placenta—Oxytocin is secreted in the *brain*. And as it's released, it triggers the release of other hormones, most notably endorphins, your body's natural pain relievers.

When a mama is induced or her labor is otherwise interfered with, however, her body doesn't always respond as it normally would. In other words, she may not produce enough oxytocin to get contractions going. When that happens, doctors have a number of ways to augment labor. One of the most common is to start you on Pitocin.

Pitocin is a synthetic version of oxytocin, but as should be obvious, it is *not* the same thing. It's unclear, for example, if the synthetic stuff ever makes it to mama's brain—and if it does, exactly how her brain might respond. In fact, it's thought that an influx of the artificial hormone may signal her body to stop producing the real stuff. Research suggests that women who are given Pitocin during labor secrete significantly less oxytocin when breastfeeding.

The other problem with Pitocin? It can make your contractions much more intense, much closer together, and therefore much more painful. The intensity of these artificially augmented contractions can also lead to fetal distress—baby doesn't have enough time to recover between contractions, and the prolonged reduction of blood flow and oxygen may cause his heart rate to drop. And since you'll be hooked up to an electronic monitor, your doctor will be hyperaware of each and every deceleration, which only increases your chance of winding up in the operating room. Use of Pitocin is also associated with lower APGAR scores, as well as unexpected admission to the NICU. Despite these risks, use of Pitocin—just like induction of labor—has doubled since 1990.

Potential Alternatives: It's important to point out that Pitocin does have its uses. When administered conservatively, it can give a woman whose labor has stalled just the boost she needs. It may even prevent the need for additional, more invasive interventions. Before consenting to Pitocin, however, you may want to give nipple stimulation a try instead. Stimulating the nipples (either via manual massage or with the use of a breast pump) triggers the release of mom's oxytocin. It's true that nipple massage, on its own, wasn't enough to get *my* labor going again—after twenty-plus hours, I still needed that hit of Pit—but I absolutely felt a surge in my contractions. Trust me when I say the technique is surprisingly effective.

INTERVENTION #4: EPIDURAL

Ah, the epidural. It's one of the most common interventions out there—administered to anywhere between 60 percent and 85 percent of laboring mamas—and it's not hard to understand why. I mean, who in the *world* would want to give birth without one? Some mamas know they'll opt for pain relief not long after getting a glimpse of that positive pregnancy test. Others, however, will choose to go the epidural route only after having been given Pitocin (because, again, Pitocin-induced contractions tend to be more intense, closer together, and more painful).

Unfortunately, epidurals come with their own set of side effects. As with other interventions, they can interrupt mama's natural cascade of labor-related hormones. So if after getting the epidural, you stop having efficient contractions (due to the suppression of oxytocin), you may now require Pitocin to get things going again. And that's assuming you haven't *already* been "pitted."

It's worth mentioning that epidurals are not as strong as they once were—back in the 1980s and early '90s, they typically contained a more concentrated dose of local anesthetic. Still, it's possible that you'll be too numb to push effectively when the time comes, which is why your doctor may want to "turn it down" when you're ready to deliver the baby. The problem? If you're not producing your own oxytocin, you're not releasing endorphins (your body's natural pain relievers), which means that turning down the epidural can, frankly, hurt. A lot. And that renders the point of having had an epidural pretty much moot.

On the flip side, there are cases in which an epidural can be hugely beneficial. Some women, for example, might be battling a great deal of fear, which can cause extreme tension in the body. An epidural can help these mamas relax. In other cases, a woman may just be plain exhausted after an extended labor, and an epidural may help her rest (or even sleep) so she can be reenergized for the final stage of pushing. Epidurals aren't always harmful or unnecessary. I do believe, however, that they're often relied on too early, and too often.

Savory Quiche Muffins

Suffering from unsightly swelling? I can relate. I puffed up considerably near the end of my first pregnancy, but experienced virtually *zero* swelling the second time around—seriously, even my wedding ring fit the same. The difference? Upping my protein intake, à la the Brewer Diet (flip back to page 32 if you need a refresher). Meat is an excellent source of protein, of course, but there are other options, too: Greek yogurt, cheese, legumes, nuts, seeds, nutritional yeast flakes, and eggs.

Speaking of eggs, they were demonized throughout the 1980s and '90s for their cholesterol content, but they're actually one of the world's most perfect foods. They're rich in vitamin B$_{12}$, selenium, and leucine (an important amino acid). They're also an inexpensive source of protein. But the true star player in eggs is choline, which is vital for the development of baby's brain and spinal cord. In fact, some studies suggest that choline may act like folate in protecting your child from neural tube defects. You can bake, fry, poach, or scramble 'em, of course, but try mixing it up in the morning with these savory quiche muffins.

INGREDIENTS

6 organic eggs

2 cups raw organic spinach, chopped

¼ cup organic sundried tomatoes, chopped

½ cup organic grated cheddar or Colby cheese

Salt, pepper, and hot sauce to taste

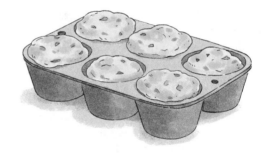

Start by preheating your oven to 350°F. Beat your eggs, then add remaining ingredients and combine. Into a greased cupcake tin (use olive oil or softened butter), pour your egg mixture, leaving a half inch of space to allow for rising. Bake for 25 minutes, or until muffins are slightly browned. Serve warm, with fresh fruit.

Potential Alternatives: We'll talk in-depth about alternative pain-relief methods in Week 34. For now, just know that if you opt for an epidural, it's not a stand-alone intervention. You'll be required to submit to continuous electronic fetal monitoring, you'll almost certainly be given IV fluids (which can reduce the likelihood of a drop in maternal blood pressure), and you may be given a urinary catheter, too.

INTERVENTION #5: CESAREAN

Any and all of the interventions described already could potentially increase your risk of eventual Cesarean. Perhaps the Pitocin-induced contractions become too stressful for baby, or the readings from your fetal monitor indicate "distress" (when really it's just a false alarm). The number one cause of unplanned Cesarean in first-time mamas, however, isn't fetal distress, poor positioning of the baby in utero, or a medical complication: it's a labor that progresses "too slowly."

Now prepare yourself for the ironic part.

Women giving birth today labor longer—2.5 hours longer, on average—than women who gave birth a half-century ago. Why? Researchers at the National Institutes of Health attribute at least some of that difference to the prevalence of birth interventions. In other words, when we interfere with a woman's natural hormonal cascade, we end up artificially *prolonging* the birth process.

We know, for example, that epidurals prolong labor—not by one hour (as previously thought) but by at least two or three, according to a 2014 study published in *Obstetrics & Gynecology*. We also know that considerably more women are induced these days (nearly 24 percent in 2010, compared to less than 10 percent in 1990), even though artificial induction is associated with a higher risk of stalled labor.

The standard physicians use to determine how long a "normal" labor should last, however—a graph called the Friedman's Curve—was published back in 1955, a time during which general anesthesia was a routine practice, but the use of interventions such as epidurals and Pitocin wasn't nearly so common. Put another way: we artificially prolong labor with the use of (often unnecessary) interventions, but then we operate on mamas when they don't progress "quickly" enough.

It's a wonder the C-section rate isn't *higher*.

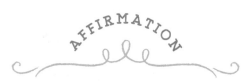

AFFIRMATION

Most babies are born perfectly healthy. Most mamas deliver without significant complications. I embrace the unknown. It's all part of the glorious design.

Interventions—from induction to fetal monitoring to Pitocin to Cesarean—definitely have their place. In fact, they can be a godsend for mamas (and babies!) who need them. The evidence is pretty clear, however, that most mamas don't need them, and they certainly don't need *all* of them *all* of the time. The crux of the issue is knowing when to accept interventions—and when not to. Sometimes that's the hardest part. (That's why I love the BRAIN acronym, on page 294!)

But fear not, Mama. As your due date approaches, we'll talk plenty more how about you can avoid the Cascade (or at least the parts that are unnecessary), whether you're giving birth at home, at a birth center, or even in a hospital.

~ mama-do list ~

- Don't want to wear a scratchy hospital gown during labor? You don't have to. Seriously—there's no law that says you have to put the thing on. If you're going to forego the gown, however, start thinking about what you *would* like to wear. My advice? Forget fashion. Go for comfort. Think: oversized cotton nightgown or tank top with stretchy skirt.

- One of the main reasons women opt for induction is because they've gone past their due date. Worried about missing yours? More on the inaccuracy of due dates—and the reasons you might want to let baby come out on his own—coming up soon!

- Some mamas *need* interventions, so don't be worried if your midwife or doctor suggests one (or several). Just know that in most cases—assuming you're low-risk and baby is healthy—you have options.

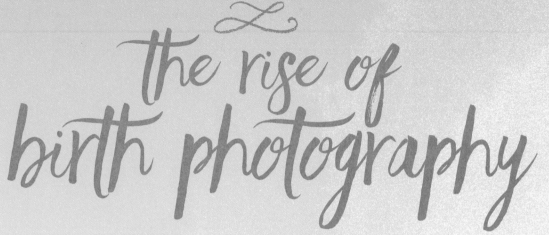

the rise of birth photography

AND OTHER WAYS TO DOCUMENT YOUR BIRTH

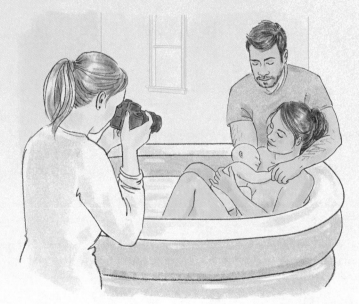

WHAT'S UP WITH *baby*?

Baby's still hovering around 17 inches long, but she's crossed the 3-pound threshold—so only a small jump in height, but a giant leap in weight over the past few weeks. This trend will only continue. She'll grow a few more inches, but she'll double or perhaps even triple her body mass. In fact, from this point forward she'll gain about half a pound per week, all the way up until D-Day. Go, baby, go! This fat she's packing on (and most of the weight gain now is fat) will help her skin appear a little smoother and a little less wrinkly. It'll also keep her warm, which means she doesn't need that coat of lanugo anymore. It's starting to shed away now—just don't be surprised if it's not *entirely* gone when you two officially meet face-to-face. A little bit of residual lanugo, even in full-term babies, is totally normal. (And totally cute!)

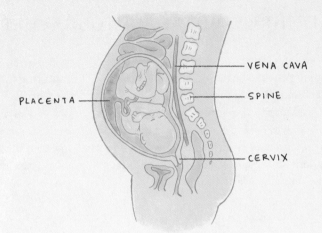

PLACENTA

VENA CAVA

SPINE

CERVIX

WHAT'S UP WITH *mama*?

If you're dealing with hemorrhoids, there's a good chance you might have noticed the appearance of varicose veins—those bulging, ropey lines that protrude through the skin—on your legs, thighs, and buttocks now, too. Why? Because all of these conditions, unfortunately, are related. The increase in blood volume causes the blood vessels to expand (making them more visible), while pressure on the vena cava increases pressure in the leg veins. Although they can sometimes cause itching or mild discomfort, the good news is that varicose veins are typically just a cosmetic issue. And while there's no "cure" per se, you can alleviate some of the discomforts by avoiding sitting or standing for long periods of time, sleeping exclusively on your left side, and elevating your feet in the evenings. Regular exercise can help, too, as it boosts circulation. Some crunchy mamas rave about an herbal formulation called CirculaTone. You might also want to purchase a pair of pregnancy support hose (the pressure stimulates blood flow back up toward the heart). These days you can actually find jazzy legwarmer-style compression socks if you feel like rocking an '80s look.

There's one aspect of each of my kids' births that you could definitely say was atypical.

And no, I'm not talking about having gone *au naturel* and drug-free, but rather the fact that both births were filmed, with the intention of sharing the footage with the world.

Such is the nature of running a natural birth and parenting website.

However, Michael and I aren't the only ones who wanted to document our big day: turns out, a growing number of parents-to-be are adding a professional photographer to their birth teams. That's right, birth photography—both still and moving images—has become another big trend in the delivery room.

WHY HIRE A BIRTH PHOTOGRAPHER?

There are few moments more intimate for a couple than the birth of their child, so it's understandable that most people—when hearing about birth photography for the first time—tend to balk at the idea. And that initial disbelief is usually followed by one pressing question: *You're going to hire a stranger . . . to point a camera . . . down there?!*

Birth photography, however, isn't about capturing the goo and gore of delivery (photographers generally don't take "crowning shots" unless you ask them to). Once you get over the initial weirdness, this is one trend that actually makes quite a bit of sense. We hire wedding photographers as a matter of course, and the birth of a child is easily as momentous of an

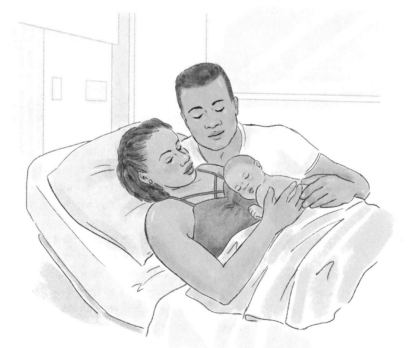

occasion. And aside from ensuring one heck of a birth announcement photo, there are some distinct advantages to having a professional in the room:

♡ Labor and delivery is a whirlwind. Ask most mamas about their birth experiences and they'll typically tell you that they don't remember many of the details—not even those who labored for eight, ten, or even twenty-seven hours (like me!). The first hour or two after baby's arrival tend to whoosh by especially quickly. And no matter how present you were at the time, there are things you just won't realize were going on, as well as moments you just won't get to see: the look on your face when you meet your son or daughter, the reaction of your friends and family when your partner bursts into the waiting room to share the news. An experienced photographer knows which moments to look out for, and the photos she takes will help to cement these life-changing moments in a more permanent way.

♡ Hiring a pro takes the pressure off your partner. Couldn't I just have my husband or partner snap a few photos or shoot some video? you may be wondering. And yes, you certainly could. But that would mean that he's saddled with a camera when he should be focused on supporting you: applying

WHAT OTHER *natural mamas* SAY

jessica: My doula doubled as our birth photographer, and she captured the most beautiful photo of me holding my son while leaning back to kiss my husband. I highly recommend having someone there to take pictures—these are moments you'll want to remember forever!

amanda: I didn't plan on having photos taken because I didn't think I'd be comfortable showing that much skin to friends and strangers. However, God intervened during my first birth. I was about 7 centimeters dilated and experiencing steady, intense contractions when my friend arrived at the hospital to say a quick hello. Literally the instant she said "hi," I felt this incredible pressure and need to push. The nurse checked me and I was at 10 centimeters and crowning. Everyone set up quickly to catch the baby, and my friend got shoved into the room—she wasn't able to get out! So she picked up my camera and started filming and photographing the big event. She got to see a whole different side of me that evening, and I got some pretty incredible pictures!

barbara: I'm probably too cheap to hire a professional photographer, but I do wish I'd taken more pictures in the first few hours after birth, especially of skin-to-skin bonding, footprinting, weighing the baby, etc.

NOT INTO BIRTH PHOTOGRAPHY?
THINK ABOUT DOCUMENTING YOUR
PREGNANCY INSTEAD

Believe it or not, you might just miss being pregnant. Strange, I know. Who would miss morning sickness, heartburn, or middle-of-the-night wake-ups?

Let me tell you, Mama. *I do.* Now that I'm on the other side, probably for good, I miss the little things. Feeling those kicks. Patting (and marveling) at my expanding belly. I loved being able to eat like a linebacker, and participating in what is truly a miracle. (And don't even get me *started* about breastfeeding!)

That's why I encourage you to document these moments. Keep track of the journey. Trust me, you'll appreciate it someday (and your children will, too!). Here are some ideas to get you started:

Maternity Photos

You might not always feel beautiful during pregnancy, but you *are*. I mean, have you checked yourself out lately? Now is a great time to capture that glow by setting up a maternity photo shoot. You can hire a professional, of course—in fact, many birth photographers offer maternity, birth, and newborn packages. You can have a talented friend get behind the lens. Or—and hear me out on this—you might think about having your partner take some

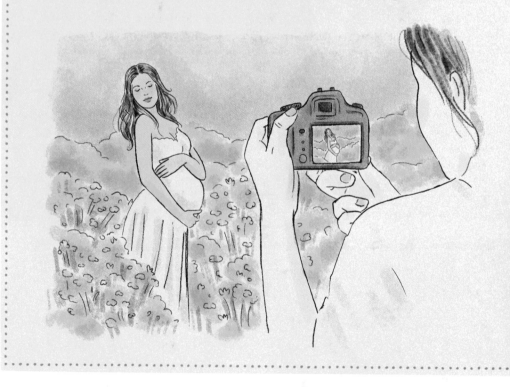

(tasteful!) nude photos. The pregnant body is all about womanhood in full bloom, and it's worth celebrating. Papa Natural took some shots of me *in the buff* right around 34 weeks, and though I cringed at the time, I'm glad to have those photos now.

Belly Casting

Ever break a bone and get a cast? *Belly casting is a similar concept*—just, you know, without the pain or the trip to the hospital. These plaster sculptures not only immortalize your baby bump, they make for some truly beautiful pieces of art. (Not convinced? Google "belly cast" and prepare to be amazed.) You can find inexpensive belly-casting kits on Amazon, or you can hire a pro—doulas and even some plaster artists often offer the service. Once your cast is complete, you can leave it plain white, decorate it with nontoxic paint, or add baby's footprints and date of birth later on.

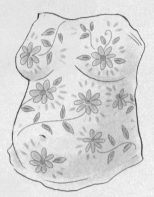

Letter Writing

Writing a letter to your unborn child makes for a super-sweet keepsake. What to say? You can write a little about your hopes and dreams for her future, what's it been like carrying her in your belly, and the kind of mother you wish to be. You can share the nickname you've coined for her or tell her how long you've waited for her. You can explain how you felt when you found out you were pregnant, too. Just be honest, as it's all meaningful!

Journaling or Scrapbooking

Perhaps an easier (or at least, less messy) way to honor this time is with a pregnancy scrapbook or journal. You can write regular entries, keeping track of your experiences week by week (no matter how great your memory, you *will* forget some of the little details), and tuck away keepsakes, such as a lock of baby's hair. You could even put together a video scrapbook, which is what Michael and I did for each of our kids.

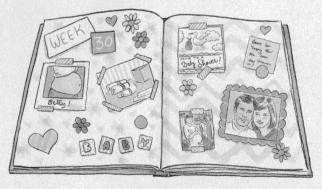

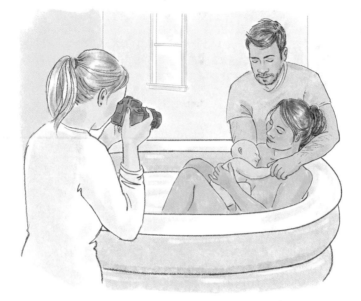

counterpressure to your back, coaching you through contractions, and cheering you on during the pushing phase. Besides, no one wants to witness the birth of his child from behind a lens or an iPhone if they don't have to. It's also unlikely that your partner is a professional. Birth photographers, on the other hand, are equipped to shoot in low light (because, obviously, they can't set up a lighting kit in the hospital), as well as in small spaces. You won't end up with blurry, shaky, or flat-out unflattering shots. No accidental fingers in the frame, either.

♡ **Commissioning birth photos can be empowering.** For many, many years, birth was a closed-door, mysterious, often fearful event—not even fathers were allowed in the room! But just hiring a professional can reframe the experience: birth becomes more joyful, something to celebrate and cherish, rather than something to be afraid of. And in the event that things don't go according to plan, having photographic evidence of how things unfolded can be, for some mamas, incredibly healing.

SO HOW DOES BIRTH PHOTOGRAPHY *WORK*?

Every photographer is different, of course, but if you decide to spring for photos (or film), the process generally goes a little something like this: a month or two before birth, you'll meet your prospective photographer for a consultation, during which you'll discuss all the specifics and logistics—you'll pick your photo

package, go over the fees (which could range from a few hundred to a few thousand dollars, just like wedding photos) and, perhaps most important, explain what *exactly* you want captured. (At most births, the photographer will stand up by mama's head, so the images can depict baby's arrival without the need to

Quinoa Pizza

To satisfy all the pregnancy cravings, I've made sure to include recipes featuring chocolate (page 176), chips (page 283), and fudge (page 214)—all healthy versions, of course! But I would be remiss if I didn't include a recipe for the ultimate comfort food: PIZZA. Instead of a typical white flour crust, this version uses quinoa, an ancient grain that supports breast milk production, so it's a great recipe for your postpartum self, too.

INGREDIENTS

1 cup organic quinoa (rinsed and soaked overnight)

¼ cup filtered water

1 teaspoon organic oregano

½ teaspoon sea salt

½ teaspoon organic garlic powder

1 tablespoon melted cooking oil such as ghee or expeller-pressed coconut oil

Preheat oven to 425°F. Drain quinoa and place in a blender. Add ¼ cup filtered water, oregano, sea salt, and garlic powder. Blend till smooth. The mixture should have the consistency of pancake batter. If it's too thick, add another tablespoon or two of water. (Batter must be pourable without being runny.)

Pour batter onto a well-oiled pizza pan. Bake for about 10 minutes or until the top of the crust looks cooked. Remove from the oven and carefully flip the crust, then bake for another 10 minutes or until the top of the crust looks cooked.

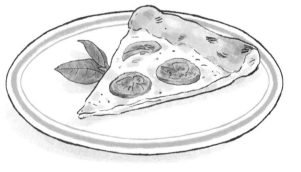

Remove from oven, add your toppings, and bake for another 10 minutes. Enjoy!

get graphic. Of course, you can request up-close-and-personal shots if you want to.) Since all births are unpredictable, you'll also want to determine how many hours the photographer is willing to make herself available. Most won't shoot the entirety of a super-long labor (think: twelve-plus hours). Instead, they may leave the hospital or birth center and return when you're further along. They'll also stay for an hour or two after the birth, in order to get footage of cord cutting, baby's first footprints, and perhaps introductions to extended family.

Alternatively, some photographers offer what's often called a "First 48" shoot—instead of photographing the actual birth, they'll arrive a day or two later to take pictures before you're discharged (a nice option for mamas who'd like to shower before having their photo taken).

Before you put down any kind of (nonrefundable) deposit, however, you'll need to double-check your hospital or birth center's photo and film policy.

Some facilities are very lax, while others may forbid photographing or videotaping of the actual delivery, or may not allow a photographer in the operating room if you're having a C-section. Keep in mind that hospitals, in particular, tend to be more wary of video than of still photos (due to liability issues). Know, too, that official hospital policy may differ from what your ob-gyn will allow.

Speaking of C-sections, there are usually lots of opportunities for photos both before and after the procedure, even if your photographer can't be in the room for the actual birth. They may also be able to follow baby while you're in recovery, capturing all those special moments you might otherwise not get to see.

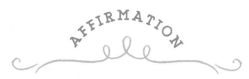

I am giving birth to my baby,
and also to my Mama Heart. I am birthing a love
that would go to the ends of the earth.

FINDING A BIRTH PHOTOGRAPHER IN YOUR HOMETOWN

In the last few years, more and more doulas (including Maura!) have started doubling as birth photographers. Generally, they're able to pick up a camera in the quieter moments of labor (when they're not providing hands-on support) as well as during delivery (when the midwife or doctor takes on a more central role). You can also check out the International Association of Professional Birth Photographers (IAPBP), which maintains a searchable database of more than 1,400 members, including links to personal websites featuring samples of each photographer's work.

mama-do list

- Want to see some truly incredible birth shots? The IAPBP hosts an "Image of the Year" contest—visit birthphotographers.com to check out previous winners, honorable mentions, and entrants.

- While we're on the subject of photography, now's a good time to decide if you're interested in setting up a newborn shoot, too. Professionals recommend scheduling them within the first ten days to two weeks of birth, since this is when brand-new babies sleep the most deeply, and their little bodies easily contort into those precious poses.

- Guess what else it's time to start doing? Looking for a pediatrician. (Crazy, right?) Choosing a doctor for your child *before* you give birth, however, will only make your life easier once baby arrives. Ask for recommendations from family and friends, and don't hesitate to set up a few consultations. It's perfectly appropriate to interview pediatricians, just as you interviewed your doctor or midwife!

HOW WOULD YOU LIKE YOUR
placenta served?

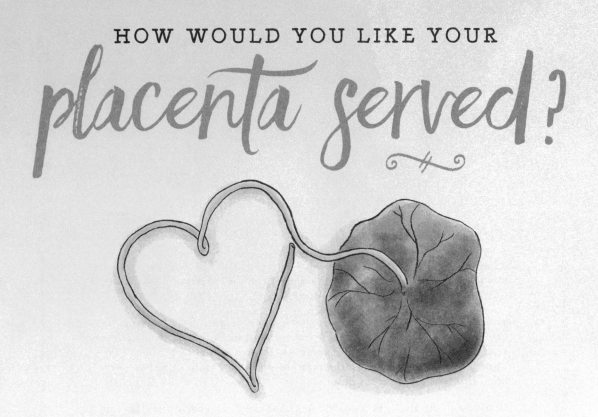

WHAT'S UP WITH *baby*?

Baby is all the way up to three and a half pounds this week and, I must say, looking more and more like a proper newborn. Of course, his newfound chunk is part of the reason you wanna squeeze those cheeks and attack him with kisses (and you will, soon!). But remember way back in Week 15, when I told you his skin was so thin you could practically see through it (if you could actually see inside your uterus, that is)? Well, the accumulation of fat also means that his skin is starting to appear less translucent and more opaque. By baby's birthday, he'll have a reddish-pink complexion (regardless of your or your partner's skin color). Over the course of several weeks or months, however, he'll adopt a more permanent pigment, once his production of melanin kicks in.

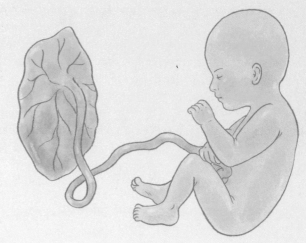

WHAT'S UP WITH *mama*?

Heartburn? Check. Out of breath? Yup. Hemorrhoids? Unpleasant, perhaps, but manageable. But what's a mama to do if she springs a leak!? That's right, leaky boobs are pretty common in the third trimester, as your body has started preparing itself for breastfeeding. That substance dripping from your nipples isn't milk, however, it's colostrum, a thick, yellowish pre-milk that's rich in protein, vitamin A, immune cells, and important antibodies baby isn't getting while in the womb. In fact, colostrum provides exactly what baby needs in the hours after birth—nothing more, nothing less—and will sustain him until your "true" milk comes in a few days later. You don't have a whole lot of use for it *now*, though. So tucking a nursing pad inside your bra can protect your clothes (and your dignity). But if you're not leaking at all, don't worry—it doesn't mean you won't produce enough milk when the time comes.

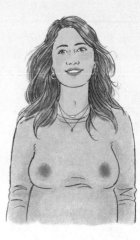

I'm leaking where?

"Please tell me you're joking."

Michael was staring at me, wide-eyed in disbelief, his spoon frozen in mid-air above his bowl of morning oatmeal.

"We're the only mammals who *don't* eat it . . ." I replied (in the most convincing tone I could muster).

"Right," he sighed. "But we're *also* the only mammals who drive cars and leave tips at restaurants."

Oh, my poor husband. Papa Natural had come so far after the birth of our son. From wearing our newborn in a baby carrier to scraping poop off cloth diapers, he'd embraced just about every crunchy practice I'd brought into our home. But now I was pregnant with Baby #2 and eating my placenta, I guess, was just too much for him.

I couldn't blame him.

To be honest, the idea had been a little too much for me during my first pregnancy.

I mean, sure, I'd heard that placentophagy was supposedly an ancient practice—dried human placenta has been used in traditional Chinese medicine for centuries. And humans really *are* some of the only mammals that don't consume the placenta immediately after birth. (Granted, some experts believe it's only eaten to hide traces of birth from predators in the wild—admittedly not something I'd have to worry about at the birth center.) I also knew that popping "placenta pills" had become all the rage in pop culture. Stars, including January Jones and Kim Kardashian, raved about surges of energy and increased breast milk production, sparking a *major*, worldwide trend. All of a sudden, placenta recipes were flooding the internet. New mamas could even flip through one of several placenta-themed cookbooks!

But is the placenta *really* a postpartum "miracle drug," or is eating it just . . . gross? This time around, I had to find out.

WHY WOULD ANY WOMAN *EAT* HER PLACENTA?

During pregnancy, baby will pull all the nutrients he needs from his mother—whether she has enough to spare or not. This is, of course, why adequate nutrition is so vitally important for mamas-to-be (growing a baby is really tough work). Unfortunately, and as I've mentioned before, our depleted soils yield produce that's less healthy than it once was. Feedlot cattle, chickens, turkeys, and pigs, meanwhile, are less nutrient-dense than pasture-raised animals. Add in the prevalence of processed, fried, and refined foods, and it's no wonder many women have some level of nutritional deficiency even *before* they get pregnant. And once they do give birth, the demands on their bodies are nowhere near over. (Breastfeeding alone, for example, burns up to 500 calories a day.) Some experts actually believe the demands of pregnancy are so intense that women are nutritionally depleted for at least a year following delivery. (One physician out of Australia, Dr. Oscar Serrallach, thinks it's more like a decade; he coined the term *postnatal depletion*.) Even the World Health Organization recommends spacing pregnancies between two and five years apart, so that mama has adequate time to rebuild her energy stores.

For these reasons and more, some people swear by human placentophagy. It's thought that eating the placenta after childbirth can provide:

♡ **A Hormonal Boost.** During pregnancy your body is chock-a-block full of surging hormones, but almost immediately after birth,

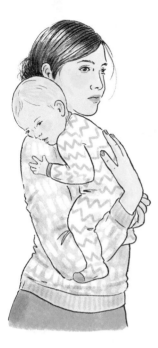

those hormones plummet. Progesterone and estrogen, in particular, remain low until the return of your menstrual period—and that could take months or even years, as some women don't begin menstruating again until they've stopped breastfeeding. These hormonal highs and lows are the reason some new mamas feel tired, sluggish, weepy, emotional, or just plain bummed out after birth (we generally refer to this as the "baby blues"); they also may be a contributing factor in the eventual onset of postpartum depression.

The placenta, however, is full of hormones, including estrogen and progesterone (which are produced by the placenta), as well as oxytocin (which crosses the placenta during labor). It's thought that ingesting the organ, then, may alleviate some of that hormonal whiplash. The placenta also contains prolactin, the hormone that triggers breast milk production, which is likely why mamas who eat it often experience a surge of milk and faster letdown.

♡ **A Nutrient Boost.** In addition to hormones, the placenta contains vitamins and minerals, including iron and vitamins B_6 and B_{12}, as well as amino acids and essential fats, which makes perfect sense when you think about it, since one of the main functions of the placenta is to deliver nutrients to the baby while in utero. It's thought that ingesting the placenta, therefore, might replenish some of the nutrients that were depleted during pregnancy and childbirth.

♡ **A Healing Boost.** Preserving or "banking" the blood from a newborn's umbilical cord has become a routine part of childbirth for a growing number of parents, but cord blood isn't the only source of life-giving stem cells. The placenta is loaded with these biological building blocks, too, which is one reason why the practice of placentophagy may speed up healing of the uterus after childbirth, as well as decrease postpartum bleeding.

OKAY, BUT HOW DOES IT *TASTE*?

Apparently—and thankfully—the placenta tastes like whatever you eat it with (you could say it's a bit like tofu in that way). Some women prepare it just as they would any other organ meat: sautéed with onions and bacon, baked into lasagna, or pan-fried on the stovetop in order to make placenta tacos or a Bolognese-style pasta sauce. Others toss a few frozen chunks into a blender with some fruit and yogurt for a refreshing placenta smoothie.

The majority of mamas, however, go with the more popular and *palatable* option: placenta encapsulation.

In the crunchy community, the idea that placentophagy is ancient—that women from all sorts of cultures from all over the world

THE PROCESS OF
PLACENTA ENCAPSULATION

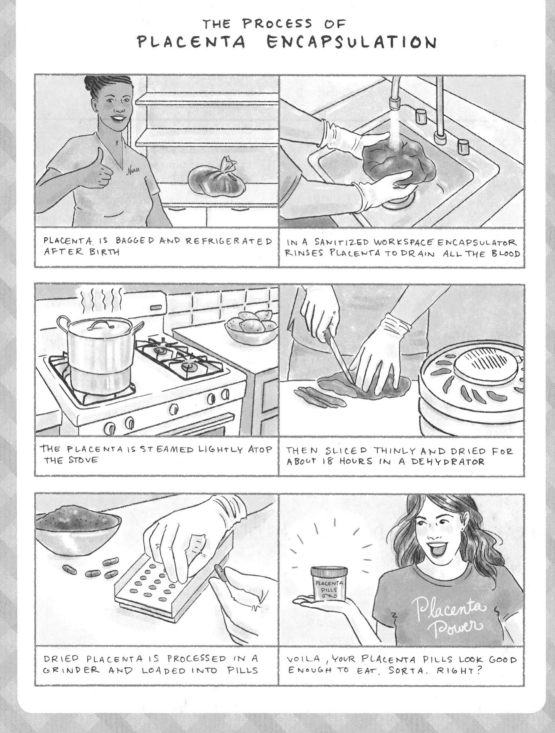

PLACENTA IS BAGGED AND REFRIGERATED AFTER BIRTH

IN A SANITIZED WORKSPACE ENCAPSULATOR RINSES PLACENTA TO DRAIN ALL THE BLOOD

THE PLACENTA IS STEAMED LIGHTLY ATOP THE STOVE

THEN SLICED THINLY AND DRIED FOR ABOUT 18 HOURS IN A DEHYDRATOR

DRIED PLACENTA IS PROCESSED IN A GRINDER AND LOADED INTO PILLS

VOILA, YOUR PLACENTA PILLS LOOK GOOD ENOUGH TO EAT. SORTA. RIGHT?

have been eating their placentas for thousands of years—is a popular one, but the research to back that claim up is pretty slim. It's true that the Egyptians, the Navajo, and the indigenous Maori tribe in New Zealand, for example, considered the placenta to be somewhat sacred. The Navajo and the Maori had a tradition of burying the placenta in the ground after birth. It's also true that there are references to the human placenta in traditional Chinese herbal medicine (although the placenta in question was not necessarily the mother's own, nor was the placenta consumed specifically for post-partum benefits). But the practice of eating one's *own* placenta is a decidedly modern practice. In fact, the first real recorded evidence we have that placentophagy had become a sort of cultural custom comes from the 1960s and '70s, when it was trending among women living in hippie communes. And the practice didn't

PLACENTA ENCAPSULATION TIPS
FROM NURSE/DOULA *Maura*

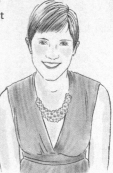

True, there's very little research to confirm the supposed benefits (or, conversely, the potential risks) of placentophagy, but one small report published in *Ecology of Food and Nutrition* in 2013 has always stood out: in a survey of 189 women who consumed their placentas after birth, 95 percent rated their experience as either "positive" or "very positive," and a whopping 98 percent intended to repeat the experience after subsequent births.

I have to say, I'm not that surprised. The placenta is beautifully complex even though it's only a temporary organ, meant to sustain just a single pregnancy. The precision and care your body takes to grow the placenta is just as awe-inspiring as the work that goes into growing a baby. And, sure, I'm a little biased. The placenta, which is said to resemble a "tree of life," is my favorite organ, and I'm a professional encapsulator. But I can tell you that all of my clients have been happy they ingested their placentas. I noticed amazing results, too, after the births of each of my children. In fact, my husband could tell when I *forgot* to take my placenta pills!

If you're interested in giving placentophagy a go, make sure you're hiring a *professional* who's received formal training. (Believe it or not, there are some rogue encapsulators out there who learned the technique via YouTube.) An easy way to separate the pros from the amateurs? Ask your prospective encapsulator about her experience working with blood-borne pathogens, and see if she'll give you a quick rundown of the process she uses to clean her equipment. Bonus points if the service she provides comes with several options: For example, is she proficient in both raw and traditional preparations? Does she offer add-ons, such as tinctures? Will she prepare the placenta in your home? None of my clients have ever regretted having their placenta encapsulated. Find a professional near you, and I bet the same will hold true.

go mainstream until *really* recently. A woman named Jodi Selander (founder of a business called Placenta Benefits) developed a proprietary method of drying, grinding, and encapsulating the placenta; she then coined the phrase "placenta encapsulation" in 2006. Ingesting the placenta in pill form has only gained traction since then, and when I found out that my doula was a certified encapsulator, I figured I'd give it a shot.

And the process, it's worth mentioning, is fascinating; just check out page 314. My encapsulator made about one hundred pills from

my placenta, as well as a placenta tincture, a.k.a. a concentrated alcohol-based infusion with a *really* long shelf life. (Some mamas use the tincture to relieve symptoms associated with menopause.)

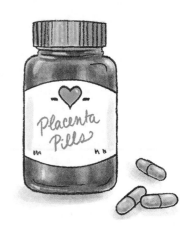

Placenta cocktail, anyone?

OKAY, SO IT TASTES FINE—BUT ARE THE BENEFITS *REAL* OR JUST PLACEBO EFFECT?

When I was pregnant with my first child, placenta encapsulation was just taking off, so I *thought* about having pills made but ended up opting out. I figured the human body expelled the organ for a reason, and I wasn't sure we were meant to ingest it. It wasn't until I'd heard from so many other natural mamas—women who had struggled with postpartum depression or low milk supply or low energy or insomnia, who raved about the miracles of placentophagy—that I opened my mind (and eventually my stomach) to the idea.

Could such claims really be true?

Unfortunately, it's hard to know for sure, because the evidence we have to support such claims is almost entirely anecdotal. There is virtually no *scientific* or *clinical* evidence that women who consume the placenta will reap a hormonal or nutritional benefit, and the practice has plenty of detractors. Since the placenta is a filtration organ, for example, responsible for removing waste and preventing toxins from reaching baby while in utero, it's possible that

it may *retain* toxins, just as it retains vitamins, minerals, and nutrients. (Though you could argue the opposite, too, since it's the placenta's job to send waste to the kidneys and bowel for removal.) Certainly, there's no regulation of placentophagy by the FDA. Some doctors and other experts have raised concerns about possible contamination by bacteria or viruses if the placenta is not handled and stored properly (as would be necessary with any raw protein). But the flip side of that coin? There's no evidence that consuming the placenta is *bad* for you, either.

I started taking my placenta pills about a week after the birth of my daughter—two after each meal, as instructed. Within twenty-four hours, I noticed my milk production substantially increase. (So they *do* work!) But while this might have been great for a woman struggling with low supply, it was not so great for me. Paloma was already overwhelmed by my fast letdown, and now she was only getting more frustrated. So was I. I was *engorged*—leaking everywhere, soaking through shirts and sheets and bras. A day or so later, another new and unfamiliar feeling took hold: the blues. I'd never experienced any kind of depression or sadness after my son's birth, but a kind of black cloud had settled over me. As an experiment, I decided to stop taking the pills. And sure enough, within twenty-four hours, my mood brightened. Within forty-eight hours, my milk supply seemed to chill out. I felt like my old self again. (I gave the pills one more shot a few days later, but when I started to feel down again, I gave them up for good.)

So, does this mean eating your placenta is a *bad* idea? I definitely don't think so. Even though my body didn't respond great to the hormones, and even though some mamas do report similar, somewhat negative symptoms (usually moodiness or weepiness), the vast majority of women who consume their placentas seem to love it. And who knows? Had I suffered from postpartum depression or had difficulty breastfeeding, perhaps those pills would have been just what I needed. In the end, I was just glad to have tried it out.

If you decide to give placentophagy a try, I think it's important—as with any supplement—to listen to your body. If you feel more energized and your milk supply is where you'd like it to be—great! If you start feeling negative side effects, however, you can always try adjusting your dose or stop taking the pills altogether. That's the beauty of it!

WHAT OTHER *natural mamas* SAY

kimberly: I've had my placenta encapsulated after each of three pregnancies, and I would definitely recommend it. The first time around it really seemed to help with mood swings and depression. As time went on, however, I did have to stop taking the pills because the hormones made me a bit dizzy.

felicity: I had my placenta encapsulated after the birth of my first (and only) baby. True, I have nothing to compare it to, but my energy, mood, milk supply, and recovery were all amazing—I attribute lots of that to taking my placenta pills.

clair: I had to cut back on the number of pills I was taking because I started to become engorged, but once I made the adjustment, I felt great!

leslie: I was in the hospital for five days postpartum because my son was in the NICU, so I didn't get my pills until day 5—and honestly, I didn't notice much of a difference. However, I do take the pills from time to time when I need a boost of energy or know that my day is going to be stressful, and they really help!

OKAY, I'D LIKE TO GIVE PLACENTOPHAGY A TRY: WHAT'S MY FIRST STEP?

Whether you're planning to whip up some smoothies or ingest the placenta in capsule form, you need to do some legwork if you're planning to take the organ home with you. Start by:

Chocolate Placenta Truffles

If you're gonna eat your placenta, you might as well do it in style, *amiright*? So close your eyes and imagine yourself a few days postpartum: unwashed hair tied up in a messy bun, lounging in a stained nursing top and pajama pants . . . and snacking on chocolate bonbons. Not too bad, eh?

Okay, maybe it sounds a little weird to eat your placenta in dessert form, but you won't taste it this way, thanks to the bittersweet flavor of the chocolate. And if you don't plan on consuming your placenta, no problem—you can still enjoy these delicious treats, sans birth organ.

INGREDIENTS

8 ounces organic dark chocolate

½ cup heavy cream (or full-fat coconut milk)

1 tablespoon honey or maple syrup

½ teaspoon vanilla extract

¼ cup crushed almonds (may substitute walnuts or some other nut or seed)

1 tablespoon dried placenta powder (just empty it right out of the capsules)

¼ cup cacao or cocoa powder (optional)

¼ cup shredded coconut (optional)

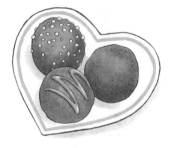

In a double boiler (over low heat) melt dark chocolate and cream or coconut milk, stirring until smooth. Remove from heat, allow to cool slightly, then add honey, vanilla, crushed almonds, and dried placenta powder. Mix well and pour into a bowl; cover and chill until firm (about two hours). Using a melon-baller, scoop individual truffles from the hardened batter. Roll in shredded coconut, cocoa powder, or crushed almonds. Chill for an additional 30 minutes, then store in an airtight container in the fridge. One or two truffles a day postpartum should help balance your mood and give you a breast milk boost. Also worth noting: this may be the one time in your life that no one else wants to eat your chocolate! Yay!

Researching Your Hospital or Birth Center's Placenta Policy. As placentophagy becomes increasingly popular, more and more hospitals across the country have begun to facilitate safe transport of the organ. Laws have been passed allowing mamas to take possession of their placentas after birth (albeit in only three states). Some alternative birth centers may even package up your placenta *for* you. But don't just show up on D-Day and expect that there will be no issues. Your hospital may outright refuse to let you take it, may require you to sign a liability waiver first, or may only allow you to take the organ after having secured a court order. The point is, you need to know *before* you go.

Find an Encapsulator. More and more birth doulas are becoming trained in placenta encapsulation through a slew of national agencies. Ask your doula if she's received training, or visit PlacentaBenefits.info or prodoula.com to find a specialist near you.

Add "Save My Placenta" to Your Birth Plan. Hospitals and birth centers dispose of the placenta as they would any other biohazard-ous medical waste, so you'll want to make sure everyone involved knows not to toss yours in the trash!

Arrange for Safe Storage. The placenta can breed bacteria if it's not handled properly. As quickly as possible after birth, it should be sealed in an airtight plastic bag, placed inside a food-grade plastic storage container, and refrigerated or put on ice (which means you might need to bring a mini cooler with you to the hospital or birth center). It should be transferred to the encapsulator within two to three days (you can wait a bit longer if it's been frozen).

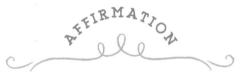

My body is a miracle. I have confidence in my strong and capable body. I allow my body to do its job.

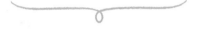

- Add "nursing pads" (available in both disposable and washable, reusable varieties) to your shopping list this week if leaky boobs have started to bother you. Speaking of breastfeeding, right around now is a good time to get measured for your first nursing bra.

- Have you started writing your birth plan yet? (Just checking!)

- Research your hospital or birth center's placenta policy. Better to know now if taking your placenta home (in the event you want to give placentophagy a go) will require some advance planning.

turning a breech baby

WHAT'S UP WITH *baby*?

With roughly eight weeks to go, baby is closing in on 4 pounds in weight and 18 inches in length. She's been working *hard* to pack on those pounds! But upstairs, her brain has been working overtime, too. Her gray matter is bustling with neurons (or brain cells)—by birth, she'll have more than 100 *billion* of them. This week, she's also busy establishing literally trillions of connections, or synapses, between those brain cells—by birth, she'll have around 50 trillion of those. Within the first

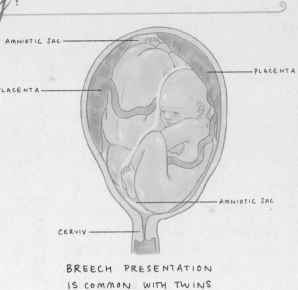

AMNIOTIC SAC

PLACENTA

PLACENTA

AMNIOTIC SAC

CERVIX

BREECH PRESENTATION IS COMMON WITH TWINS

three months of her life, however, that number will increase twenty times over. We're talking 1,000-trillion synapses by age one. Some quick perspective: it would take you more than thirty thousand years just to count to *one* trillion. Mind. Blown.

WHAT'S UP WITH *mama*?

Right around now, baby's kicks, rolls, and punches may start to feel a bit less intense. It's because she just doesn't have space in her increasingly crowded room (er, *womb*). But what happens if baby abruptly stops moving? Around this point in my first pregnancy, Griffin gave me a scare. I was out of town on business, and by early afternoon I realized I hadn't felt him move all morning. Feeling freaked, I called my midwife, who told me to drink a glass of orange juice and lie down. Thankfully, my little Rocky perked up and was back to slugging away within 20 minutes. (Thanks, Cynthia!) It is *incredibly* important to be aware (without being neurotic) of baby's movements in the third trimester, though, since sudden changes can indicate serious health problems. So after your next meal (assuming baby is awake), find a quiet spot where you can concentrate and get comfortable. Count each of baby's movements (kicks, rolls, *and* wiggles) until you get to ten; keeping in mind this might take just 10 minutes or close to an hour. Do this every day, around the same time. If you notice a significant change or decrease in movement, try to perk baby up by drinking some juice or taking a quick walk. If you still don't feel much movement, it's time to call your midwife or doctor. He or she will want to perform an emergency non-stress test or BPP—which could be lifesaving.

Few words can strike terror in a natural mama's heart like: "Your baby is breech." And right around 32 weeks, after a quick ultrasound confirmed her suspicion, my midwife informed me that, yes, my son's head was up by my ribs rather than down near my pelvis.

I was shocked. I was scared. I was also, frankly, a little bit miffed.

What about my plans for an unmedicated vaginal birth? Was all that preparation—everything I'd been working on for the previous seven months—out the window?

Doesn't a breech presentation equal an automatic C-section?

Not necessarily. It's certainly *possible* to deliver a breech baby vaginally; it's just that most doctors today won't do it. Vaginal breech births are tricky, in part, because baby's head—the largest part of her body—could theoretically get stuck within the maternal pelvis. (When the head comes out first, the cervix is adequately stretched and the soft bones of the fetal skull are able to mold to fit the shape of the birth canal.) Breech presentations also carry an increased risk of cord prolapse, a condition in which the umbilical cord drops (or prolapses) through the cervix, where it might become trapped against or compressed by baby's body during delivery, resulting in a prolonged loss of oxygen. The increased risks, coupled with liability issues and a decline in training (these days, attending a vaginal breech birth has become a bit of a lost art) have driven the Cesarean rate for breech babies to something approaching nearly *100 percent*.

So, Mama? If you're aiming for a natural childbirth and your little bundle is breech, it's pretty imperative that we figure out a way to flip that baby.

BUTT FIRST (SORRY, COULDN'T HELP MYSELF) WHY IS MY BABY BREECH?

Throughout your pregnancy, baby has been flipping and rolling and even walking around in your uterus. By the midpoint of the third trimester, however, she's grown big enough that she no longer has much room to maneuver, which is why babies typically settle into a more permanent position sometime between 32 and 36 weeks. Usually, that position is head-down (this is also called "cephalic" or "vertex"), but some babies present as butt-first or feet-first—a.k.a. breech. Ready for some good news? The vast majority of babies classified as breech *before* 37 weeks will manage to turn themselves around, all on their own. In fact, only 3 percent to 4 percent will still be headed the wrong way by the time they're considered full-term. We don't know exactly why some stubborn babies just refuse to flip, but we do know that there are quite a few risk factors, including:

♡ **The Shape of Your Uterus.** A congenital abnormality affecting the size or shape of the womb, a previous uterine infection, uterine fibroids, or excess scar tissue from previous C-sections might mean baby doesn't have enough space to flip himself before birth.

♡ **The Position of Your Placenta.** A low-lying placenta that covers the cervix (placenta previa) may prevent baby from assuming a head-down position.

My baby is in a great position for birth.
My baby is part of me, and made to fit my body.
My body will open, and my baby will descend with ease.

♡ **The Volume of Your Amniotic Fluid.** Too little fluid can make it difficult for baby to swim around in there, while too much fluid might encourage him to keep flipping right up until D-Day.

♡ **A Previous Breech Baby.** For some reason, women who've had one breech baby are more likely to have another, as are women with a family history of breech presentations.

Our modern and increasingly sedentary way of life may be another factor in breech presentations. We know that the hours and hours we spend sitting at desks or driving in cars, for example, can throw the pelvis out of alignment. On the other hand, the more active you are, the more limber and balanced your pelvic floor will be. This may encourage baby's head to descend downward.

NATURAL TECHNIQUES TO FLIP A BREECH (OR POSTERIOR) BABY

Hopefully, you've been staying active and doing your pelvic exercises over the course of the last few months. But if you haven't, it's not too late to get started! Switch out your regular desk chair for a birthing ball, make walking around the block part of your regular morning or evening routine, and when you feel baby wiggling around in there, drop to your hands and knees and knock out some pelvic rocks. If you've gotten the okay from your midwife or doctor, you can try a daily Puppy Pose, too. If that baby still won't budge, however, you may be ready to try some more advanced methods:

THE WEBSTER TECHNIQUE

As your pregnancy progresses, the more your center of gravity is pulled forward by the weight of your belly. Relaxin, meanwhile, the hormone that's been relaxing all your joints and ligaments, can make your bones a little shifty, too. This makes a pregnant woman's pelvis ripe for misalignment, which may result in a malpositioned baby. And that's where chiropractic care comes in. As a reminder, the Webster technique is a type of chiropractic care that focuses on reducing strain on the ligaments supporting the uterus, as well as improving pelvic alignment, which may encourage baby to flip. Visit the International Chiropractic Pediatric Association's website (icpa4kids.org) to find a Webster-certified provider near you.

JOCKEYING FOR POSITION:
DIFFERENT POSES BABY MAY STRIKE IN UTERO

When it comes to baby's position in the womb, there's a lot more to it than just head up or head down. The orientation of baby's back in relation to your spine, and of her head in relation to your pelvis, can make a difference on labor day. Here are some ways baby may situate herself in the weeks before birth.

Left Occiput Anterior (LOA)

When a baby is head-down, favoring mama's left side, and looking inward toward mama's spine, she's said to be left occiput anterior. This is the optimal position for childbirth, as it encourages baby to tuck her chin to her chest, so that smallest part of her head (the occiput) enters the birth canal first.

Right Occiput Anterior (ROA)

Baby is head-down, facing inward, favoring the right side of mama's belly. While the LOA position is much more common than ROA, both positions are considered to be favorable.

Left Occiput Posterior (LOP)

Baby is head-down, favoring mama's left side but facing outward toward her belly—in other words, the occiput (the back of her head) lines up with mama's posterior (the rear or spine). OP babies are sometimes referred to as "sunny-side up," and while they can absolutely be delivered vaginally, childbirth may be a bit more difficult. These labors may be more likely to stall, and a bit more painful, because OP babies don't always tuck their chins. This results in uneven pressure on the cervix (making for slower dilation) and a propensity for back labor. OP deliveries are also associated with higher intervention rates, which is why

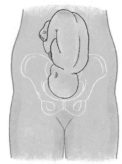

LEFT OCCIPUT ANTERIOR

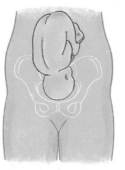

RIGHT OCCIPUT ANTERIOR

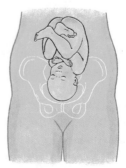

LEFT OCCIPUT POSTERIOR

you'll want to rotate baby to the anterior position, if possible. Keep in mind that babies can rotate themselves during labor, and many moms, especially those who have labored before, can deliver OP babies without issues.

Right Occiput Posterior (ROP)

Baby is head-down, facing outward, and favoring the right side of mama's belly. Pretty sure this is how my son was situated, which could be the reason I needed that hit of Pit.

Transverse

Rather than head-up or head-down, baby is sideways in the womb, almost as if he's relaxing in a hammock. While a full-term transverse presentation is rare (especially for a first-time mama, whose uterus hasn't been, shall we say, *pre*-stretched), it means a mandatory Cesarean; a sideways baby just will *not* fit through the vagina.

Oblique

Instead of lying vertically or horizontally in the womb, a baby can occasionally (and rarely) settle into an oblique or diagonal position; in this case, baby's head will essentially point toward one of mama's hips. These babies can make a head- or feet-first descent during labor.

What Position Is Your Baby In?

Ask your midwife or doctor to perform Leopold's Maneuvers so you can better understand your baby's positioning (see page 329 for more information).

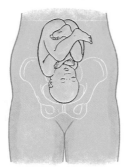
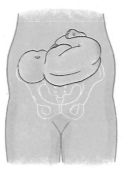
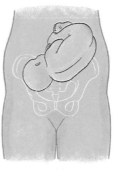

RIGHT OCCIPUT POSTERIOR   TRANSVERSE   OBLIQUE

Five Versions of Breech Presentation

✻ **Frank breech.** This is a true butt-first position, as baby's knees and feet are up by his ears. The majority of breech babies (around 65 percent to 70 percent) fit this category.

✻ **Complete breech.** Baby is butt-first, but he appears to be sitting cross-legged in the womb; his knees are bent, and his feet are lower in the pelvis.

✻ **Footling breech.** Instead of leading with his bottom, a footling baby leads with his feet—either one (called a single footling) or both (a double). Footling presentations are rare in general, but more common among premature babies.

✻ **Footling-frank.** Baby is butt-first, with one leg straight (like a frank breech) and the other bent (like a complete breech)—how awkward!

✻ **Kneeling breech.** This one's pretty much what it sounds like: baby is essentially kneeling in the pelvis. Kneeling presentations are so rare that they're sometimes not even considered to be a true breech category.

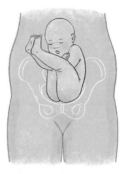

FRANK BREECH

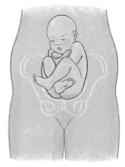

COMPLETE BREECH

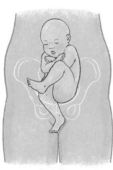

FOOTLING BREECH

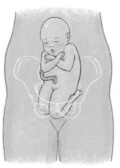

KNEELING BREECH

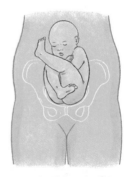

FOOTLING-FRANK BREECH

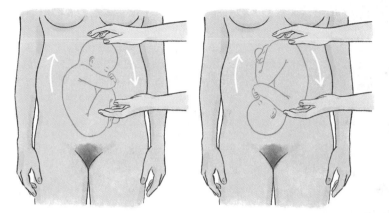

EXTERNAL CEPHALIC VERSION (ECV)

One of the few *clinically* proven techniques to turn a breech baby—with a success rate hovering a little under 60 percent—external cephalic version is the manual manipulation of baby's position by a midwife or doctor. In other words, your healthcare provider will use his or her hands to push against your belly to flip baby from a butt-first to a head-down position. (In some cases, you may be given medication to relax the uterus and prevent contractions. Your doctor may want to monitor the fetal heart rate both before and after the procedure, just to make sure baby tolerates the pressure.) The procedure can be uncomfortable, or even painful, but it also might make the difference between a vaginal birth or a Cesarean.

When my midwife determined that Griffin was breech, she performed an ECV and flipped him *in a snap*. (She said it was easy because it was early, and still quite roomy in my womb.) My son, however, did not stay in a head-down position after the version—and that's not unusual. It's best to undergo an ECV closer to D-Day, usually between 36 and 38 weeks. The procedure is generally considered safe, but do know that there are a few risks: twisting or squeezing of the umbilical cord, compres-

sion of the pla[...]
rupturing or te[...]
amniotic sac. A[...]
complications [...]
you'll want to speak with your healthcare provider to determine if an ECV is a good option for you.

MOXIBUSTION ACUPUNCTURE

Admittedly the *weirdest* technique I tried, moxibustion is an ancient practice that involves inserting acupuncture needles in various points on your feet while incense (made from mugwort, a type of herb) is burned near the outside of your pinky toes. (Look, I told you this was weird.) It's thought that the combination of smoke, heat, and acupressure stimulate the release of prostaglandins, which may trigger gentle contractions, which may encourage baby to move. Does it work? My acupuncturist certainly seems to think so; he claims that only two babies have failed to flip for him (one of whom, it was later discovered, had the cord wrapped around his neck). From a clinical standpoint,

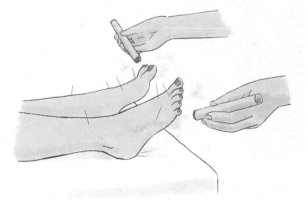

here is some evidence (albeit from a few small studies) to suggest that moxibustion—when combined with acupuncture—can be effective; the results, however, are certainly not conclusive. Keep in mind that moxibustion isn't a one-time treatment. To be most effective, research suggests it should be repeated once or twice daily for a week to two weeks.

Looking for a more DIY approach to flipping a breech baby? Consider experimenting with some of these old wives' remedies:

♡ Place a cold compress or a frozen bag of peas up near your rib cage—the idea is that baby doesn't like the cold.

♡ Shine a bright flashlight between your legs (some mamas are convinced their babies flipped toward the light). Or try experimenting with noise, whether that means having papa coax baby with his voice, or playing some Beethoven down near your pelvis. (Weird, I know.)

♡ Some mamas swear that performing repeat headstands in water can encourage baby to flip.

♡ Finally, certain homeopathic remedies may be effective, in particular Pulsatilla. Talk to your healthcare provider about dosing and frequency.

WHAT OTHER *natural mamas* SAY

kimberly: My obstetrician scheduled a C-section—and scoffed at my efforts to seek help—after discovering our baby was breech. In the final few weeks, however, baby turned after several adjustments from my chiropractor.

amanda: My baby wasn't breech, but he wasn't in an optimal position for birth, either: he was occipital posterior, and his chin wasn't tucked. My doula helped me stretch during a contraction in order to move him down—I don't know what she did exactly, but it worked! Had it not been for her, I'm pretty sure I would've had a C-section.

kelley: We discovered that my second child was breech at 35 weeks. I was devastated at the thought that I wouldn't be able to have a natural birth, and I tried all the natural methods. I even scheduled an ECV, but I was really nervous because I'd heard it can be painful. Desperate, I made an emergency appointment with my prenatal chiropractor. As she was palpating my abdomen, she told me she thought my baby's foot was stuck too low. She had me take a deep breath and count to three—on three, she unstuck his foot, and I felt him move! With her help, I immediately did an inversion, and I felt different right away. I showed up for my scheduled ECV and, sure enough, baby was in the right position, ready for birth!

CAN'T MAKE HEADS OR TAILS OF BABY'S POSITION? LEO CAN HELP!

No, not Leo DiCaprio, although that would be nice. I'm talking about Leopold's Maneuvers, which was developed by gynecologist Christian Gerhard Leopold back in the late 1800s.

Leopold's Maneuvers is a systematic way to determine baby's position and presentation in utero. The maneuvers consist of four distinct "grips," and while not diagnostic in nature, it can help determine baby's position and is an alternative for moms who want to avoid extra ultrasounds.

Your midwife and/or ob-gyn may perform Leopold's Maneuvers regularly once you hit your third trimester. It's even an effective tool during labor to help midwives determine where to place fetal monitors.

At your next prenatal visit, ask your provider to talk you through each grip so you can understand how baby is resting inside you. Keep in mind that these maneuvers are to be performed by trained professionals only.

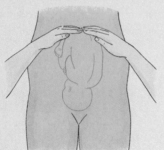

FUNDAL GRIP

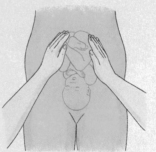

UMBILICAL GRIP

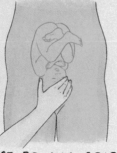

1ST PELVIC GRIP

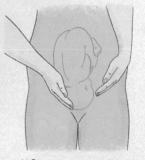

2ND PELVIC GRIP

Salmon Cakes

Since baby's brain development is taking center stage this week, let's focus on foods you can eat to support his smarts, like omega-3 fatty acids. Or, more specifically, docosahexaenoic acid (a.k.a. DHA).

Now that's a mouthful.

DHA is a primary component of brain tissue, and it's especially vital in the last three months of pregnancy. Unfortunately, many mamas don't get enough from their diet, and if *you're* not getting enough, baby's not getting enough, either, and that's a problem. Low levels of DHA during pregnancy have been linked to premature birth, low birth weight, and hyperactivity in children. So where can you find this miracle nutrient? Marine animals such as tuna, sardines, and anchovies are especially rich sources, but salmon is one of your best bets. In fact, this pink fish is one of the most nutrient-dense foods on the planet. Sink your teeth into a baked or grilled salmon filet for dinner this week (heck—*every week!*) or try whipping up these super-simple salmon cakes.

INGREDIENTS

One 14.75-ounce can wild salmon

2 pastured eggs

1 tablespoon coconut flour

½ onion, finely chopped

½ organic red pepper, finely chopped

2 tablespoons Dijon mustard

2 tablespoons fresh dill, minced (optional)

1–2 tablespoons olive oil

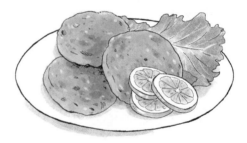

Drain your salmon (the drier, the better). In a medium-size bowl, whisk your eggs. Add in the coconut flour and stir until dissolved. Add remaining ingredients except the oil and mix well. With clean hands, form the mixture into small cakes. Heat the oil in a large skillet over medium-high heat, then add several cakes and cook for a few minutes on each side, until browned. Serve with lemon wedges and fresh tartar sauce. YUM!

SHOULD I BE WORRIED ABOUT BABY'S UMBILICAL CORD?

With all this talk of flipping babies, mamas might have some concerns about the umbilical cord—in particular, the idea that it might become knotted or wrapped tightly around baby's neck. Mercifully, true cord accidents are rare. In fact, knots in the cord (which occur in about 1 out of every 100 births) are typically loose enough that they don't restrict blood flow to the baby.

Having the cord wrapped around baby's arm or leg or—yes— even neck doesn't usually present much of a problem, either.

In fact, most cord issues aren't even visible via ultrasound and therefore aren't usually discovered until baby emerges from the vagina at the moment of birth. What providers are focused on, instead, are major decelerations in baby's heartbeat during labor. A very tightly knotted or wrapped cord, though rare, can restrict oxygen to the baby. In the event that baby's heart rate plummets, your provider will make multiple attempts to correct it, up to and including emergency C-section. The most common symptom of a cord issue in the weeks *before* birth, however, is a slow-down in baby's movements in utero. Keep up with your daily kick count, and let your provider know if you sense a change in baby's in-womb activity.

mama-do list

- Even if your baby's in the head-down position, keep up with your pelvic exercises. They can encourage baby to get down and *stay* down. To learn more about baby positioning, midwife Gail Tully's website spinningbabies.com is an excellent resource.

- Keeping track of baby's "kick count" during the third trimester is so effective at preventing stillbirth even the American College of Obstetricians and Gynecologists recommends it (*especially* for high-risk mamas). Make the process even easier by downloading an app on your smartphone. You can read more about fetal movement in the last few weeks before birth at countthekicks.org.

- It *is* possible to deliver a breech baby vaginally. We'll talk more about how to do so safely in Week 39.

I make milk— what's your superpower?

WHAT'S UP WITH *baby*?

We're approaching four and a half pounds this week, Mama, and somewhere around 18 or 19 inches in length. Baby's lungs are continuing to grow and mature, and his fat layers are filling in nicely. He's also started to receive maternal antibodies, which will protect him from certain bacteria and viruses (including chicken pox, assuming you've had them) once he's outside the womb. This is called passive immunity—since he'll be relying on your antibodies, rather than producing his own—and it only lasts for a few weeks

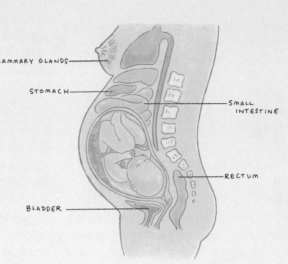

MAMMARY GLANDS

STOMACH

SMALL INTESTINE

RECTUM

BLADDER

BABY IS SITTING RIGHT ATOP YOUR BLADDER NOW

or months. Hmm. If only there was a way to extend this immunity? Oh, wait. There is: it's called breastfeeding. Breast milk (and especially *pre*-milk, a.k.a. colostrum) is rich in antibodies, which can keep baby safe from sickness and infection until his immune system grows a bit stronger.

WHAT'S UP WITH *mama*?

Back when we were discussing the many ways that pregnancy might interfere with your ability to get a good night's sleep, I mentioned restless leg syndrome. It's a little-understood disorder that affects roughly 15 percent of mamas-to-be and is characterized by a creeping, crawling, tingling feeling in the legs and feet, coupled with an *intense* desire to kick and thrash around. In short, it's crazy-annoying, especially since it tends to show up at nighttime when it's time to sleep! RLS is also most common in the third trimester so it might be showing up right about . . . *now*. We don't know exactly what causes it, although some research suggests that it may be genetic, a neurological issue, or stem from a nutritional deficiency. If you find yourself with a strong urge to karate kick make sure you're staying well hydrated, getting plenty of electrolytes (try drinking coconut water or bone broth) and—perhaps most important—upping your intake of magnesium. You could opt for a supplement, or apply topical magnesium oil directly to the legs. Some researchers believe there's a link between RLS and iron deficiency, so try eating more red meat, dark leafy greens, and pumpkin seeds, too.

When I was seven or eight years old, my mother's friend came over to the house with her brand-new baby in tow. She turned out to be one of those super-blatant, whip-out-a-boob-at-the-slightest-peep-from-her-baby type of mamas. You know, the kind of woman who's not afraid to breastfeed any time, any place, no matter who's around or who's watching. God bless her.

I remember being fascinated. Shocked at first, then intrigued, then moving in for a closer view.

So *this* was how mothers fed their babies, I marveled.

And what I know now, many years later, is that this woman actually gave me quite a gift: She normalized breastfeeding for me. At a young, impressionable age, I learned how the process worked, saw that it was utterly normal, and ever since then I just assumed that one day I'd do the same. Of course, my opinions were also shaped by my own mother, who I know nursed me for almost a year, even though formula feeding was all the rage back then.

Unfortunately, many women don't get these kinds of normalizing experiences early on; they never get to see it up close and personal.

Instead, breastfeeding remains mysterious, secret, and foreign. (Kinda like natural childbirth!)

So, is it any wonder that more than *90 percent* of new moms, according to researchers at UC Davis Medical Center, have trouble breastfeeding when the time comes?

So much trouble, in fact, that only 13 percent manage to breastfeed exclusively for six months, the length of time recommended by the American Academy of Pediatrics, the World Health Organization, and a slew of other medical groups.

And lest you think that I—with all my childhood wonder—took to breastfeeding right away, let me set the record straight. I had my fair share of problems, too. My daughter, for example, had what's called a shallow latch, and as a result my nipples turned some pretty intense shades of black and blue.

Turns out that breastfeeding is not nearly as intuitive as you might think. But the good news, Mama, is that you're getting this info early. In fact, you've got a little more than six weeks or so to prepare. So let's get to it!

THE BENEFITS OF BREASTFEEDING YOU *HAVEN'T* HEARD

It's no secret that "breast is best." That little slogan, introduced back in the late 1990s, has become the backbone of pro-breastfeeding campaigns launched by the government, internal health organizations, advocacy groups, parenting magazines, and local hospitals around the country, and for good reason. Breast milk is loaded with vitamins and nutrients, as well as those protective antibodies I mentioned, which

boost baby's delicate, still-maturing immune system. You've likely heard that breastfeeding is a major help when it comes to dropping the baby weight (the act alone can burn up to 500 calories a day), and that breastfed babies have lower rates of asthma, ear infections, respiratory illness, and intestinal distress. Breast milk is also, ya know, *free*. (Ever notice how they keep the infant formula locked up in glass cases at the grocery store? I mean, seriously, this stuff is *expensive!*)

My guess, however, is that there are plenty of benefits to the boob that you haven't yet heard of, even if this isn't your first baby.

BREASTFEEDING KEEPS YOU PUMPED UP WITH IRON

During pregnancy, baby receives—and stores—iron from his mama; in fact, the steady drain on your reserves is why iron-deficiency anemia is such a common pregnancy ailment. You'll only grow more depleted after birth, however, as you'll be losing iron-rich blood for at least four to six weeks, or as long as your lochia lasts. (Remember, lochia is the technical term for the bleeding and discharge that all women experience, whether they deliver vaginally or via C-section.) But while a bottle-feeding mama can expect her period to return after a month or two—sometimes menstruation returns just as the lochia is tapering off—women who breastfeed exclusively often go much, much longer without a period. Some may not have another period at all until they completely stop breastfeeding. And the longer you go without bleeding, the better able your body is to replenish its iron stores. (It took me fourteen months, if you're wondering.)

BREASTFEEDING LOWERS THE RISK OF SUDDEN INFANT DEATH SYNDROME (SIDS)

For reasons that aren't entirely clear—it may be the protective benefits of breast milk itself, the hormonal changes that occur in mama's body when she breastfeeds, or the boost from so much skin-to-skin contact—exclusive breastfeeding appears to reduce the risk of crib death. And not just by a little, but by as much as *50 percent*, according to a large Germany study published in *Pediatrics*.

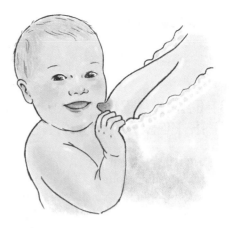

BREASTFED BABIES HAVE FEWER DENTAL ISSUES

Children who are exclusively breastfed have fewer instances of malocclusion (a.k.a. mis-alignment of the teeth), fewer overbites, and may have a lower chance of needing braces and other mouth hardware in the future. Why? It has to do with the way a baby must move her tongue and jaw when suckling at the breast. The repetitive motion molds both her palate and the oral cavity, laying the proper founda-tion for tooth alignment.

BREASTFEEDING HAS LONG-TERM HEALTH BENEFITS FOR MAMA, TOO

Turns out that delaying the return of your period doesn't just help you replenish your iron stores. The reduced exposure to repro-ductive hormones like estrogen also lowers your risk of developing breast, uterine, and ovarian cancer in the future. How much? When it comes to breast cancer, specifically, by as much as 4.3 percent for every twelve months you breastfeed, according to a study published in the medical journal *Lancet*. Risk of ovarian cancer, meanwhile, drops by as much as 63 percent among mamas who breastfeed for at least 13 months, according to a study by Australian researchers published in the *American Journal of Clinical Nutrition*. And the longer you breastfeed, the more protection you get.

IF BREASTFEEDING IS SO GREAT, WHY IS IT SO FREAKING HARD?

When I was pregnant the first time around, I figured breastfeeding would be a breeze. I mean, it certainly seemed easy for my mother's intrepid breast-baring friend. Just pop baby on boob and you're done—there's not much else to it, right?

Oh, how wrong—and naïve—I was! To work effectively (and painlessly) there are actually quite a few components to breastfeeding that you have to get right. It's tricky; it takes practice; and learning the ropes is time-consuming. What's particularly troubling, however, is that the majority of new mothers—right around 80 percent, according to the CDC—start out breastfeeding, probably with the highest of hopes. But most of them stop as soon as the going gets tough. By month three, only around 40 percent are still breastfeeding exclusively. By six months, that number drops down to less than 20 percent.

What this tells us is that most mamas *want* to breastfeed, but that far too many aren't getting the support and the education they need.

And after my own experiences, I totally understand why so many women throw in the towel and switch to formula. I ended up breastfeeding my son for two years, but after struggling through the first few weeks, I wasn't sure if I'd make it past month two.

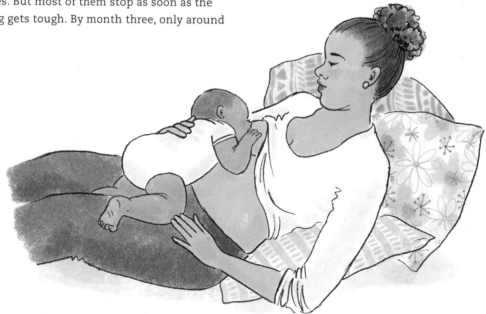

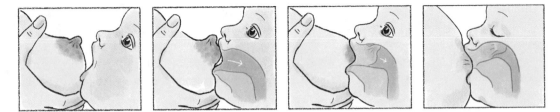

A GOOD LATCH IS A "DEEP" LATCH, WHERE BABY TAKES A BIG MOUTHFUL OF BREAST TISSUE

The key is not to get discouraged if you don't get the hang of it right away. And don't give up.

Here's a look at some of the most common barriers to breastfeeding. Keep in mind that we'll talk even more about breastfeeding in the Special Delivery section, coming up soon.

THE LATCH

The position of your baby's mouth on and around the nipple—a.k.a. the latch—isn't random; it's a foundational component of successful breastfeeding. In fact, I suspect that latch issues are one of the main reasons mamas give up on breastfeeding before they've really gotten started. Because the wrong latch can turn what should be a pleasant experience into something completely and utterly painful.

Ideally, both the nipple and the areola should fit deeply within baby's mouth. This forces the nipple back toward the soft palate, encouraging baby's gums to compress the breast tissue and his tongue to do the milking. When baby has a shallow latch, on the other hand, his gums directly compress the *nipple*. (Ouch!)

Artificial nipples, meanwhile, don't need to be inserted quite so far, nor do they require the same jaw and tongue coordination. The difference between an artificial nipple and the real thing is what leads to "nipple confusion," one of the many reasons you want to breastfeed exclusively, preferably for four to six weeks, before introducing a bottle or pacifier.

What You Can Do: Enlist help early! Habits (both good and bad) form quickly, so it's vital to get the latch figured out ASAP. I was blessed that the birth center where I delivered had a phenomenal lactation consultant on staff. Midwives and nurses can be of great help, too. If something doesn't feel right—ask! And keep in mind that breastfeeding should never be painful. I also *highly* recommend hiring a certified lactation consultant for one-on-one support. (Look for the initials IBCLC after her name.) She can spot things like tongue or lip ties, which can make a good, deep latch nearly impossible. I was blown away at the amount of knowledge I got from a single in-home visit. These ladies are so helpful, in fact, that I call them Breast Whisperers. Finally, there are loads of free resources available online: check out La Leche League, the Academy of Breastfeeding Medicine, and Breastfeeding Inc. for instructional videos and tutorials. Even better, drop by a free Le Leche meeting or seek out a Breastfeeding USA chapter in your own town.

OVERSUPPLY AND ENGORGEMENT

In the immediate days after birth, the milk your baby receives isn't really milk at all: it's colostrum, the thick, yellowish liquid that's super-rich in nutrients and antibodies. True breast milk doesn't "come in" until day three, four, or five, at which point your breasts may

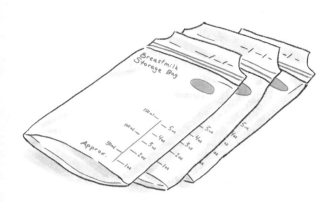

flow should regulate itself. This is why it's so important to keep at it. Skipping a feeding, for example, will only worsen engorgement, making things more difficult. In the meantime, swollen breasts can be soothed by warm baths and light massage.

SORE NIPPLES

Breastfeeding can become positively toe-curling if you're suffering from sore or cracked nipples. Since I experienced no pain with my son, however, I didn't really understand this problem until my little Paloma came into the world. I thought the discomfort I was starting to experience had something to do with the fact that she was nursing every hour, *on the hour*. What I didn't realize—even as a second-time mama—was that she had an extremely shallow latch. (That's why she was nursing so often; she wasn't getting enough milk with each feeding.) By day three, my soreness turned to violent pain. I had blood blisters on both nipples, and was nearly in tears at the mere thought of another breastfeeding session. Once again, though, a lactation consultant came to my rescue. First, she pointed out that Paloma had a lip tie, which we addressed right away with a laser treatment. (Everyone has a connective membrane, called a frenulum, behind the upper lip that attaches to the gums. Sometimes, however, a frenulum is especially

suddenly become swollen, hard, and—frankly—*enormous*. Breast engorgement is not only uncomfortable it can make breastfeeding difficult for two main reasons.

First, engorgement sometimes goes hand in hand with a fast letdown, or milk that comes out too fast, which can overwhelm and frustrate baby. Second, you may struggle with oversupply, which can sometimes result in a baby consuming too much *foremilk* (which is lactose-rich, great for hydration and quick energy) and not enough *hindmilk* (which is more satiating due to a higher fat content). Babies who receive too much foremilk can suffer with excess gas—so, lots of belching, hiccups, and toots.

What You Can Do: Breast milk production is a supply-and-demand system, so as you and baby settle into a nursing pattern, your milk

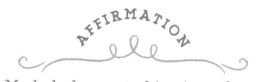

My body has everything it needs to
nourish and feed my baby.
My body is already preparing to breastfeed.

WHAT IF I REALLY CAN'T BREASTFEED?

In the study from UC Davis I mentioned, 40 percent of mamas surveyed worried they weren't making enough milk to feed their babies. And I'm not surprised. Research indicates that perceived low milk production (also called perceived insufficient milk, or PIM) is the number one reason mamas discontinue breastfeeding and/or begin formula supplementation. But that's just it: their low supply is only *perceived*. Lack of experience reading a baby's cues, knowing sleep-wake patterns, and feeling like the breasts aren't full or large enough can all undermine a new mama's confidence. This is why education and support are so important, not to mention empowering, because the majority of mamas *are* producing enough milk, and low production can usually be boosted without much trouble—by pumping between feedings, limiting the use of artificial nipples and pacifiers, and continuing to breastfeed. A lot.

Some mamas, however, really do produce too little milk (usually this is due to some hormonal issue or insufficient glandular tissue) or are unable to breastfeed for other reasons (perhaps due to taking a medication that's not baby-friendly, or a job that makes regular pumping difficult, if not impossible). Still others would just prefer to formula feed. All mothers, however, want to give their babies the very best nourishment possible. So, what to do? Is conventional formula your only option?

Definitely not.

Option 1 is to consider giving your baby donor milk, that is, breast milk from another woman. It's important to mention that there are always risks associated with feeding baby anything but his own mother's milk, directly from the breast. Parents have to weigh the benefits of optimal nutrition against the possibility of disease or pathogen transmission. Check out Only the Breast, MilkShare, and Eats on Feets, all of which have their own recommendations regarding the screening of donors and safe handling and storage of donor milk.

Option 2 is to explore organic formulas. In the United States, the FDA mandates that all infant formula—even organic brands—contain certain nutrients, some of which can only be created synthetically. This is why I actually prefer two brands of European formula, HiPP Organic Infant Milk and Holle Organic Infant Formula (they don't contain as many artificial ingredients). You can read loads more about organic formulas, both American and European, as well as homemade varieties, at mamanatural.com.

Finally, some especially crunchy mamas actually make their own formula. Seriously! (For example, the Weston A. Price Foundation carefully crafted a homemade formula, which thousands of babies have thrived on.) Certainly, you need a careful blend of the right nutrients; lack of the right ingredients (or inclusion of the wrong ones!) could render a DIY formula very dangerous. Always consult your child's pediatrician about what to feed baby.

Lactation Cookies

It's a wee bit early to be worried about milk supply, but it's great to have a recipe for lactation cookies on hand—and there's no rule that says you have to wait for baby's birth to try them. In fact, I've fed these scrumptious cookies to my husband, my son, and some friends that came over to visit, and nobody started lactating but me (everybody *loved* the cookies, though!). The secret to a good lactation cookie is lots of "galactagogues," which is a fancy word for substances that promote the formation and flow of breast milk. True, there aren't any definitive studies to support the effectiveness of food or herb-based galactagogues (as opposed to pharmaceutical varieties), but the benefit reaped by many, many natural mamas is proof enough for me. I like to freeze a few batches of dough and bake as necessary. The best part? We're eliminating all the junk—gluten, refined sugar, etc.—that gets tossed into store-brought brands.

INGREDIENTS

2 cups organic rolled oats

¼ tapioca flour (or substitute organic cornstarch)

½ cup organic coconut sugar

¼ cup brewer's yeast flakes

1 tablespoon fennel seed, ground

1 teaspoon aluminum-free baking powder

½ teaspoon baking soda

½ teaspoon sea salt

½ cup almond butter

¼ cup plus 2 tablespoons coconut oil, melted

2 eggs

2 tablespoons raw honey

½ teaspoon organic vanilla extract

Preheat the oven to 350°F. Add rolled oats to a food processor and pulse until you've achieved a flour-like consistency. Combine oats, flour, and all other dry ingredients into a large bowl. In a smaller bowl, combine the almond butter, coconut oil, eggs, honey, and vanilla. Add the wet ingredients to the dry ingredients, mixing 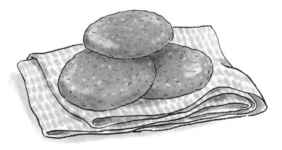 *well with a spoon or clean hands. Form flat cookies about the size of a silver dollar and place them on a greased (with coconut oil) sheet pan. Bake for 15 to 20 minutes, checking for the slightest bit of browning at the edges.*

tight, and it essentially holds the upper lip in place. Tongue ties are common, too.) Next, I had to correct her shallow latch, which she defaulted to due to the lip tie and my oversupply. Eventually we got it all worked out, but in the meantime, I needed something to soothe the pain.

What You Can Do: There are loads of nipple creams on the market. Many natural mamas use just plain ol' coconut oil. And while both of those provided some relief, I knew there had to be a better solution. After some tinkering, I came up with a concoction that's pretty close to magical. In my experience, this simple routine will reduce any pain within a feeding or two, and end discomfort completely within twenty-four hours. It's also a good way to ward off infections like thrush, as well as give baby a probiotic boost, so it's a win-win. (One caveat: If you have a premature or immune-challenged newborn, it's best to just stick with coconut oil.) Here's what you'll need:

♡ 1 tablespoon raw apple cider vinegar

♡ 1 cup filtered water

♡ Raw coconut oil

♡ Powdered infant probiotics (I like Klaire Labs)

♡ Organic cotton balls

Start by mixing the apple cider vinegar and water (you can keep your solution in a peri bottle or Mason jar). After each feeding, use a cotton ball to apply the vinegar solution to each nipple and areola (this kills any harmful bacteria or yeast). Next, apply a small amount (less than ¼ teaspoon) of the coconut oil to the breast. Pour a small amount of probiotic powder into the palm of your just-washed hand, and sprinkle it directly onto the oiled nipple. Finally, cover the nipple with a small piece of paper towel—this creates a barrier between your breast and bra, preventing staining and rubbing. Repeat for twenty-four hours or keep up the routine as a preventive practice.

mama-do list

- Want to test your breastfeeding knowledge? Head over to mamanatural.com to take a quick quiz.

- Didn't score so well? You don't have to wait for birth to learn more about breastfeeding. Consider meeting with an International Board Certified Lactation Consultant (an IBCLC) now and you'll have tips you can put into practice right away—not to mention a pro to call if you run into any problems. The best part? Most insurance plans cover the cost.

- If you work full-time and are planning to breastfeed, you've likely thought about purchasing a breast pump. However, plenty of stay-at-home mamas pump too: to encourage milk supply, to relieve engorgement, or to let their partner tackle a few middle-of-the-night feedings via bottle. Now is a good time to buy one. Luckily, most insurance plans will cover the cost of your pump, too.

a little something for the pain

WHAT'S UP WITH *baby*?

We have reached the six-week mark! No, we haven't traveled back in time—you've got six weeks left to go (give or take) in this pregnancy! You've also got more *baby* inside you now than amniotic fluid. This fluid is still serving some important purposes, however: cushioning her from bumps and thumps, preventing compression of the umbilical cord, and giving her tiny muscles a daily workout—in fact, you could say floating around in there is a bit like water aerobics. Baby is also continuing to drink the fluid, as well as replenishing the supply (through urination) at a rate of roughly two cups a day. To help her with this process, make sure you're staying well hydrated. About 4 percent of mamas-to-be will be diagnosed with oligohydramnios, the technical term for too little fluid, which can cause complications in the latter stages of pregnancy; treatment often includes IV infusion or induction. So drink up!

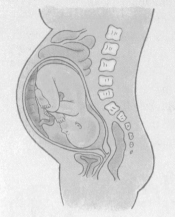

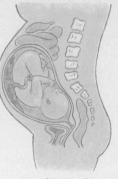

ANTERIOR
PRESENTATION

POSTERIOR
PRESENTATION

POSTERIOR PRESENTATION CAN CONTRIBUTE TO "BACK LABOR,"
OR INTENSE LOWER BACK PAIN DURING CONTRACTIONS.

WHAT'S UP WITH *mama*?

Baby's not the only one with a constant need to urinate—just when you thought you couldn't pee any more, you're back in the bathroom! Of course, that's because baby is sitting *right on top* of your bladder now, which leaves the organ with a lot less, shall we say, storage space. (Don't be surprised if you leak a little when you sneeze, too.) Be advised that the urgency and frequency with which you need to go may only increase in these final few weeks before birth. Resist the urge to cut down on your water intake, thinking that'll provide some sweet relief (remember: stay hydrated!). Do consider reducing your nighttime fluid consumption to help reduce middle-of-the-night pit stops. And if you're feeling the urge to pee but having difficulty urinating, touch base with your midwife or doctor, as this could be a sign of a UTI.

There's an old joke about childbirth: if anyone could remember the pain, no one in the world would have more than one kid.

There's just no getting around it: childbirth can hurt. Although for many women, it's not so much *painful* as it is intense. Unfortunately, horror stories about "awful" childbirths abound on the internet. As we've discussed already, birth is almost always depicted as comically horrifying in the movies. Even childbirth "reality" shows feature a disproportionately large number of "emergency" deliveries (because, *hello!*, ratings).

The result? Many women are terrified—and I do mean terrified—of giving birth. Even mamas who would like to go natural often sign up for drugs before the contractions get going, because they're just not convinced they can handle the pain.

One thing that may prove helpful is to reframe pain as a *positive* part of the birthing experience.

Each and every contraction, after all, only brings you closer to meeting your baby. But it's also important to point out that childbirth isn't uncomfortable for no good reason. In fact, pain has a crucial role to play in the process:

♡ In the wild, intensifying contractions tell mama it's time to hunker down in a safe space away from predators—for us humans, it's how we know it's time to get to the birth center or hospital. Without a bit of pain, a lot more women would be delivering in cars and at the supermarket.

♡ Labor pains also indicate *how* best to birth your baby. Being uncomfortable can signal us to change positions, which helps baby descend through the birth canal. Laboring flat on your back, on the other hand, not only compresses the pelvis, but it also prevents you from following your body's natural cues. It's no wonder that women who remain mobile tend to have shorter, less painful deliveries.

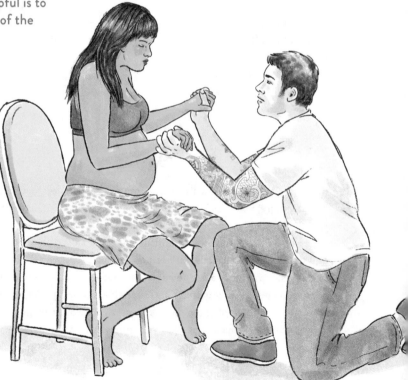

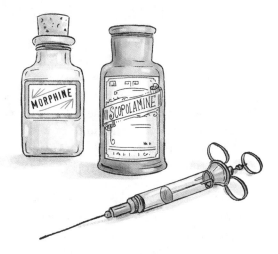

♡ Pain is part of a delicate dance within the body: It signals your brain to release more oxytocin, for one thing, so that contractions become more efficient and effective. It triggers the release of endorphins, which help to relieve pain and, at the moment of birth, create a sense of euphoria. It also provides a measure of protection: pain can indicate when it's time to back off from pushing or shimmy to a new position to prevent tearing.

Pain, in other words, is just your body's way of talking to you. So, you could say that masking it or completely numbing it is akin to sticking your fingers in your ears and shouting "I can't hear you!" Epidurals and narcotic pain-relief drugs, when administered indiscriminately, can have unintended consequences.

THE EPIDURAL DILEMMA

Have you ever heard of "twilight sleep"?

Invented by German doctors back in the early 1900s, twilight sleep emerged as a way to completely eradicate (supposedly) the pain associated with childbirth. Laboring women were injected with a small dose of morphine (for the pain) mixed with scopolamine, which wiped out all memory of the main event. That's right. Women woke up with zero memory of birth and a cute little baby in their arms.

The problem? I mean, *besides* the fact that mamas couldn't immediately hold, bond with, or breastfeed their babies, nor could they remember anything about the births of their children? *Besides* the fact that the drugs depressed baby's central nervous system, which often contributed to difficulty breathing?

Women undergoing twilight sleep also went a little bit nuts.

Turns out the hit of morphine wasn't enough to actually dull the pain—women were still very much in pain—they just had no memory of it. They were so drugged up during the procedure, however, that they acted like crazy people. Patients thrashed and screamed and clawed and scratched. They had to be strapped down like mental patients to keep from hurting themselves. In fact, it's widely believed that if husbands had been allowed in delivery rooms back then, the practice never would have been allowed to continue, and certainly not for as long as it did. But the really surprising part about twilight sleep? It was *women* who demanded it be made available.

The issue of pain management during childbirth has a long, weird, and winding history, which far precedes the invention of the morphine-scopolamine cocktail. Before twilight sleep, ether and chloroform were commonly used for anesthesia. Before that, nitrous oxide, bloodletting, alcohol, and various herbal concoctions were all popular pain relief methods. But it really wasn't until the mid-1800s that the issue turned political. Physicians, inspired by the increasingly sophisticated opiates and anesthetics at their disposal, began to medicate more and more births. That caused a bit of a backlash among religious and conservative thinkers, who believed that pain during childbirth was divine punishment: Eve's curse for eating the forbidden fruit. In other words, seeking pain relief during labor amounted to sinning against God.

We could talk for hours and hours (or should I say, pages and pages) about the feminist implications of pain relief during labor, but the short version of the story is this: Mamas-to-be began to advocate for anesthesia during childbirth as a woman's right. In 1847, Fanny Longfellow, wife to the poet Henry Wadsworth Longfellow, became the first American woman to undergo anesthesia during the birth of her third child. She later wrote to her sister-in-law: "I did it for the good of women everywhere." When American doctors failed to adopt the German practice of twilight sleep (incidentally, most American physicians were against the practice), women formed the National Twilight Sleep Association and campaigned to make the procedure more widely available. To meet the growing demand, however, more and more doctors (with less and less training) began offering fixed—rather than individualized—doses of morphine and scopolamine, which led to more and more complications, injuries, and side effects. Twilight sleep eventually fell out of favor by the late 1960s, which is right around the time a new form of pain relief, the epidural, was coming on the scene.

The practice has modernized considerably over the years, but these days "epidural" may actually refer to one of three different procedures:

Epidural Anesthesia: The name is sort of misleading (for laypeople, at least), since "epidural anesthesia" doesn't knock you unconscious, nor does an "epidural" denote

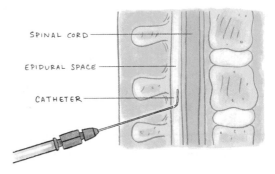

EPIDURAL ANESTHESIA

a particular kind of pain relief drug; rather, it's a part of the body. Women undergoing an epidural during labor will first have their lower back numbed with a local anesthetic. Then, a slightly larger needle will be inserted into the "epidural space" (which lies between a membrane that envelops the spinal cord and the vertebral wall) through which the anesthesiologist will thread a hair-thin catheter. In fact, an epidural is a little like having an IV inserted into the small of your back—the catheter (not the needle) will remain in place, and the medication will be delivered continuously or via periodic injection.

As for the medication itself (as well as the *amount* of medication you're receiving), that will vary from hospital to hospital. Typical numbing agents include local anesthetics like lidocaine or bupivacaine, but they may be delivered in combination with narcotic drugs, like fentanyl, morphine, or Demerol. Some hospitals allow mama to control the dosage of the drugs herself (via one of those little bedside buttons). Interestingly, a study from researchers at Long Beach Memorial Medical Center indicates that when allowed to control the dosage, women use less medication (and have lower C-section rates).

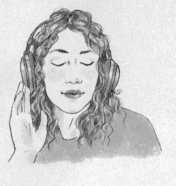
Spinal Block: Unlike an epidural—which allows for the continuous administration of pain relief drugs—a spinal block is a one-time injection of either narcotic or anesthetic directly into the spinal fluid. Spinals typically last for up to two hours, which is why they're generally used when your doctor has a clear indication of exactly how long you need to be numb; for example, if you're being wheeled in to deliver via Cesarean.

Combined Spinal-Epidural (CSE): Also called "walking epidurals," CSEs are essentially what they sound like: a spinal (a.k.a. a onetime dose of drugs) combined with the administration of an epidural (a catheter than remains in the lower back). When and if the initial spinal injection wears off or becomes inadequate, the epidural kicks in. The advantages of CSEs are that they may allow more sensation in the legs and more freedom of movement, but—despite the name—it's unlikely that you'll be up and walking around.

Obviously, the modern epidural is a heckuva lot safer and more effective than twilight sleep—none of that troublesome screaming and thrashing. Epidural anesthesia allows mamas to stay awake and present for the births of their babies. It has grown much more sophisticated with time (typically, because less anesthetic is injected, allowing for greater mobility and movement). Today, epidurals are the number one most-requested form of pain relief during labor, administered to anywhere from 60 percent to 85 percent of mamas.

WHEN AN EPIDURAL MIGHT BE *EXACTLY WHAT YOU NEED*

Sure, you may be imagining a blissful, peaceful, "orgasmic" vaginal birth, but Mama? Not all of us get that experience. I certainly didn't the first time around! Birth is messy. It's unpredictable. And it won't always bend to your wishes. Which is why we're so lucky that interventions do exist. In some cases, an epidural can actually *save* you a trip to the operating room:

✣ By relaxing a tensed-up mama, an epidural can help to open the pelvic passage.

✣ For mamas who end up laboring for what seems like days, an epidural may allow them some much-needed rest before it's time to push the baby out.

✣ Birth can be overwhelming—physically, emotionally, mentally, and even spiritually. For some mamas, an epidural offers a way to cope, bringing about a sense of calm.

It's important to remember that epidurals aren't the enemy; it's just good to understand their uses and side effects.

Opting for an epidural? Ask your practitioner if he or she has access to a "peanut ball," which is a birth ball shaped like—yes—a large peanut. Placing one between your legs during labor (even when you're confined to a bed) helps keep the pelvis open and encourages baby to descend. In fact, a small study published in the *Journal of Perinatal Education* suggests that peanut balls can help shorten epidural-aided labor by nearly two hours!

Nitrous oxide, a.k.a. laughing gas, has been used for centuries as a form of pain relief, although you're more likely to see it at the dentist's office than a birth center. However, that may be changing.

In 2011, the American College of Nurse-Midwives announced that there's adequate research to support the reasonable safety and efficacy of nitrous oxide during labor, recommended that midwives be trained to administer nitrous, and suggested that mamas-to-be should be educated about it as an option during childbirth.

Nitrous oxide presents a lower risk than epidurals or narcotics because the half-life is short. (As soon as mama takes off the nitrous, the gas leaves her system.) Talk to your midwife or doctor for more info.

But as with all previous forms of pain relief, epidurals are not without side effects.

♡ One of the most common is a drop in maternal blood pressure, which could disrupt the flow of oxygen-rich blood to the baby. To prevent that, you'll be started on IV fluids before receiving the epidural, and your blood pressure will be routinely monitored. In the event of a sudden drop, you may be given medications, more fluids, or supplemental oxygen.

♡ Epidurals require the use of continuous electronic fetal monitoring to ensure that baby's heart rate isn't affected; you'll likely have to spend the remainder of your labor in bed or close to bed. You may need a urinary catheter, too.

♡ Generally speaking, a modern epidural shouldn't completely restrict your ability to push the baby out when the time comes. Because not all epidurals are created equal, however—and because not all mamas react to them the same—there's always a chance that you won't have enough sensation to push effectively when the time comes. In these circumstances the flow of drugs may need to be "turned down" or halted. (Since your body hasn't been producing endorphins, turning down an epidural can be pretty painful.) Epidurals also tend to space out or weaken the strength of contractions, which is why so many women will require Pitocin to get things going again. Together, these interventions up your chance of needing an eventual C-section or instrument assistance (such as forceps or vacuum extraction).

♡ Rarer side effects include headache, severe "spinal headache," fever, ringing in the ears, shivering, itching, drowsiness, nausea, infection, bleeding, and nerve damage.

♡ Any narcotics administered during labor can cross the placenta and reach the baby. Exactly how baby might be affected, however, is difficult to determine—again, the type of medication, the dosage, and the baby's tolerance will vary from hospital to hospital and from birth to birth. According to the American Pregnancy Association, there is evidence to suggest that babies may become lethargic in utero, and that epidurals can cause respiratory distress and/or decreased fetal heart rate.

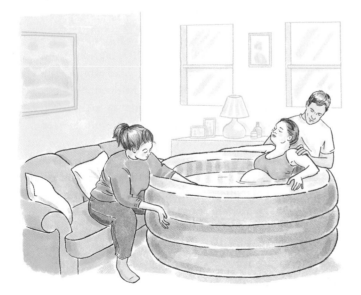

♡ The most important time for establishing a breastfeeding relationship is in the minutes and hours after birth; epidurals, however, can make baby lethargic, and sleepy babies don't tend to breastfeed well. Epidurals have also been linked to problems "latching on" and a depressed sucking reflex.

♡ Finally, we know that epidurals extend labor—by at least two to three hours, according to a study published in *Obstetrics & Gynecology*.

ALTERNATIVE PAIN RELIEF THAT *WON'T* DISRUPT YOUR LABOR

Something else interesting happened alongside the rise of twilight sleep. Although it was women who advocated for access to the morphine-scopolamine combo, being rendered completely unconscious meant that childbirth underwent a *major* shift: instead of control resting in the hands of women (both the mother and her midwife), it fell into the hands of men (after all, there weren't many female physicians in the early 1900s). A desire to reverse that trend, combined with concerns about the effects of such heavy anesthesia, is partly what gave rise to the natural childbirth movement. Whereas first-wave feminists claimed pain relief drugs as a right, second-wave feminists called for a return to nonmedicalized, low-intervention birth.

Birth without anesthetics or narcotics, however, doesn't mean birth without pain management *at all.*

The 1970s brought us the first of several programs geared toward nonmedical pain relief, including the Lamaze and Bradley methods. Slowly, mamas began to reclaim some control in the birth process. And the big benefit of nonmedical, alternative pain relief? It won't disrupt the progress of labor. Non-narcotic interventions don't interfere with your body's natural chemical cascade, don't artificially prolong the birth process, and don't jeopardize the health of mama or baby.

But the best part about alternative pain relief is that you can mix and match as many of these methods as suit you.

HYDROTHERAPY

Water births are on the rise, and rightfully so—a Cochrane review of existing studies confirms that immersion is not only an effective pain-relief technique, but that it actually reduces the need for an epidural. (Although, I don't find this surprising—I mean, who among us hasn't soaked in a tub to soothe tired and achy muscles?) But there are some benefits associated with hopping in a birth tub other than pain relief: The buoyancy helps keep you in an upright position (so that you're working *with* gravity, rather than against it), as well as eases the feeling of pressure. A warm bath is also relaxing; the less tense you are, the less likely you are to secrete fear-based hormones that might stall your labor.

Of course, you can reap the benefits of hydrotherapy even if you're not planning to give birth in a tub. I spent some time in the shower during my first birth, letting the water beat down on my back, which helped considerably. You might also try sitting down on a shower stool and directing the showerhead where you need the most relief.

CHANGING POSITIONS

Your labor pains will guide you into the positions that are best for delivering your baby. If baby is coming too fast, for example, many mamas will instinctively lie down. When babies need the help of gravity, mamas often prefer to stand, sit or squat. Laboring on your hands and knees can help when a baby is not in the exact right position for birth. Walking around can help baby settle into the pelvis and speed dilation. Birthing balls, bars, and stools can all help support you in whatever position *feels* right. Labor tends to be quicker and less painful when you're free to work with gravity to encourage baby's movement and rotation.

BREATHING, UNICORNS, AND
FINDING YOUR HAPPY PLACE

In any birth class worth its salt, you'll hear about "breathing" as a way to cope with the pain. And I'll be honest: I used to categorize that right alongside leprechauns and fairies—which is to say, I figured there's no way *breathing*, of all things, could possibly help me in the heat of labor.

I've been proven wrong, though—not only by my own experience, but by a boatload of medical research.

A study from St. Joseph's Hospital and Medical Center, for example, found that women with painful conditions such as fibromyalgia experienced less pain when they focused on controlled breathing at a slow rate. (Why? Probably because focused breathing calms the sympathetic nervous system, which is responsible for—you guessed it—pain.) On the flip side, other studies have demonstrated that focused breathing actually *increases* our pain threshold.

Your breath has a rhythm that's actually quite similar to a birth contraction. There's a peak (the top of inhalation) and then a release (exhalation). If you can stay "on top of your breath"—that is, stay in charge of the pace of your breathing—then you've got a good shot that your labor will be completely manageable. And while there are plenty of breath patterns you can learn about and research, I think simplest is best: steady inhale through your nose for a few seconds, steady exhale for a few seconds. Try breathing consciously for at least 5 minutes each day (right before bed is a *great* time to do this). Notice how relaxed you feel? With regular practice, you can carry this calm and centered breathing right into your birth. The Pelvic Power Pose (page 234) is great for this, too.

Okay, so you're breathing, right? Good. Now go to your happy place.

It's natural to close your eyes when you're doing breath work, which makes it easy to add in some visualization. Some mamas like to picture a peaceful scene in their minds and then "visit" that place during the tough parts of labor. Just as your body will release stress hormones and adrenaline if you're watching, say, a scary movie, it will release positive endorphins when you're focused on a peaceful mental image.

So figure out your happy place. Bring in as many sights, sounds, smells, and sensations as you can to make it real. Get it all nicely prepared, and then go there when you're doing your breath work and, of course, during childbirth.

Clove Rice Pudding

Everybody knows the spicy flavor of clove, probably from sipping warm apple cider in the dead of winter. But did you know that cloves are a centuries-old pain-relief remedy? Forget Novocain; ancient dentists used cloves to numb an aching tooth. (Try it yourself: chew a clove and you'll experience a slight numbing sensation.) The clove is also a rich source of antioxidants, as well as a powerful digestive aid, and one of my favorite ways to use it is in this creamy, comforting clove rice pudding.

INGREDIENTS

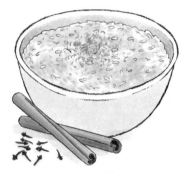

1 cup organic long-grain brown rice (preferably sprouted)

2 cups filtered water

2 cinnamon sticks

1 teaspoon whole cloves

¼ cup raisins

2 tablespoons maple syrup

1 cup whole coconut milk

A dash each of ground cinnamon, nutmeg, and sea salt

2 eggs (optional)

Into a saucepan, add rice, water, cinnamon sticks, and cloves. Let soak at room temperature overnight. In the morning, bring to a boil, then reduce heat to low. Carefully remove cinnamon sticks and cloves with a slotted spoon. Cover and let simmer for 45 minutes, or until the rice is fully cooked and the water has evaporated. Add raisins, maple syrup, and coconut milk and simmer uncovered for an additional 15 to 20 minutes. If you like, you can stir in the eggs in the last 5 minutes for extra protein. Serve warm, with a dash of cinnamon, nutmeg, and sea salt, and a dollop of butter.

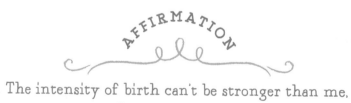

AFFIRMATION

The intensity of birth can't be stronger than me,
because it *is* me.

kimberly: I've given birth five times, and it's always been intense. What helped most was a birthing ball, squatting, pushing on my hands and knees, and my husband telling me that he loved me and couldn't wait to meet our baby. I actually tried an epidural with my fifth baby and wound up laboring on my back, stuck in bed. I hated it! It ended up being the longest labor of all five deliveries, and I am now the biggest advocate for natural birth!

amanda: My labor was a bit unique in that my baby was transverse cephalic (head down, but facing sideways) and didn't want to turn. Because of that, my labor was crazy-long—forty-seven hours!—and much more intense than I'd expected. Eventually, I was given an ultimatum: get an epidural so my body could have a break, or end up with a Cesarean. I had to grieve the decision; for a while I felt like I'd done this horrible disservice to my baby by not following through without drugs. But I think natural moms need to understand that epidurals weren't necessarily invented only for pain relief, but rather for situations like mine: when mom needs some help in order to avoid further complications and interventions. It's still really hard for me looking back. I still sometimes think, *What if I'd just waited one more hour?* But as determined as I was to go natural, babies can't be born sideways—it just doesn't work that way.

patricia: The pain of labor was much less intense than I expected it to be. I had more fear than anything; because it wasn't that bad, I kept thinking it would get worse. But it didn't!

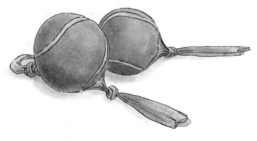

MASSAGE

You don't need a professional masseuse to reap some serious benefits from healing touch. The key to effective massage during labor, however, is that the movements should be slow and repetitive to stimulate the production of oxytocin (intense or aggressive deep tissue massage, on the other hand, won't provide the same hormonal payoff). Have your partner or labor support person practice before your labor begins, so you can help him learn what's most relaxing to you.

To take your massage to the next level, let me introduce you to an easy-to-make but remarkably effective little device: the tennis ball back massager. A Bradley childbirth instructor turned me on to this, and while the contraption looks kinda awkward, I couldn't *believe* how good it felt. To make one, you'll need two tennis balls, scissors, and a pair of old nylons.

Start by cutting one leg off the pantyhose. Then, about four inches from the tip of the toe, tie a knot. Drop one of the tennis balls into the nylons, pushing it down so that it rests firmly against the knot you've tied, then tie another knot directly on the other side of the ball (the knots should hold the ball firmly in place). Drop the second tennis ball into the nylons, create another knot, then tie your loose ends together. (Confused? We have a video demo on mama natural.com.) Have your partner roll the tennis balls across your lower back as if using a rolling pin; the targeted counterpressure, provides excellent pain relief.

ACUPRESSURE

Acupressure is a form of traditional Chinese medicine that involves the application of direct, firm pressure to specific points on the body. Using your fingers, thumbs, knuckles, or elbows, try applying steady pressure (or having your partner apply steady pressure) to the following areas—just don't give this a go until you're at least 37 weeks along, and keep the pressure light until you're actually in labor:

♡ The fatty pad between the base of your thumb and pointer finger. (In the world of acupressure, this point is referred to as Large Intestine 4, or LI4.) Putting some pressure on this point can be helpful in the earliest stages of labor, as well as during the pushing phase.

♡ Have your partner press on your lower back on either side of the spine (just above the glutes). Pressure to the lower-back points can be soothing if you're experiencing back labor or when you're in the middle of an intense contraction.

♡ There's a point on your inner calf, about four fingers up from the ankle, that should feel tender to the touch—that's known as Spleen 6, and pressure here may be especially helpful in the case of stalled labor.

♡ In the middle of the foot, located in the depression just beneath the ball, is Kidney 1. Pressure here is said to pull energy downward, and may help to calm stress and anxiety.

ACUPRESSURE POINTS DURING LABOR

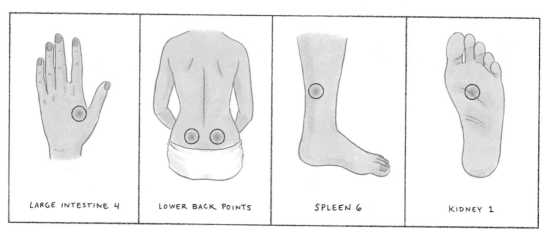

| LARGE INTESTINE 4 | LOWER BACK POINTS | SPLEEN 6 | KIDNEY 1 |

HOMEOPATHIC REMEDIES

Homeopathic medicine is made from diluted substances derived from plants, animals, and minerals; it's very gentle, as well as generally safe to take during childbirth. If you're not familiar with homeopathic remedies, however, you may want to consult a naturopath and/ or your midwife or doctor. Here's a look at the remedies I tucked into my birthing bag:

- ♡ Caullophyllum or Cimicifuga: for cervical dilation

- ♡ Gelsemium and Pulsatilla: for slow or stalled labor

- ♡ Arnica: for pain and fatigue during the pushing phase

- ♡ Kali Carbonicum: for back labor

- ♡ Kali Phosphoricum: for overall exhaustion

mama-do list

- ○ Want to see the Tennis Ball Back Massager in action? Head over to mamanatural .com to watch a quick how-to video.

- ○ Here's another quick tip for labor pain relief: stay hydrated. Sounds simple, I know, but have you ever gotten bad leg cramps after a hard workout? Some of that's due to electrolyte and glucose deficits. Truth is, our muscles need glucose to contract and relax effectively. When a mama goes hours on end without food and drink, she can unknowingly make her contractions worse. So have your coconut water or sweetened red raspberry leaf tea on hand!

- ○ Have you installed baby's car seat yet? Have you had your installation job *inspected*? Visit seatcheck.org to find a qualified inspector near you. Local police and fire stations sometimes have a certified installer on-duty, too. Call ahead to inquire.

- ○ Consider visiting a naturopath if you'd like to try some homeopathic remedies during labor.

WEEK 35

are you positive?

GBS-POSITIVE, THAT IS

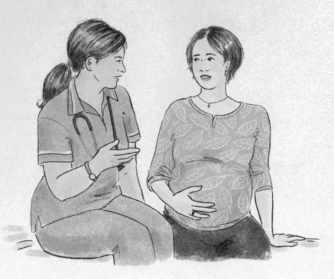

WHAT'S UP WITH *baby*?

Five-and-a-half pounds and near 20 inches long, Mama—can you believe how big Baby Natural is getting? (Judging from the size of your belly, the answer is probably: *Uh, yes.*) If you're having a boy, big things are happening this week: His testicles are migrating from his abdomen (where they've been growing all this time) to his scrotum. And since we're talking about, well, boy parts, now is as good a time as any to talk about circumcision. Some people wish to circumcise (or not to) for religious reasons. Others just think baby should "match" his father. When we discovered we were having a boy, my husband's initial thought was "of course he'll be circumcised." But after doing a bit of research, we decided to leave our son intact. Two things to keep in mind . . . Circumcision is not medically necessary—in fact, some of the claims (that circumcised penises are somehow "cleaner") are a little dubious. It's also not as common these days as most people think. You'll find more info on page 447.

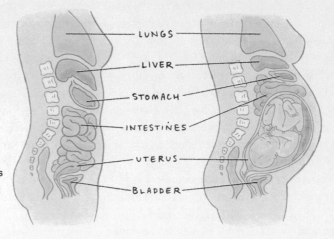

LUNGS
LIVER
STOMACH
INTESTINES
UTERUS
BLADDER

HOW YOUR ORGANS MOVE DURING PREGNANCY

WHAT'S UP WITH *mama*?

The closer I got to my due date, the more I felt like I couldn't breathe. Sure, I was nervous about the impending delivery and the inevitable changes that come with having a newborn, but that wasn't the reason I was gasping for air—it felt like my son was doing the Harlem shake *right on top of my lungs*. Some women experience shortness of breath as early as the first or second trimester, which is usually the result of rising hormones triggering your body to breathe more deeply. (Baby's lungs are filled with fluid, remember, so you're technically "breathing for two" during pregnancy.) Shortness of breath in the *third* trimester, however, is caused by a far more obvious culprit: your growing uterus has started to squish your internal organs, including your lungs. Ready for some good news? Any time over the next few weeks, your baby will likely begin to drop down into the pelvis. The phenomena is called "lightening," and it'll relieve some of that pressure, making it easier to take deep, satisfying breaths.

Over the last few months, you've been poked and prodded (and asked to pee—a lot!) in order to complete a variety of prenatal screenings and diagnostic tests. And though you've likely been enjoying a bit of a reprieve from all stuff, soon you'll be called to do the Group B Strep test. You'll be asked to wipe yourself with a cotton swab from the vulva, across the perineum, to the anus. (In other words, front to back—just like wiping.) In many cases, your provider will perform the test for you. So, the procedure itself is simple.

What you'll choose to do with the results, though? Not so much.

WHAT IS GROUP B STREP?

Group B Streptococcus (also known as Group B Strep or GBS) is a particular type of bacteria—*not* the same bacteria that causes strep throat, by the way—that exists naturally in the intestinal tract, urinary tract, vagina, and/or rectum. Roughly 25 percent of women are carriers, although the bacteria may come and go, almost always without triggering any symptoms or health issues. In fact, most women will never even realize it's there. It is a bacterium, however, so there are risks associated with exposure to those who are vulnerable. Think: elderly people, those with chronic medical issues, and—you guessed it—newborn babies.

It's thought that a baby is most likely to be "colonized" with GBS bacteria when passing through the birth canal, although the majority of these babies—just like their mothers—will never develop any symptoms or health issues. A baby is most at risk of developing a GBS *infection*, however, after the amniotic sac ruptures, especially if there's a long delay (more than eighteen hours) between the rupture of membranes and birth. In these cases, the infection is usually the result of bacteria migrating up from the vagina into the amniotic fluid, which baby may then swallow or aspirate.

And GBS infections? They're not good. Complications range from fever and respiratory issues to pneumonia, sepsis, and meningitis (an infection of the fluid surrounding the brain and spinal cord). In short, GBS infections have the potential to cause life-threatening illness, which is why all pregnant women in the US are tested—via vaginal and anal swab—usually sometime between 35 and 37 weeks. Occasionally, GBS is detected even earlier, during a routine urine test, in which case mama will be categorized as a "heavy colonizer" and considered to be GBS-positive for the remainder of her pregnancy.

OKAY, I'VE TESTED POSITIVE FOR GBS: NOW WHAT?

GBS infections emerged (for reasons unknown) back in the early 1970s; and at the time, an infected baby's prognosis was dire—as many as 50 percent of them died. In the face of such grim statistics, the medical community got right to work. Clinical trials and observational studies commissioned throughout the 1980s demonstrated that treating "high-risk" women (that is, women at high risk of transmitting GBS to their children) with antibiotics during labor could prevent infant infections. By the mid-1990s, the CDC had issued new guidelines, giving obstetricians and midwives one of two choices: either follow a risk-management approach (meaning, administer antibiotics during labor only to women who exhibit certain risk factors) or perform a recto-vaginal culture and give antibiotics to any woman who tests positive.

In 2002, the CDC deemed universal screening superior to risk-management and revised its guidelines.

Which brings us to today. If you test positive for GBS at any point in your pregnancy—whether via swab or urine culture—the majority of midwives and doctors will follow the recommendations of the CDC and suggest treatment via IV antibiotics during labor. This approach, it's important to point out, seems to have worked: GBS infections have plummeted since the 1990s, dropping from 1.7 cases per 1,000 births down to 0.25. Put another way, .025 percent of children born in the United States will develop a life-threatening GBS infection.

Universal screening, however, is by no means a perfect solution, and what we don't tend to hear about are the risks associated with widespread antibiotic use.

Here's what you need to know about GBS:

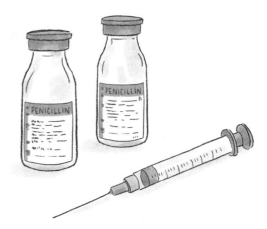

♡ Infections are mercifully rare, even among babies born to women who receive no treatment. Roughly 50 percent of GBS-positive mamas will pass along the bacteria, but only 1 percent to 2 percent of those babies will develop a serious infection. The current mortality rate for infected infants is between 1 percent and 2 percent, although it's significantly higher for premature infants born before 33 weeks.

♡ GBS screening is not foolproof. Because GBS bacteria can come and go, your colonization status may change even after you've had the screening. For example, a mama who tests positive at 35 or 36 weeks might become negative by the time she gives birth (in which case, she'd be receiving antibiotics unnecessarily). Conversely, a mama who tests negative might develop GBS bacteria by the time she goes into labor, yet receive no treatment. In fact, in a review of more than 800,000 live births published in the *New England Journal of Medicine*, the highest percentage of GBS-infected babies (61 percent) were born to mamas who had previously tested negative. Just 18 percent were born to women who received no screening.

♡ Antibiotics do not appear to lower the rate of infant mortality. Most of the information we have to support the use of antibiotics during labor comes from those clinical trials and observational studies performed back in the 1980s. A recent Cochrane review of those trials, however, determined that while the number of GBS *infections* dropped significantly with the administration of antibiotics, the number of infant *deaths* remained unchanged.

♡ Antibiotics come with their own set of side effects. Minor risks include an elevated occurrence of yeast infections in both mothers and babies, as well as the (admittedly rare) possibility of allergic reaction. The much bigger concern, however, is the potential for creating antibiotic-resistant strains of GBS and other bacteria due to such widespread antibiotic use. A separate *New England Journal of Medicine* study, for example, indicates that while GBS infections have fallen in recent years, E. coli infections may be on the rise.

♡ Antibiotics may affect the gut microbiome. We know that babies who are born vaginally pick up protective bacteria with long-term benefits. We also know that babies who are given antibiotics shortly after birth appear to have lower levels of these protective bacteria. However, we know very little—next to nothing, in fact—about the potential effect IV antibiotics administered during labor may have on the formation of baby's microbiome. This is still an emerging field of medical research.

THOUGHTS ON GBS TESTING
FROM MIDWIFE *Cynthia*

I have a love-hate relationship with GBS screening. On the one hand, the risk of a baby getting sick from exposure to the bacterium is very small, but if baby *does* get sick? The outcome is often catastrophic. GBS sepsis, for example—a condition in which the bacterium enters baby's bloodstream, causing multiple infections and multi-organ failure—can be fatal.

As a provider, have I seen babies get sick due to GBS exposure? Yes.

Have I seen babies die from GBS infections? Yes.

Does it happen very often? No.

And there's the rub.

Like many midwifery practices, mine follows the recommendations for screening and treatment put out by the CDC: Mamas are given a urine culture at the beginning of their pregnancy, and at any point from then on if they develop symptoms of a urinary tract infection (UTIs can be caused by GBS). If GBS bacteria is present in the urine, mama will be considered GBS-positive for the remainder of her pregnancy. Otherwise, she'll be screened sometime between 35 and 37 weeks via vaginal culture. For women who test positive, we recommend IV antibiotics in labor.

Some holistic providers do recommend alternative treatments. But while these methods may decrease the colony count of GBS bacteria in the vaginal canal, studies indicate they do nothing to improve newborn outcomes. From a clinical standpoint, the same number of babies will get sick whether a mama chooses an alternative treatment or opts for no treatment. This is why I recommend antibiotics. If a patient declines, however, she'll be treated with the risk-management approach.

HOW TO PERFORM PERINEAL MASSAGE—
AND WHY YOU'D WANT TO

It's one of the great mysteries of childbirth: How will I squeeze something the size of a watermelon out from between my legs without being split in two?

The short answer is that your body is capable of miraculous things. One way or another, you *will* deliver that beautiful baby of yours.

The longer (admittedly less pleasant) answer is that childbirth can definitely take its toll. Vaginal and perineal tears are fairly common, especially among first-time mamas. (The perineum is the soft skin between the vagina and anus. Because of its proximity to the birth canal, as well as the pressure exerted during the pushing phase of labor, this delicate area can undergo a fair amount of trauma during birth.) Not all tears are the same, mind you—some are small and superficial, while others require stitches or sutures to close and take several weeks to heal. And that just begs the question: Is it possible to *prevent* tearing?

Yes! Well, probably. Okay, *maybe.*

It's called "perineal massage," which is exactly what it sounds like: massaging the perineum. It's thought that gently stretching the skin in the weeks before birth may increase flexibility, thereby lessening trauma. And yes, there is some research to support the practice. A 2013 Cochrane review of four separate clinical trials found that once- or twice-weekly massage—performed from 35 weeks onward—reduces the risk of a tear requiring sutures by around 10 percent in first-time mamas. (Among more experienced mamas, regular massage doesn't seem to have much effect on tearing, but it is associated with less perineal pain in the months following delivery.)

My thought is, it's certainly worth a shot! Here's how to do it:

- First, you'll want to prepare your body—soak in a warm bath or use a warm washcloth to soften the area (about 10 minutes or so should do). Then, lie back in a comfortable position with your feet flat on the bed or floor, knees bent. Prop up your back with pillows and use a mirror if necessary.

- Onto clean hands, apply a small amount of nonirritating massage oil (coconut or olive oil are good options). Next, insert the tips of your thumbs into your vagina, and apply firm yet gentle pressure on the perineum, pushing down and away from the body.

- Allow the perineum to stretch gradually for a few minutes. Then move your thumbs along the sides of the vagina for a minute or two, stretching it from side to side.

- Repeat once or twice a week until you go into labor.

Still not sure what you're doing down there? You can find a handy-dandy instructional video (don't worry—it's an *animation*) over at mamanatural.com. There are also detailed instructions in case your partner does the massage for you.

DO I REALLY NEED ANTIBIOTICS?

Statistically speaking, 200 GBS-positive mamas will need to receive antibiotic treatment in order to prevent a single infant infection—that's a lot of antibiotics to dispense "just in case." It's perhaps understandable, then, that some natural mamas may choose to decline IV therapy. (You can always decline the routine GBS screening, too. However, you *will* need antibiotics if you develop signs of infection—more on that in a bit.) Other mamas may prefer to try an alternative remedy. Still others will be more comfortable opting for antibiotics if at any point they've tested positive. (After all, it doesn't matter how low the rate of infection is—it's 100 percent if it's *your* baby!) The risks of GBS infection are serious, and every woman should do her own research, as well as discuss the pros and cons of potential methods of treatment with her midwife or doctor.

NOM OF THE WEEK

Mango Lassi

I remember the first time Michael and I went out for Indian food. I ordered a mango lassi—basically, a yogurt-based milkshake or smoothie—and my taste buds exploded. It was sweet, it was tangy, and I immediately went home and started tinkering with a make-at-home version. The result? This lassi is high in vitamin C, beta-carotene, and calcium, but it'll give you a hefty probiotic boost, too (excellent news if you're trying to ward off GBS).

INGREDIENTS

1 cup whole-fat yogurt

½ cup whole milk

1 cup frozen mango, cubed

1 heaping tablespoon raw honey

Dash of cardamom

Probiotic capsule (I like Klaire Labs or BioKult)

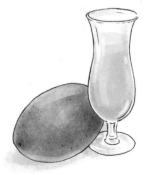

Add yogurt, milk, mango, and honey to a blender and mix until smooth. Pour into a large glass, then open your probiotic capsule and add to the smoothie. Stir well, finish with a dash of cardamom, and enjoy.

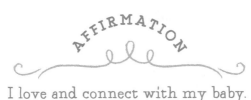

In the event that you opt for antibiotics during labor, you'll likely be given penicillin. Current guidelines suggest your first dose should be administered at least four hours before birth, with subsequent doses given every four hours until delivery of baby. (In between doses, you'll typically be given a saline- or heparin-lock, which—unlike being tied to an IV pole—won't inhibit your mobility.)

If you're interested in alternative methods of treatment, however, here's a look at your options:

THE RISK-MANAGEMENT APPROACH

Although universal GBS screening is standard in the United States, other countries (in particular, the UK) still used risk-based management. Rather than obtaining vaginal swabs during the ninth month of pregnancy, women are given antibiotics during labor *only* if they develop one or more of the following risk factors:

- ♡ If GBS is present in the urine at any point during pregnancy. (Heavy colonizers are more likely to pass along GBS bacteria to their babies.)

- ♡ If you go into preterm labor. (Babies born shy of 37 weeks have a much higher risk of contracting an infection.)

- ♡ If at any point during labor you develop a fever (a classic sign of infection).

- ♡ If your water has been broken for more than eighteen hours.

- ♡ If you've previously given birth to an infant with a GBS infection.

It's worth mentioning that the administration of antibiotics—regardless of the risk factors present—sometimes just isn't possible. (For example, if you arrive at the hospital just before birth, labor is super-short, and there's just not enough time.) In these cases, you may be surprised to discover that the CDC does not recommend an immediate dose of antibiotics for the newborn, but rather close monitoring for signs of infection. All mamas should familiarize themselves with the symptoms of GBS disease, but for mothers who decline or aren't able to receive antibiotics, being able to recognize these symptoms is *especially* important.

HIBICLENS

One of the most popular alternative treatments among more holistic-minded midwives is something called chlorhexidine, which is a topical disinfectant, as well as the active ingredient in an antiseptic skin cleanser known as Hibiclens. Simply put, chlorhexidine kills bacteria. And to treat GBS, many midwives recommend douching with a diluted Hibiclens solution.

You'll want to get the okay from your provider first, of course, but the process is simple: Dilute 2 teaspoons of Hibiclens (4 percent chlorhexidine solution) in 8 ounces of water in a periwash bottle, and use to rinse both the inside of the vagina as well as the exterior of the rectum, keeping in mind that these areas should always be washed separately—you don't want to cross-contaminate!

The trouble with Hibiclens is that a vaginal douche can't possibly remove any GBS bacteria residing in the intestinal tract, so the vagina and rectum are likely to be recolonized. For this reason, the douche must be performed at the onset of labor, and repeated every four to six hours until birth. (Kinda similar to the dosing of antibiotics.)

As for whether it's really effective, well, the jury is still out. Studies have shown that chlorhexidine *does* reduce the risk of a baby being colonized. There is no clinical evidence, however, to suggest that it reduces the number of GBS *infections*. Something else you'll want to consider are the possible side effects of an antiseptic douche on the formation of baby's microbiome. If Hibiclens can kill off "bad" GBS bacteria, it can kill off the good bacteria, too. We just don't have enough research to know the implications of this yet.

GARLIC

Garlic, well known for its antifungal and antibacterial properties, has been used in advance of routine GBS screenings for years. Standard protocol is to insert one peeled clove directly into the vagina before bed (same as if you were treating a yeast infection), remove in the morning, and repeat for five to seven consecutive nights in advance of your GBS test.

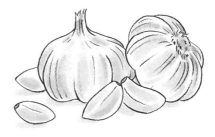

What's important to understand about the garlic method, however—about all alternative methods, really—is that the results (if any) are almost certainly temporary.

Even antibiotics have been shown to be ineffective when administered during pregnancy, rather than during labor. GBS bacteria, remember, come and go, so if you're attempting to kill it off with garlic, you may want to consider continuing treatment one or two nights a week until labor begins, even if you received a negative GBS screening.

PROBIOTICS

High doses of probiotics are another remedy that's gaining popularity in the natural world. It's thought that by flooding the system with good bacteria, our bodies naturally balance out the bad. Several studies, in fact, do indicate that higher levels of probiotics may inhibit the growth of GBS, although there is virtually no research on probiotics and colonization or infection in infants yet. This is one remedy I'd recommend regardless, however, as probiotics have loads of other great benefits.

You can talk to your midwife or doctor about taking a probiotic supplement, of course, but make sure you're getting a daily dose of fermented foods, too, including homemade sauerkraut (find the recipe back on page 275), kefir, kvass, pickles, and yogurt. Alternatively, you can target the GBS locally by using a probiotic capsule as a vaginal suppository.

ADDITIONAL IMMUNE SYSTEM SUPPORT

A strong immune system is thought to ward off unfriendly bacteria, which is why daily vitamin C supplementation (opt for food-based forms like citrus fruit and camu camu powder), a dose of raw apple cider vinegar, and several cloves of smashed garlic (eaten any way you like) may boost the effectiveness of probiotics and other natural remedies. Be sure to flip back to Week 12 for more immune-boosting strategies.

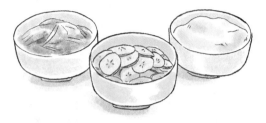

FERMENTED, PROBIOTIC-RICH FOODS

mama-do list

○ Spend some time educating yourself about the pros and cons of antibiotic and alternative treatments for GBS bacteria, and have a frank discussion with your midwife or doctor. Keep in mind that GBS screening and treatment is the same whether delivering vaginally or via C-section.

○ Is your crib, co-sleeper, or sleeping space set up and ready for baby?

○ Are you keeping up with your kick counting?

○ Looking for more ways to eat raw garlic? Check out the Pistachio Pesto recipe on page 226.

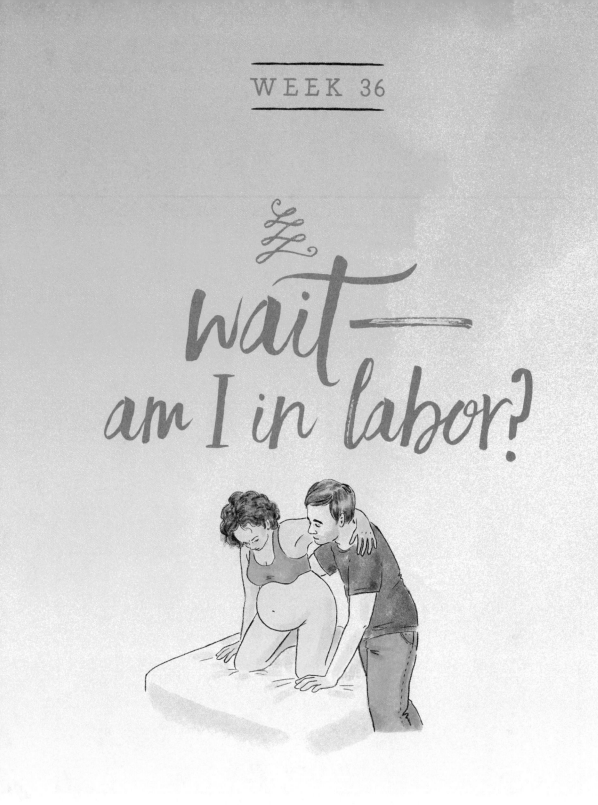

wait—
am I in labor?

WHAT'S UP WITH *baby*?

BOOM! It hardly seems possible, but we've hit six whole pounds! And if she hasn't already, there's a good chance that baby may be flipping to a head-down position this week. (If she's still breech by 37 weeks, however, you might want to start discussing with your provider the pros and cons of an external cephalic version.) Though her kicks and jabs are likely much less forceful than they once were (there's just not a lot of room left in there) you may notice some movement and flutters lower down in your tummy. Like, *way* down low. In fact, it may feel at times like she's just going to fall right out. For most mamas, that's totally normal, but if vaginal pressure gets really intense, give your doctor or midwife a call. And remember: just because her movements may be lower and more muffled, doesn't mean they should be any less frequent.

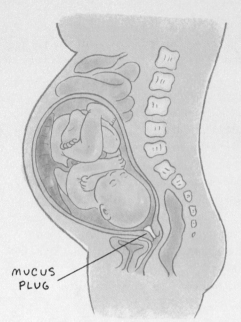

MUCUS PLUG

WHAT'S UP WITH *mama*?

Guess what, Mama? We've not only crossed the six-pound threshold, we've hit the nine-month-mark, too! That means baby is likely to be here in as little as three to five weeks. But it also means that plane travel, as well as extensive travel by car—like a last-minute cross-state-lines road trip—are pretty much not recommended. (If you *must* travel, remember that most airlines will require a note from your doctor. You'll also want to bring along copies of your medical records, as well as your midwife or ob-gyn's contact information.) Luckily, most mamas feel like staying close to home anyway. Blame it on the nesting instinct!

Something was happening.

Four days before my daughter's due date, I woke up and felt a tightening in my uterus. The sensation wasn't what I'd call a *contraction*—my muscles never really *un*-clenched, nor did the feeling come and go in waves. The tightening wasn't at all painful, or even particularly uncomfortable, either. In fact, I spent the morning shopping and grabbing lunch with my mom, even though that crampy feeling lingered for hours.

The next morning I woke up and felt the exact same thing. I figured this was perhaps my body's way of gearing up for delivery, so again I went along with my regular routine. But the following day around dinnertime, as I was standing in the middle of Whole Foods, I felt a tightening, followed immediately by a loosening.

Now that must have been a contraction, I thought to myself.

Right?

Here's the thing: It's common to feel some crampiness in the uterus or a dull achiness in your groin and back in the days and weeks before birth. Braxton Hicks contractions, meanwhile, more commonly known as "fake" labor pains or "false" labor, can start as early as Week 20 for some mamas. So if you *do* start to feel something going on down there, who's to say it's the real thing? Should you call your midwife or doctor right away? Should you just ignore those first twinges and flutters?

Could you go into labor and somehow *not* know it?

Relax, Mama. This week we're talking about the stages of labor, as well as the symptoms of pre-labor—which you could start experiencing any day now!—so you'll know when it's officially show time (and *not* just a mere dress rehearsal).

LABOR AND DELIVERY IN THREE ACTS

Even though every woman's pregnancy and birth experience is unique, labor unfolds in a surprisingly predictable fashion. So unless you deliver via scheduled C-section, you can expect to progress through each of three stages:

Stage One. Without question the longest—but not necessarily the most arduous—Stage One of labor has three distinct parts. During the first phase, a.k.a. "early labor," your cervix will gradually begin to thin (efface) and open (dilate), all the way to 6 centimeters. Contractions during *very* early labor may be extremely mild, as well as wildly irregular—anywhere from 5 to 30 minutes apart. What do they feel like? It's different for every woman, but mine felt like a concentrated force of pressure and

tightening, a little like an extra-intense menstrual cramp.

Once "active labor" kicks in—the second phase of Stage One—your contractions will become much stronger, much longer, and much closer together, lasting anywhere from 40 to 60 seconds at a time, occurring anywhere from 3 to 5 minutes apart. Meanwhile, your cervix will continue to dilate, from 6 to 8 centimeters.

"Transitional labor" marks the final phase of Stage One. It's typically the shortest phase, as well as the most intense. During transition, your contractions will *really* pick up, usually with very little to no rest in between, and your cervix will continue to dilate, expanding rapidly from 8 to 10 centimeters.

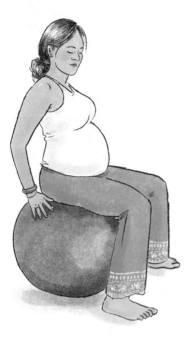

FIRST STAGE OF LABOR

Stage Two. Often called the "pushing stage," Stage Two is when it's time to do some work. Luckily, your body will have a strong, natural urge to push—in fact, first-timers are often surprised at just how intense and urgent (and involuntary!) the need is to bear down. Mean-while, your baby will begin to move through the pelvis and into the birth canal. His progress will be measured in "stations" (more on that soon) until the moment his head appears at the vaginal opening, which is called "crowning."

Stage Three. The final stage of labor begins right after your baby makes his or her debut, and ends with the delivery of the placenta.

Seems pretty straightforward, right? Long before any of this happens, however, your body will have already started preparing itself for the big day. In fact, the physical changes associated with pre-labor might precede baby's birth by as much as a full month—or for some mamas, just hours. In other words, the *stages* of labor may be predictable, but exactly how long it'll take you to progress through those stages is anyone's guess. Here's what you can expect in the weeks, days, and hours before baby's birthday.

Be sure to check out the Labor Playbook (page 422), which contains more detailed descriptions—and helpful suggestions!—for every stage of labor.

RECOGNIZING THE SIGNS OF PRE-LABOR

A *few weeks* before labor kicks in, you may experience:

A Surge of Energy. Although not every woman will succumb to the nesting instinct—you know, the compulsive desire to scrub and straighten everything in existence. For those who do, it tends to peak during the third trimester, and can *sometimes* be a sign (although an unreliable one) of impending labor. Feel free to use this newfound energy to finish up some last-minute baby prep. Just don't *overdo* it—save it for birth!

Lightening or Dropping. During your final prenatal appointments, your healthcare provider will begin to monitor you for signs that D-Day is approaching, and one of the things she's looking for is whether or not your baby has "dropped" and "engaged." Dropping, a.k.a. lightening, is when baby begins to drop down into the pelvis (usually a relief, since it'll be easier to take full, deep breaths). You may have dropped long before stepping into the delivery room. It's possible, however, for your baby to drop without yet having *engaged*.

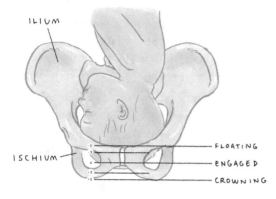

ILIUM

ISCHIUM

FLOATING
ENGAGED
CROWNING

BIRTH STATIONS

If you were to look at it straight on—in fact, check out the illustration above—you'd see that your pelvis looks a bit like a butterfly. Up top, two round bones (called ilium) curve away from the base of the spine; down below, two smaller bones (the ischium) curl back toward one another. Looks like butterfly wings, right? Well, when the top of your baby's head reaches the midpoint of the pelvis he's said to be "fully engaged" or at "zero station." At this point, he's pretty much locked into place and ready for birth, and it's unlikely that he'll flip or change positions from here on out. Then, once labor begins in earnest, his progress through the pelvis and into the birth canal will be measured in 1-centimeter intervals. You might hear that you're "complete and +2," for example, which means you're dilated to 10 centimeters and baby's head is 2 centimeters below the midpoint of the pelvis. Once you reach the final station, +5, your baby's head will be crowning.

A negative number, on the other hand—ranging from -5 to -1—means your baby is settling into the pelvic rim, but he isn't fully locked into place yet. In this case, you might be told that your baby's head is still "floating." It's important to remember that every pregnancy is different—some babies don't drop or engage at all until contractions kick into high gear;

others drop and engage weeks in advance. For this reason, being "fully engaged" isn't a reliable indicator of impending labor, but it's definitely a sign that you're getting close—or at least *closer*—to baby's birthday.

Dilating and Effacing. Most *first-time* mamas will begin to gradually dilate and efface in the days and weeks before birth, so your health-care provider may begin monitoring your cervix—via internal exam—during those final prenatal appointments, too. But what exactly is a cervical exam? And how can a midwife or doctor really tell if your cervix is opening up and thinning out?

Allow me to explain. During pregnancy, your cervix is somewhere around 2 or 3 centimeters long and protrudes down into the vagina. As you get closer to delivery, however, it will begin to shorten in length. When it's about half its usual size, you're said to be "50 percent effaced." When it's paper thin, you'll be "100 percent effaced." And, yes, these are rough estimates rather than an exact science. In other words, your practitioner is just guesstimating.

When it comes to dilation, your midwife is determining whether or not she can insert a finger into the cervical opening. One finger equals 1 centimeter dilation, two fingers equals 2 centimeters, and so on. Again, every pregnancy is different. Some first-timers may already be a centimeter or two dilated in the weeks before birth; more experienced mamas may not dilate at all until contractions begin.

A few days before labor kicks in, you may experience:

Diarrhea or Loose Bowel Movements. Prostaglandins are hormonelike chemical compounds that soften (or "ripen") the cervix and help the uterus contract—but they *also* have a cramping effect on the bowels, which is why some women may experience loose stools or fre-

CERVICAL DILATION AND EFFACEMENT

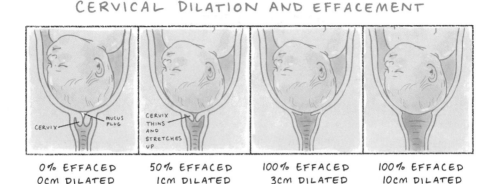

0% EFFACED
0CM DILATED

50% EFFACED
1CM DILATED

100% EFFACED
3CM DILATED

100% EFFACED
10CM DILATED

quent bowel movements shortly before going into labor. (Ever notice that diarrhea seems to be a common side effect of having your period? You can thank prostaglandins, which trigger your uterus to contract during each menstrual cycle, for that too.) While it's certainly true that nobody wants to spend hours on end in the bathroom, this development is actually a really good thing. Emptying out your bowels now means you won't have to deal with the discomfort of constipation during labor. It also makes you significantly less likely to poop in the delivery room.

Loss of the Mucus Plug. During pregnancy, your womb is sealed off from bacteria, pathogens, and even semen by a thick plug of gelatinous mucus. As your cervix begins to dilate and efface, however, the mucus plug will no longer be held firmly in place. In fact, it will eventually fall out—usually a few days, but perhaps several weeks, before birth. It may fall out all at once, or in chunks over a period of days. You might not notice it at all, but if you do, it'll probably look like a glob of thick, snotty discharge.

In fact, the mucus plug looks a bit like— forgive me for this—a giant booger.

For most women, there's no need to do anything when you pass the mucus plug—you might want to let your midwife or doctor know, but there's no need to grab your go-bag and head to the hospital or birth center. Your baby will still be protected by the amniotic sac, and your cervix is constantly producing *new* mucus (yes, the plug can actually regenerate itself). Losing the plug before 37 weeks, however, can *sometimes* be an indication of premature labor. If that happens, you definitely want to give your midwife or doctor a call, just to be on the safe side. And if you never notice losing it? That's fine, too.

Unless they're medically necessary, you might want to consider declining cervical exams in your final month of pregnancy. Some studies have linked them to infection and premature rupture of membranes. Plus, knowing that you're, say, 3 centimeters dilated (or none at all) can sometimes set up unrealistic expectations heading into birth.

DIY Date Bars

If I told you there was a particular food that's associated with a lower risk of induction, premature rupture of membranes, and the need for Pitocin to boost contractions, you'd eat it—right? Well, a small study published in the *Journal of Obstetrics & Gynecology* suggests that dates *are* that miracle food. More specifically, eating six dates a day from 36 weeks onward appears to result in shorter, easier labors. (Apparently, dates have an oxytocin-like effect on the body; they're also rich in fatty acids, the building blocks of prostaglandins.)

How lucky are we that this labor-inducing superfood isn't, like, mayonnaise? Or turnips? Or goat brains?

On the contrary, dates are delicious and extremely versatile, so you can enjoy them a number of ways: straight up, stuffed with almond butter (just slice 'em open and smear with a teaspoon of the sticky stuff), or blended into 2 cups of whole-fat milk (or almond milk) to make a sweet, creamy shake. One of my favorite recipes, however, is for homemade date bars. If you're watching your sugars, this is an especially great way to hit your daily date goal, since you'll be consuming them alongside protein-rich foods such as nuts and seeds, which may prevent a spike in blood sugar.

INGREDIENTS

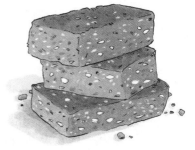

1 cup pitted, dried dates

1 cup nuts of your choice (I like walnuts and almonds)

½ cup seeds of your choice (hemp hearts are particularly delicious)

½ cup nutrient-dense additions, like coconut flakes or goji berries

1 tablespoon coconut oil

1 tablespoon raw honey

Toss all ingredients into a food processor and blend until the mixture forms clumps. Scoop mixture onto a plate. With clean hands, roll into balls or form into bars and chill to set. Store in an airtight container. Recipe makes 4 to 6 servings.

Intensifying Braxton Hicks Contractions. Named for the English doctor who "discovered" them (way back in the late 1800s), Braxton Hicks contractions are essentially practice contractions. A way for the muscles of your uterus to practice contracting in preparation for childbirth. They can begin as early as Week 20 for some mamas, and they may pick up in both frequency and intensity as you near your due date. (It's common for first-time mamas not to *feel* Braxton Hicks contractions, even when a non-stress test picks them up, so don't worry if you don't experience this phenomenon.) You might notice a mild tightening near the top of your uterus (as opposed to lower down in the pelvis, like with menstrual cramps). Some women may notice that their usually round belly looks a bit contorted during a Braxton Hicks contraction. And, yes, this is likely what I was experiencing in those days immediately preceding my daughter's birth.

But how do you tell the difference between practice contractions—a.k.a. fake labor—and the real thing?

Unlike "real" contractions, Braxton Hicks typically go away if you change positions—so try getting up if you've been sitting for a while or lying down for a bit if you've been walking around. (Try drinking a glass of water, too.) They also tend to be infrequent, irregular, and unpredictable; in other words, they have no discernible rhythm or pattern. On the other hand, if your contractions *don't* go away after moving around, lying down, or having a drink, and if they become progressively stronger, longer, and closer together, then, Mama? You're likely in labor.

Prodromal Labor. Unlike Braxton Hicks contractions, which are practice contractions that aren't generally painful, some mamas may experience painful or uncomfortable contractions in the lower pelvis. This is called Prodro-

mal Labor. The contractions will not stop or slow down if you drink some water or put your feet up—but they won't pick up in frequency, either. (Some midwives think prodromal labor contractions occur if baby is poorly positioned, or if mama's uterus is a little irritable—and yes, *irritable uterus* is an actual medical term.) While prodromal labor can be maddening for some mamas, it can sometimes result in a shorter *actual* labor, since your body has done so much "pre-work" before D-Day.

A few hours before labor kicks in, you may experience:

The Bloody Show. There's always been some confusion about whether or not the mucus plug and the bloody show are the same thing. The answer? Not necessarily. The bloody show (horrible name, I know, but a totally normal part of pre-labor nonetheless) is the passing of a small amount of dark red or brown blood, usually combined with a small amount of discharge or mucus—hence the confusion. See, some women pass a clear, white, off-white, or yellowish mucus plug, and then notice a bit of blood in their underwear or on toilet paper a few days later. Others notice that their mucus plug is tinged with blood—so they may be experiencing both phenomena at the same time. In either case, the blood is just the result of small blood vessels breaking as the cervix thins and dilates. So long as you're not experiencing significant blood loss (more than a tablespoon or two) and the discharge isn't bright red, you can relax—but not for long. The bloody show tends to be a more reliable indicator of impending labor than passing the mucus plug alone.

The Breaking of Waters. How many movies have you seen in which the pregnant protagonist seems to be going about her day—grabbing lunch, running errands, chatting with her

IS THIS AMNIOTIC FLUID . . . OR URINE?

When your water eventually breaks—whether you're days away from delivery or mere moments from needing to push—don't expect a dramatic, Niagara Falls–worthy gush of fluid. Most women will notice only a slow leak, or perhaps a few small gushes with each contraction. In fact, the sensation is a little like having peed your pants, which is why amniotic fluid is so often mistaken for urine. Here's how to tell the difference: amniotic fluid may be odorless or have a slightly sweet smell (whereas urine has a far more pungent aroma, akin to ammonia). You can also try squeezing the muscles you'd use to stop the flow of urine mid-stream: if you *keep* leaking, it's amniotic fluid.

If your water breaks before 37 weeks, this is considered preterm premature rupture of membranes (or PPROM), and you should contact your provider immediately. (Thankfully, this experience is uncommon, occurring in less than 3 percent of pregnancies.) If your water breaks and you're already having contractions, you've got nothing to worry about—you can call your midwife or doctor just to check in, but you can (and should!) continue to labor at home until it's time to head to the birth center or hospital. If, however, the fluid has a greenish-brown color, call your healthcare provider right away, as this usually indicates the presence of meconium (a.k.a. baby's first poo). In and of itself, meconium is not a definitive indicator of fetal distress—there's no need to panic—but your midwife or doctor will want to monitor you and your baby very closely, just in case.

co-star, when out of nowhere, *BAM!*, her water breaks. Too many to count, right? Well, rest assured, Mama, this scenario is more fantasy than reality. In fact, the vast majority of women—around 85 percent to 90 percent—are *well* into active labor by the time the amniotic sac ruptures. (During my second birth, for example, my water didn't break until my daughter was crowning!) Sometimes, the amniotic sac *never* breaks.

Believe it or not, some babies are born inside a perfectly intact sac—it's called birth en caul.

Every now and then, however, the sac might rupture twelve to twenty-four hours *before* labor begins. Rarer still, the amniotic sac ruptures and labor doesn't seem to kick in . . . at all.

Here's the thing about the amniotic sac: it's the last line of defense between the outside world and your baby. So, if your water breaks and you're *not* yet in labor (called PROM or premature rupture of membranes), you'll want to give your midwife or doctor a call. You'll also want to keep the vaginal area clean and dry, and avoid putting anything inside the vagina—that means no tampons and no fingers (don't reach in there to see if you can feel baby's head). Sex is off-limits now, too.

Why? Because the longer it takes for labor to kick in, the greater your risk of possible infection. Keep in mind that many natural-minded practitioners will happily let you wait anywhere from twenty-four to forty-eight hours (in some cases, up to seventy-two hours) to see if contractions begin naturally—because

in 90 percent to 95 percent of cases, *they will.*
"Expectant management," the technical term
for waiting it out, is considered a perfectly
safe option by the American College of Nurse-
Midwives, so long as your pregnancy is uncomplicated and low-risk, you're experiencing no
signs of infection (including fever), you're not
GBS-positive, and the fetal heart rate remains
normal. In the meantime, your midwife will
likely want to monitor baby's well-being via
a non-stress test. (Vaginal exams, however,
should be kept to an absolute minimum—
preferably avoided entirely until labor begins—
because they significantly increase the risk of
infection.)

Unfortunately, despite the evidence to support expectant management, many ob-gyns
and practitioners working in more conservative
hospitals will want to induce labor within six
to eighteen hours, if not sooner. In fact, some

RUPTURED
AMNIOTIC
SAC

AMNIOTIC FLUID
LEAKS OUT
THROUGH CERVIX

WHAT IF MY CONTRACTIONS KICK IN BEFORE 37 WEEKS?

Labor that begins before 37 weeks is considered preterm, and while there are a number of
risk factors—including alcohol and drug use, vaginal infections, preeclampsia, and twin
pregnancies, to name but a few—sometimes we just don't know what causes it. Luckily,
the majority of women who experience symptoms of preterm labor will actually *not* deliver
a premature baby—instead, they'll manage to carry another few weeks. But the key is to
recognize the symptoms early.

If at any point before 37 weeks you experience: consistent contractions (not Braxton
Hicks contractions, mind you, but rather contractions that will not subside by changing
positions or drinking some water), bright red blood or discharge, the bloody show, leaking
of amniotic fluid, or increasing pelvic pressure and/or strong menstrual-like cramps, call
your midwife or doctor ASAP. Potential treatments for preterm labor symptoms include bed
rest, IV fluids, antibiotics (in the case of uterine or vaginal infection), and medications to
stop contractions—although these are usually only administered if baby is *extra*-early, like
less than 34 weeks.

will want to induce almost immediately after your water breaks. It's important to point out that induction—in this case, at least—is considered an "evidence-based" option (meaning, there is clinical evidence to support the practice). Also important to note: induction after the premature rupture of the amniotic sac is *not* associated with higher rates of eventual Cesarean or instrument-assisted birth. Either method—expectant management or induction—may be an appropriate choice for you, and you should discuss the pros and cons with your midwife or doctor. If at any point, however, you experience symptoms including fever, chills, elevated pulse, a change in the color or smell of vaginal discharge, or a reduction in fetal movement, report it right away. We'll talk plenty more about induction in weeks 40–42.

OUCH! THESE AREN'T PRACTICE CONTRACTIONS: WHEN SHOULD I HEAD TO THE BIRTH CENTER?

The first phase of Stage One labor—a.k.a "early" or "latent" labor—begins with the gradual effacement and dilation of the cervix, a process that might take mere hours for some women. For others, however, it'll take *days*. So, provided you're not experiencing any sort of complication, there is absolutely zero reason to hop in the car at the first sign of a contraction. In fact, some doctors won't even admit you until you're in (or approaching) "active" labor—that is, until your contractions are consistently 3 to 5 minutes apart and you've dilated at least 4 or 5 centimeters. Unfortunately, we as a society are so conditioned to think of childbirth as a medical event that some women feel like they simply *must* rush right off to the hospital.

Mama? Don't do that.

Spending the majority of early labor at home isn't just more comfortable (there's nothing like having access to your own bed and bathroom!), it actually tends to be more *productive*.

In the wild, animals search out safe, secluded spots in which to give birth, but at the first sign of danger—a lurking predator, perhaps—they release a stress hormone called catecholamine, which shuts down labor (presumably so they can safety relocate). Turns

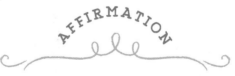

I focus on each breath to find comfort.
Breath comes and goes. Peaks and valleys. In and out.
Labor won't last forever, but my love for my baby is everlasting.

christina: My doctor told me that my water wouldn't break prior to the start of labor—in fact, that "only happens in the movies" were his exact words. So I prepared myself for mild contractions to begin sometime during the night, build until I couldn't take it anymore, and then I'd arrive at the hospital minutes before my baby was born. Imagine my surprise when I walked into a movie theater and my water broke.

megan: I got sent home from the birth center—twice—for only being 2 centimeters dilated. I wish someone had told me beforehand to go about my normal day when early labor kicked in.

leeza: I felt a sudden twinge that was just different than all the others. Since my previous labor didn't follow any patterns, I called my doctor and went in. I was dilated to 7, even though my contractions were still very random.

tasha: I was huge when I was pregnant, but I could always walk normally. So when I started waddling and my belly felt like it was tightening, I was sure I was in labor. I went to the hospital the following morning, only to find out I wasn't even at a 1. They said I could be induced or go home and wait longer. I went home, had contractions throughout the night, and returned to the hospital the next morning—but I was still only dilated 1 centimeter, so I agreed to some Pitocin. Obviously, I did not know when to head to the hospital.

out that when we *mamas* feel stressed out or scared—when our privacy is threatened, when we're forced to fend off unwanted interventions, we release the exact same hormone. In other words, the lack of privacy in a hospital setting, the bright fluorescent lights, and the anxiety-inducing *beep-beep-beep* of machines and monitors, actually can be stressful enough to slow your progress.

Which is exactly why you want to stay home as long as possible.

Ideally, you want to arrive when you're well into active labor, and at least 5 to 6 centimeters dilated.

Everyone's labor is unique, however, and judging how far along you are is easier said than done, especially for first-timers. So, if you're near your due date, and those contractions start coming, here's what to do:

Could they be Braxton Hicks? Have you been on your feet for a while? Take a load off. If you've been sitting for a few hours, get moving. Have a glass of water or a small snack. Does the tightening sensation stop? Then it's not time yet.

Are they growing stronger, longer, and closer together? If not, you may be experiencing prodromal labor. Still not time.

Have they settled into a regular pattern? As you move through the earliest phases of labor, your contractions will become closer and closer—*and closer together*—so start timing them (by measuring the length of time from the start of one contraction to the start of another). When they're consistently 4 minutes apart, each lasts for a full minute, and they've held that pattern for an hour—this is known as the "4-1-1" rule—it's probably time to pack up the car. Other hints that you need to get moving:

♡ You're finding it difficult to talk during a contraction.

♡ You're using all of your energy to cope with contractions.

♡ Your doula says it's time to go in!

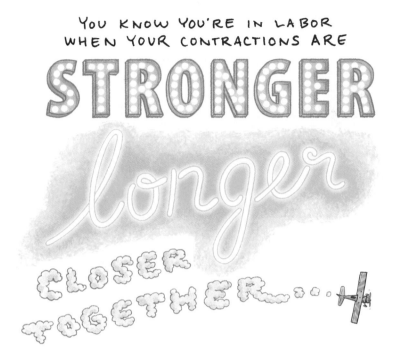

YOU KNOW YOU'RE IN LABOR
WHEN YOUR CONTRACTIONS ARE

STRONGER

longer

CLOSER TOGETHER....

mama-do list

- Rather than using a wristwatch or a wall clock to time your contractions, consider downloading an app on your phone (so high-tech!). There are loads of free and low-cost apps to choose from, but I like the aptly named Contraction Timer and Full Term.

- Want to know what a mucus plug really looks like? Head over to mamanatural .com to see a couple of photos.

- If you're not sure whether you're in labor—no matter how many times you've read this chapter—don't hesitate to give your doula, doctor, or midwife a call, even if it's three o'clock in the morning, just in case. It's always better to be safe than sorry. And trust me, you will *not* be the first mama who wasn't sure.

what to pack
FOR THE BIG DAY

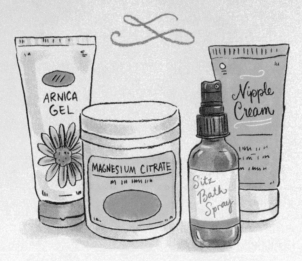

WHAT'S UP WITH *baby*?

He may be at nineteen inches and
nearly six-and-a-half pounds, Mama,
but baby is still growing (if you can
believe it), at a rate of roughly one
ounce per day. Were he to be born
anytime this week, however, he'd
likely thrive. In fact, it wasn't all that
long ago when babies were considered
to be full-term at 37 weeks. The definition was changed in 2013 (in a decision endorsed by both the American
College of Obstetricians and Gynecologists and the Society of Maternal-
Fetal Medicine) in order to reduce
medically unnecessary inductions and
C-sections. These days, babies aren't
technically full-term until they reach
39 weeks. Research shows that the
bun in your oven will do better if he's
allowed to cook just a little bit longer.

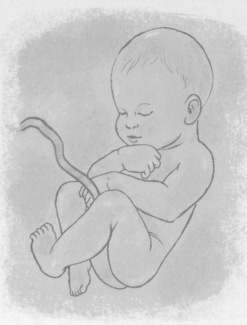

WHAT'S UP WITH *mama*?

By 37 weeks, most mamas are no longer putting on much weight (even though their babies
are certainly still growing). In fact, I didn't gain so much as a pound during the final month
of my pregnancy, and I remember feeling pretty freaked out—that is, until my midwife
confirmed that it was all good. Turns out, you have less amniotic fluid, not to mention less
room in your stomach, thanks to baby's expansion. If you're continuing to put on the pounds
though, know that that's normal, too. And if you're worried about how much weight you've
gained since all this started, try not to. I packed on 40 pounds with my first child and about
35 with my second. My sister-in-law, on the other hand, gained 60, and she managed to
bounce back in record time. So don't stress if you're a little over or under the averages.

What's the most exciting trip you'll ever pack for?

I'll give you a hint: it's baby's birthday!

Do yourself a favor and get your hospital or birth center go-bag packed up (or your house stocked if you're planning a home birth) sometime this week—it'll give you one less thing to think about when those contractions start coming. Here's everything a natural mama might need:

YOUR PAPERWORK

You've worked so hard on your birth plan, the last thing you want to do is forget to print it out and bring it with you, so pack several copies. (Nurses usually work eight- to ten-hour shifts, so you may meet a few of them before baby makes his debut). You can also contact your hospital or birth center—now—in order to fill out pre-registration papers and provide your insurance information. The last thing a mama in active labor wants to deal with is paperwork and red tape!

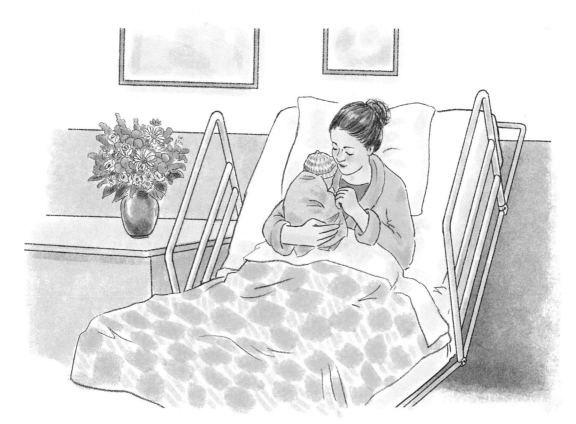

CLOTHES (FOR YOU *AND* YOUR BABY)

First-time mamas are often under the impression that their bellies will deflate immediately after giving birth—kind of like letting air out of a balloon. News flash, Mama: it will not. It takes several days for the acute swelling to go down, and several weeks for the uterus to contract to its pre-pregnancy size. You'll also be bleeding—lochia is the technical term for the vaginal discharge (a mix of blood, mucus, and uterine tissue) that women experience for anywhere from one to eight weeks postpartum. Exactly how much you pack in your go-bag will depend, of course, on how long you plan to stay at the birth center or hospital. I brought enough clothes for at least two nights. But whatever you bring, make sure it's comfortable and oversized. Consider packing:

♡ A labor outfit. Obviously, you can wear a hospital gown if you'd like, or bring your own. We had so little time before the birth of my daughter that I delivered in the shirt I arrived in—and that's it. But if you're planning to wear your own clothes, choose something that you don't mind potentially throwing away, and that can be easily removed after birth for skin-to-skin bonding. Some mamas opt for just a nursing or sports bra and a cheap, flowy skirt; some wind up naked by the end. It's entirely up to you.

♡ A bathing suit top or sports bra (if you're planning a water birth and don't want to go topless)

♡ Loose-fitting, button, or snap-front shirts for easy breastfeeding

♡ Yoga pants and/or sweatpants

♡ A sweatshirt, robe, hoodie, or cardigan—hospitals can be arctic!

♡ Pajamas (if you don't feel like sleeping in regular clothes)

♡ 1–2 nursing bras and some nursing pads

♡ Socks. Bring a cozy pair for lounging in bed, and a crummy pair (preferably with treads) for wandering the floors of the birth center or hospital.

♡ Slip-on, comfortable shoes

♡ Underwear. Most hospitals and birth centers supply new mamas with some very large disposable mesh panties (yes, *mesh*). They're breathable, nonbinding, and big enough to hold the enormous maxi pad you'll be wearing in the days and weeks after birth. Some mamas love them. In fact, plenty of mamas will suggest you *hoard* the panties, the way you might stockpile those mini bottles of shampoo from a fancy hotel. But others? Not so much. Personally, I'm a fan of disposable Depends FIT-FLEX Incontinence Underwear, which are like panties and a giant pad for postpartum bleeding all in one. Super-crunchy mamas may want to opt for heavy-flow cloth pads and some giant maternity underwear (at least one size up from normal) that they don't mind sacrificing to the cause. Whatever you choose, keep in mind that you'll be swollen and sore, so you want something airy and comfortable. Mamas recovering from C-sections, meanwhile, will want underwear that doesn't rub or aggravate the incision as it heals.

FOR BABY

♡ A going-home outfit. A onesie and footed pants are a fine option (no need to bring anything fancy). If you're delivering in the dead of winter, though, make sure you've got warm clothes and a hefty blanket. Hospitals will generally supply you with a hat and a receiving blanket or swaddle, but you may want to bring your own.

♡ Cloth or nontoxic disposable diapers and wipes. Hospitals will, of course, supply your little one with diapers, too—actually, plenty of mamas hoard hospital diapers like they do mesh panties (they're free!). Bringing your own is only necessary if you prefer to use an eco-friendly or nontoxic brand. Remember that baby's first few bowel movements will be sticky and tar-like (that's the meconium we've been talking about); we chose to use "green" disposable diapers for the first ten days before switching to cloth for that very reason.

WHAT OTHER *natural mamas* SAY

lynsey: I was most glad to have brought Greek yogurt and a healthy protein bar to the birthing center with me. These snacks gave me strength during labor, and they also tasted good to me when few other things did.

irene: Olive oil! This came by way of our childbirth education instructor, who gave all the couples a miniature-sized bottle at the end of classes. You rub it on baby's bottom very soon after birth (and after every diaper change thereafter) so that the tar-like meconium wipes right off!!

rhianna: A water bottle with a straw was helpful so I could drink in any position—my husband would just hold it up and encourage me to take small sips in between contractions.

chelsey: Deodorant—I didn't shower until the day I left the hospital.

annika: I wish I'd packed food for my husband—the hospital didn't feed him, and he didn't want to leave. When he did manage to sneak out, everything was usually closed!

DRINKS AND SNACKS

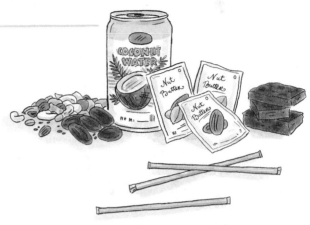

I can't stress how important it is to replenish during labor, whether you're planning a natural birth or not. I went nearly nine hours without food and drink the first time around, and I'll never forget the surge of energy I got when my doula finally gave me some apple juice. Liquid nourishment tends to be best—it's easier on the body, and you won't feel like eating a proper meal between contractions.

Planning on giving birth at a conservative hospital, where you know you won't be allowed to eat and drink? Bring food anyway.

You'll certainly be allowed to eat *after* you deliver, and if that happens to be at two in the morning, you don't want to be stuck scrounging something from the vending machines. I made sure to bring:

- ♡ Red raspberry leaf tea. Freeze some in an ice cube tray (a *great* option if you'll be allowed only ice chips during labor).

- ♡ Coconut water

- ♡ Dates and date bars

- ♡ Honey sticks. They're like Pixy Stix for natural mamas—the simple sugar makes

for a quick pick-me-up when you don't feel like eating.

- ♡ Nuts, nut butters, and/or trail mix.

If you think you might be in for a longer stay (say, two to three days), you may want to consider packing some more substantive meals in a mini cooler. Hospital cafeterias aren't exactly known for serving top-notch, restaurant-quality cuisine, nor are they always great at catering to patients with dietary restrictions or who are health nuts. Keep in mind that plenty of takeout joints will deliver to hospitals—which is what Michael and I opted for after each of our kids' births.

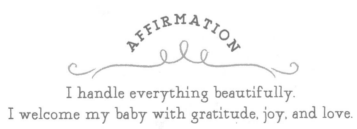

AFFIRMATION

I handle everything beautifully.
I welcome my baby with gratitude, joy, and love.

Lasagna Bolognese

The tradition of bringing easy-to-heat-up meals to new mamas is one of the great acts of service—and so needed. It takes a while to build up your depleted nutritional reserves, but you'll be so tired and busy with baby that cooking (for most mamas, at least) takes a backseat. But you *will* be hungry. Breastfeeding mamas, in particular, tend to have appetites like linebackers. So here's a tip: Don't just rely on friends and family. Start preparing and freezing several weeks' worth of nutrient-rich meals now. One of my all-time favorites is classic lasagna Bolognese with a power-packed twist: beef liver. Liver is loaded with iron, vitamins A, B, C, D, and E, trace elements and minerals, and the essential fatty acids EPA and DHA. It is truly one of nature's most incredible foods. But don't worry. You won't even taste it. I promise.

INGREDIENTS

BOLOGNESE SAUCE

2 tablespoons olive oil

1 large onion, chopped

4 cloves garlic, minced

1½ pounds grass-fed ground beef

½ pound beef liver (ask your butcher to grind it for you; otherwise, mince)

Two 16-ounce jars organic marinara sauce

Two 6-ounce cans organic tomato paste

LASAGNA

1 box gluten-free lasagna noodles

2 pounds organic ricotta or cottage cheese

2 eggs

¼ cup parsley, finely chopped

2 pounds organic Swiss cheese, sliced

1 cup grated Parmesan

To make the Bolognese sauce, add olive oil to a large stockpot and warm over medium heat. Add the onion and garlic and cook until translucent. Add the ground meat and liver and cook until browned. Reserve 1 cup of the marinara sauce; add remaining sauce and all the tomato paste to the pot. Mix well and simmer on low.

Heat the oven to 350°F. Fill a large stockpot with water and bring to a rolling boil. Add the lasagna noodles and cook for about 10 minutes, or until they're just shy of al dente. Drain the noodles and drizzle with olive oil (to prevent sticking). Meanwhile, in a large bowl, combine ricotta cheese, eggs, parsley, and salt and pepper to taste.

To assemble the lasagna, oil a 13 X 9-inch baking dish, then spoon one ladle of Bolognese sauce into the bottom of the dish. Layer with lasagna noodles, then meat sauce, then ricotta, then Swiss cheese. Repeat until all of the layers are formed, ending with the plain marinara sauce you reserved and the Parmesan. Bake for 55 to 65 minutes, until the lasagna is bubbling and golden brown on top. Allow to cool completely before portioning and freezing.

GADGETS, GIZMOS, AND BOREDOM BUSTERS

It seems weird to think that you might actually get a bit *bored* during D-Day, but it's impossible to predict how long your labor will last—best to be prepared for quite a wait:

- ♡ Childbirth affirmations
- ♡ Music. As much as I loved my soothing birth affirmation soundtrack, I found that I needed some rockin' tunes, too. Load up your smartphone or MP3 player with different types of music.
- ♡ Books, magazines, or movies (mostly for your partner)
- ♡ Camera
- ♡ Chargers—for your cell phone, camera, laptop, Kindle, iPod, or any other electronics you may be bringing.

LABOR TOOLS, AFTERCARE PRODUCTS, AND HOMEOPATHIC REMEDIES

You already know that my daughter was easy to birth. Delivering my placenta, however, was not so simple. I had to hand over my beautiful newborn, get into a squatting position, and really focus to push that sucker out. To move things along, my midwife suggested clary sage essential oil—and luckily, I just so happened to have some.

Homeopathic remedies are a great alternative to conventional medicine and may reduce or eliminate your need for certain (albeit minor) interventions. How much of this you choose to bring is, of course, entirely up to you, but here's a peek at my stash of natural childbirth products:

LABOR TOOLS

- ♡ DIY tennis ball back massager (pages 353–354)
- ♡ Rice socks (page 404)
- ♡ Rebozo (page 423)

> ### NEED MORE INSPIRATION?
> Visit mamanatural.com for a video showing what I packed for the big day, plus a hospital bag checklist.

ESSENTIAL OILS

- ♡ Clary sage to support healthy contractions (warning: this stuff is *strong,* and should not be used before you're in active labor).
- ♡ Orange or lemon for energy
- ♡ Lavender for relaxation
- ♡ Peppermint for tummy trouble
- ♡ Frankincense to focus the mind and elevate the mood
- ♡ Black pepper for muscle support (back labor)
- ♡ A diffuser or personal inhalers

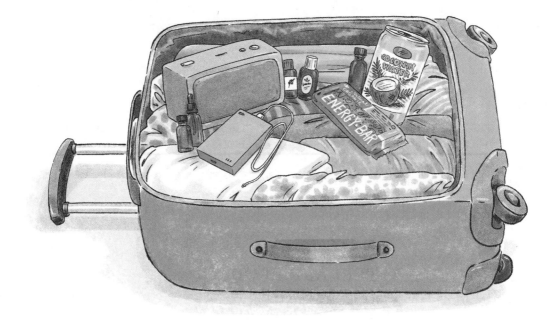

HOMEOPATHIC REMEDIES (OPTIONAL)

- ♡ Caullophyllum or Cimicifuga for cervical dilation

- ♡ Gelsemium and Pulsatilla for slow or stalled labor

- ♡ Arnica for pain and fatigue during the pushing phase

- ♡ Kali carbonicum for back labor

- ♡ Kali phosphoricum for overall exhaustion

AFTERCARE PRODUCTS

- ♡ Sitz bath spray. A sitz bath is great for soothing inflammation of the vagina, hemorrhoids, or stitches (in the event that you have any tearing), but you won't always be able (or willing) to hop in and out of the tub at the birth center or hospital. Motherlove Sitz Bath Spray is an amazing alternative. Seriously, I *love* this stuff. Just spray after birth to relieve any soreness.

- ♡ For repeat mamas, AfterEase—a non-GMO, gluten-free herbal tincture to relieve after-birth contractions and cramping (which actually tend to be more painful the second time around—this stuff was my life saver!).

- ♡ Nipple cream or salve

- ♡ Arnica cream (great for sore muscles)

- ♡ Natural Calm magnesium supplement. There's a tendency for brand-new mamas to develop constipation—partly due to trauma in the region and partly due to anxiety. That first bowel movement after having a baby just *feels* weird, and sore mamas can be (understandably) hesitant about, well, pushing. This is why I start on magnesium citrate right away—it helps to keep things moving, and is gentler than what most hospitals offer.

PERSONAL TOILETRIES

Hospitals and birth centers will provide basic toiletries (soap, shampoo, toothpaste, etc.), but many women prefer to pack their own—it's the little things, after all, that often bring us the most comfort! Even a bare-essentials kind of gal, however, will want to tuck these additional items into her go-bag:

♡ Lip balm. Hospitals are notorious for the dry air. Meanwhile, all that heavy breathing you'll be doing during labor can dry out your lips, too.

♡ Hair ties or headbands

♡ Dry shampoo can be a lifesaver if you're not up to showering.

♡ Baby nail clippers. Hospitals won't stock them for liability reasons, but you'd be surprised at how long and how sharp a newborn's nails can be—and how easily they manage to scratch themselves.

mama-do list

● Trust me: the more meals you can prep in advance of baby's birth, the better. For more recipes, including my hearty miso shrimp with oats and leafy greens pie, head over to mamanatural.com.

● Don't forget about your partner when you're packing. Papa may want some basic toiletries, a laptop, some snacks, and/or a change of clothes. Being a labor-support person is hard work, too!

● After you've finished all that packing, think about treating yourself to a pedicure. Let's be honest—it'll likely be a while 'til your next one.

● Are you enjoing your six dates a day? (See page 372 for a refresher.)

the gentle cesarean

WHAT'S UP WITH *baby*?

Baby is hovering right around seven whole pounds and 19 or 20 inches in length, so in fruit terms, she's roughly the size of a pineapple. (In human terms, that means she's just about full-grown.) Even though her due date is right around the corner, however, these last few weeks are still vitally important for her development. Her brain, for example, is still maturing and building important neural connections. In fact, babies born just shy of 37 weeks have significantly smaller brains than full-term newborns. (A recent study in *Pediatrics* found that babies born at 37 or 38 weeks' gestation scored significantly lower on math and reading standardized tests administered in the third grade.) She's also continuing to produce surfactant, that soapy substance that'll help her lungs to drain fluid and then fill with air so she can breathe easy. So, Mama? Don't rush her! She still has work to do.

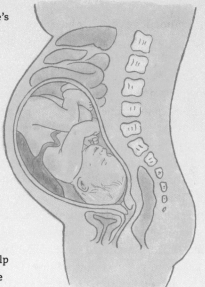

WHAT'S UP WITH *mama*?

We're in the home stretch! In fact, your cervix may *already* be dilating and effacing, your baby may have dropped and engaged, and you may be feeling . . . well, there's just no polite way to say it: as big as a house. Need even more proof that D-Day is approaching? Try hand-expressing some milk from your breast next time you're in the shower. (That's a fancy way of saying giving yourself a mini boob massage.) See? Your girls are already brimming with that magical elixir we've been talking so much about: colostrum. The female body is truly miraculous!

Thank God for the modern Cesarean.

What was once a fairly brutal procedure—okay, *totally brutal*, seeing as how mamas in antiquity weren't even meant to live through them—has become a safe, sterile, virtually painless method for delivering babies that otherwise might not survive. I was a C-section baby, and I probably wouldn't be here today had my mother not had the surgery. But for women who planned on a natural, vaginal birth, learning that you need a C-section can be disheartening, if not downright traumatic.

There are the obvious drawbacks, of course: a surgical birth requires a longer hospital stay, takes longer to recover from, and comes with a host of lifting and driving restrictions, not to mention a higher risk of long-term complication. But the bigger toll tends to be an emotional one. During a standard Cesarean, mamas are hooked up to a battery of machines, frequently have their arms strapped down to the operating table, may be cocooned in blankets up to their chins (operating rooms are kept *very* chilly), and are routinely separated from their children following the procedure. Depending on your health, your baby's health, and

protocol, you may have to wait anywhere from 5 minutes to several hours to hold, cuddle, bond with, and breastfeed your baby. Some hospitals, in fact, have a *mandatory* separation period, during which newborns may be fed with supplemental formula. It's no wonder that C-section mamas sometimes feel let down by their birth experiences!

And there are a lot of women who feel this way. As you know, 33 percent of births end in Cesarean—for reasons both necessary (e.g., fetal distress or medical emergency) and, well, *not* (larger-than-average fetal weight). In fact, C-sections are the most common surgical procedure in the United States, with more than 1.2 million of them performed each year.

Mamas can do everything in their power to avoid interventions, but here is the truth: not every baby can be delivered vaginally.

Should these women just accept their fate? Give up on their dreams of an ideal birth? Mourn the loss and move on?

Just a few years ago, the answer would almost certainly have been yes. But nowadays—thanks to changing attitudes in the OR—it looks like mamas won't have to.

NATURALIZING A SURGICAL BIRTH

Without question, there are distinct, significant, and measurable advantages to a vaginal delivery—which makes complete sense when you think about it, since Mother Nature *designed* it this way, including:

♡ Squishing through the birth canal compresses baby's lungs, for one thing, which helps him to expel amniotic fluid. This not only facilitates breathing, but may lower his risk for developing respiratory problems such as asthma later in life. (Interestingly, mamas who labor for a while before having

an eventual Cesarean give birth to babies with a lower risk of respiratory problems than if they hadn't labored at all. In other words, *any* amount of labor has long-term benefits for baby, even in cases when labor does not result in a vaginal birth.)

♡ Babies born vaginally also pick up protective bacteria from the vagina, which will colonize their skin and gut; the absence of this bacteria transfer may explain why C-section babies are more likely to develop allergies, asthma,

Turkey Chili

Still freezing meals for those first few weeks postpartum? Good, because I couldn't resist giving you another easy make-ahead recipe, this time for a super-satisfying turkey chili. Bonus points for the fact that you can eat it one-handed (with some organic blue tortilla chips)—and, trust me, you won't realize how helpful this is until you're juggling a breast-feeding newborn. It could be weeks before you sit down to the dinner table and eat with a knife and fork again!

INGREDIENTS

1 tablespoon olive oil

1 large onion, chopped

1 organic yellow pepper, chopped

1 organic red pepper, chopped

1 pound pastured ground turkey

3–4 cloves garlic, minced

One 28-ounce can diced organic tomatoes, undrained

1½ cups red kidney beans, soaked and cooked (use canned in a pinch)

1½ cups black beans, soaked and cooked (use canned in a pinch)

¼ cup chili powder

2 cups homemade chicken or beef stock

1½ teaspoon sea salt

1 tablespoon dried oregano

2 tablespoons cumin

1 teaspoon hot sauce (optional)

In a large stockpot, sauté onions and bell peppers in olive oil over medium heat until the onions are translucent. Add ground turkey and garlic, and cook until browned. Add remaining ingredients and stir well to combine. Reduce heat, cover, and simmer for 45 minutes, stirring occasionally. Serve with avocado, grated cheese, and cilantro. If you're making ahead and freezing, consider making a double batch!

certain immune diseases, obesity, and other health issues.

♡ When babies are born vaginally, they can almost always be held by their mamas right away, and that's important, since brand-new babies cannot regulate their own body temperatures. In fact, newborns can lose an enormous amount of heat very quickly, which is why they're usually swaddled and given a little knit cap to wear. Placing baby on mama's chest, however, will stabilize baby's temperature, as well as his heart rate and breathing. Immediate skin-to-skin contact (sometimes called "kangaroo care") has a host of other benefits, too: babies tend to cry less, produce less of the stress hormone cortisol, produce more of the bonding hormone oxytocin, gain more weight, and sleep better. There are several studies that suggest skin-to-skin bonding may even alleviate or prevent postpartum depression.

Unfortunately, the limitations of a surgical birth—the need for a sterile environment and the intrusiveness of all that machinery—means that C-section babies don't reap these same benefits.

Well, they *couldn't* reap these benefits. That is, until now.

One of the first physicians to question the way modern Cesareans are routinely performed was Dr. Nick Fisk, a professor of obstetrics at Imperial College in London. In response to Britain's rising C-section rate, Fisk wondered if the surgical experience could be rendered more meaningful, if there were opportunities for parents to be more involved in the process.

RESTORING BABY'S MICROBIOME WITH A VAGINAL SWAB

So, we know that babies born vaginally pick up protective bacteria with long-term benefits, and that babies born via C-section miss out on this apparent gift from natural birth.

The question is: Can we *fix* that?

A first-of-its-kind study, published in *Nature Medicine* in 2016, suggests the answer may be yes. How? By collecting a vaginal swab and wiping it on baby's skin—as well as in and around his or her mouth. Vaginal seeding, as the procedure is called, appears to contribute to the formation of a healthy microbiome (it's thought that mama's microbes help to train baby's immune system). Alternatively, a swab can be wiped on the nipples just before baby breastfeeds for the first time.

Admittedly, this is a very new practice, and additional studies are underway to confirm its efficacy. Researchers also point out that it's decidedly not a DIY procedure. In other words, don't try this at home—you could inadvertently transmit dangerous bacteria to baby (women in the study were prescreened for known pathogens, as well as given antibiotics). But it's definitely something you can discuss with your midwife or doctor. And if you are unable to do the swab, know that breast milk is brimming with live, beneficial bacteria, too.

ashley: I have some intense birth stories. With my first, I went nine days past my due date, started laboring on a Thursday morning, and finally was admitted to the hospital on Friday night. I didn't progress past 3 centimeters, so they gave me Pitocin. I labored from about 10:00 p.m. Friday to 4:00 p.m. Saturday—my daughter was sunny-side up and she was not budging at all. When her heart rate started dropping drastically after two and a half hours of pushing with no progress, I had an emergency C-section.

With my second, I went five days past my due date, but I made it through labor naturally. Everything was going great, until it came time to push. Again, it was like pushing on a brick wall—I made even less progress than with my first baby. I had another emergency C-section, and she came out blue with the cord wrapped around her neck. She went straight to the NICU with my husband for two hours.

After two Cesareans in the previous five years, my third baby was a planned C-section. However, I was the first "natural Cesarean" delivery at Baptist Hospital in Nashville. Now, when I hear a mother say she wants to go natural, I'm 100 percent supportive, but I also encourage her to consider the possibility of an emergency Cesarean. Too often, women have no idea they have a voice in the operating room. A Cesarean doesn't mean you don't have a say in the delivery process. My third childbirth was incredible and my daughter never left my side, even though I didn't have a vaginal delivery.

And in the early 2000s, he pioneered what he called the "skin-to-skin Cesarean" (alternatively referred to as the "gentle Cesarean," the "family-centered Cesarean," and "walking the baby out"). The point was to make a C-section delivery feel more like a birth and less like a surgery, as well as to mimic the circumstances of a vaginal delivery, and in the last decade, the technique has only grown more popular.

Keep in mind that the procedure will vary from doctor to doctor and hospital to hospital, but the differences between a routine Cesarean and a gentle C-section look a little something like this.

THE STANDARD CESAREAN

♡ Before receiving an epidural or spinal anesthesia, mama will be hooked up to an IV, a blood pressure cuff will be placed on her arm, and EKG electrodes (to monitor her heart rate) will be placed on her chest.

♡ Surgical drapes are set up to provide a sterile operating environment, as well as to block mama's view of the incision site (and, incidentally, the birth of her child).

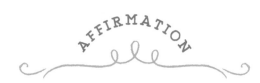

I know I will have the perfect birth for me.
All is well, and I can trust my body,
my baby, and myself.

♡ The doctor will make an incision in the skin of the abdomen, cut through layers of fat and tissue, and then make an incision in the uterus, pulling the baby out as quickly (and safely) as possible.

♡ The umbilical cord is clamped and cut immediately.

♡ Baby may be raised above the surgical drape (so mama can sneak a quick peek) before being handed off to a waiting nurse.

♡ The doctor will remove the placenta and begin to suture the incision.

♡ The baby will be taken to a nearby warmer, assessed by several nurses, weighed, and swaddled (operating rooms are kept *very* cold).

♡ Baby may be taken to the nursery while mama recovers, where he may be given a first feeding of formula.

♡ No one is allowed in the operating room other than mama and papa.

THE GENTLE CESAREAN

♡ IVs, blood pressure cuffs, and EKG electrodes will be placed in areas that don't infringe mama's ability to see, hold, or breastfeed her baby.

♡ A clear drape may be raised just before delivery so that mama can watch as her baby is born. Alternatively, some hospitals may use a surgical drape with a sealable flap, through which baby can be passed from doctor to mother.

♡ The doctor will free baby's head but allow baby's body to linger inside the uterus; this compresses the baby's torso, which helps to drain any fluid from his lungs (thus mimicking a tight squeeze through the vaginal canal).

♡ The cord is left intact for a few minutes, ensuring that baby is still receiving oxygenated blood from the placenta.

♡ The baby is swabbed with protective bacteria from mama's vagina.

- Baby is placed directly on mama's torso for immediate skin-to-skin bonding. If mama is under general anesthesia, papa may have skin-to-skin contact.

- Any and all newborn procedures (barring medical emergencies) are delayed for skin-to-skin bonding; baby's health will be assessed by nurses while he lies on mama's chest, same as after an uncomplicated vaginal birth.

- Mama is allowed to initiate breastfeeding immediately, and may continue to breastfeed while her incision is sutured.

- Mama, papa, and baby remain together throughout recovery.

- A doula (and potentially a photographer) may accompany mama into the OR.

REQUESTING A GENTLE CESAREAN

The gentle Cesarean is still a relatively new procedure, so while it is growing in popularity, it's possible that your doctor has little to no experience providing it, and/or that your hospital doesn't officially offer it. Less likely—but still possible—is that your doctor hasn't even heard of it. Mama, don't let that discourage you. Talk to the members of your birth team about allowing some or all of these measures. You can be a pioneer!

GENTLE
CESAREAN

～♍ *mama-do list* ♍～

- Read up on gentle Cesareans—even if your doctor isn't familiar with the procedure, he or she may be open to accommodating some (or all) of your requests.

- Have you washed baby's onesies and PJs yet?

- In 2015, three Richmond, Virginia-area nurses developed a patented surgical drape with a sealable flap through which baby can be passed from doctor to mother. You can learn more about their ingenious invention (as well as download a request form to pass along to your physician) at clevermedicalob.com.

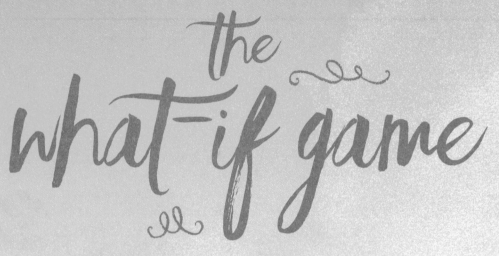

the what-if game

DISPELLING COMMON FEARS ABOUT BIRTH

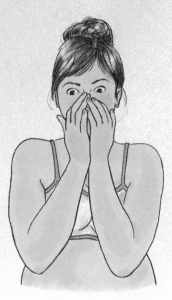

WHAT'S UP WITH *baby*?

All systems go! Yes, Baby Natural is officially "full-term" and ready for life outside the womb (as I imagine *you* are, too). He's weighing somewhere around 7 or 8 pounds and measuring about 20 inches long—and these stats likely won't change much, even if he decides to keep hibernating for another week or two. I bet you're already imaging those big, gasping cries you'll hear the moment he arrives. But here's something you won't *see* on the big day: tears. Strange as it sounds, baby's tear ducts don't become functional for at least one to three months. Who knew?

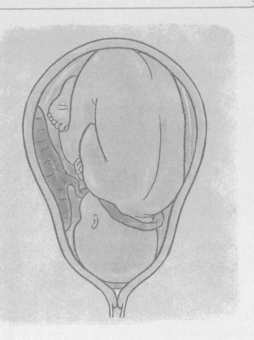

A "NUCHAL CORD," OR WHEN THE UMBILICAL CORD WRAPS AROUND BABY'S NECK, IS FOUND IN AROUND ONE THIRD OF ALL DELIVERIES AND RARELY CAUSES PROBLEMS.

WHAT'S UP WITH *mama*?

So . . . will this week be *the* week? It certainly could be, Mama, so keep an eye out for signs of impending labor: diarrhea or loose stools, loss of the mucus plug, the "bloody show," and—of course—the onset of contractions. If it turns out that baby is ready to make his debut, try not to get too wound up. Now's the time to hunker down, stay well fed and hydrated, and get some sleep. For most first-time mamas, early or latent labor may take anywhere from six to twelve hours—or perhaps significantly longer. No need to become a slave to the stopwatch (or contraction timing app) right away, either. Instead, time your contractions periodically to get a sense for where you're at, give your doula a call to check in, and make yourself comfortable—you could be in for a long wait.

Psssst. I want to let you in on a little secret.

If you're feeling a little, well, *freaked out* about all the weird or scary things that might happen during birth, you're not alone. (And I'm not just talking about the pain here, Mama!) I remember spending tons of time reading, researching, and attempting to empower myself before going into labor with my son, and still having a major case of the jitters. There were just *so* many unknowns; I wasn't sure if I'd ever be ready. Of course, it didn't really matter if *I* was ready, because that baby was gonna come out, one way or another. And so will yours. So, this week—with your due date rapidly approaching—we're gonna bust some myths, shatter some fears, and make some final preparations in anticipation of the big day. In no particular order, here are the answers to those questions you've just been too afraid (or embarrassed) to ask.

WILL I POOP IN THE DELIVERY ROOM?

As I imagine you've noticed, I've made a few passing references to the fact that pooping during delivery is a distinct possibility. Yes—horror of horrors—some women poop while giving birth, right there on the hospital gurney or in the birthing tub. And while that probably ranks way up there on your list of "most embarrassing things that could ever happen, *ever*," it really shouldn't be all that surprising: the same muscles used to push out a baby are involved in emptying your bowels.

Back in the day, women were routinely given enemas in the earliest stage of labor to prevent this from happening, but the practice has largely fallen out of favor. Why? Because it turns out that enemas provide exactly zero benefits to women in childbirth. They do not reduce the length of labor (as was previously thought), nor do they lower the risk of infection (from fecal matter contamination, that is—they may actually *increase* the risk, due to, um, anal leakage). And the *last* thing a pregnant mom wants at 40 weeks? Cold liquid shot up her butt. (Just sayin'.)

So what's a mama to do? First, know that while pooping during delivery is totally possible, it probably won't happen. As you may remember, the prostaglandins your body releases to help the cervix efface and the uterus contract also have a cramping effect on the bowels. (In the twenty-four hours before I went into labor with my son, I must have gone to the bathroom no fewer than twelve times—by the time I was ready to push, my bowels were pretty much empty.) But if it *does* happen, you probably won't even realize it. Nurses and midwives have plenty of experience quickly and discreetly cleaning up any accidents, so you stay focused on the work at hand. Seriously, these ladies have seen everything—they just wipe it up and keep on moving. I can tell you, too, that once you're in active labor, you won't give a poop about anything other than getting your baby out. I'm a pretty modest person, and I was walking around naked and growling like a tiger, and I didn't care who saw me. The intensity of birth tends to lower your inhibitions. If you're *really* worried about soiling yourself, however, you can push for a bit while sitting on the toilet; incidentally, lots of mamas find this to be super comfortable. Whatever you do, don't hold back during the pushing phase out of fear that you'll do the doo. You'll risk lengthening your labor, increasing the pain, and upping your need for interventions.

WHAT IF WE DON'T MAKE IT TO THE BIRTH CENTER IN TIME?

Every woman who's not planning a home birth has thought about it: *What if I end up giving birth in the parking lot? Or worse—in the car?!* The thought certainly crossed my mind, and the second time around my fears were almost realized: As we were driving to the birth center on the day of my daughter's birth, I very nearly instructed my husband to pull over so I could deliver our little bundle right there in the Volkswagen. Fortunately, we arrived just in time—I was "complete and +2" in case you're wondering—and very nearly delivered my baby on the gurney.

Despite these totally normal, entirely understandable fears, however, it is extremely rare that a first-timer will wait too long to head to the hospital.

In fact, it's much more likely that you'll arrive too *early*, only to find out you've barely begun to dilate. (A good rule of thumb: if you're able to be super-chatty during contractions, you're probably not even close to delivering that baby.) Worst-case scenario? Plenty of women have given birth in transit— google "birth in car" if you don't believe me— and things worked out for them just fine. So, in the *highly unlikely* scenario that baby starts coming fast and furious, here's what to do:

♡ **Remain calm.** Believe it or not, when babies come this fast, all is usually well and birth tends to proceed smoothly.

♡ **Pull over.** The last thing you and your partner need is to get into an accident on the freeway.

♡ **Call 911.** The operator will remain on the phone with you (or preferably your partner) until the baby arrives, and he or she can provide valuable instruction specific to your circumstances.

♡ **Be ready to "catch" the baby.** His head will come out first, and then there may be a pause (as your body prepares for another contraction) before his body emerges. No need to do any fancy maneuvers here—certainly don't *pull* the baby out. Just let nature take its course, and make sure baby doesn't slip out of your grasp when he pops out.

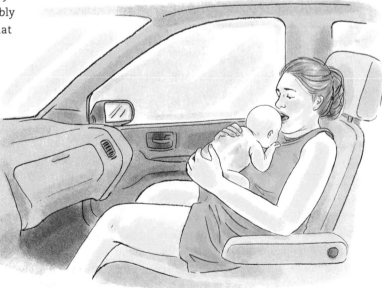

- **Do not pull on the head, the body, or the umbilical cord** (if you happen to notice it wrapped around baby's neck). Instead, carefully unwrap the cord once baby has been delivered.

- **As soon as baby makes his debut, place him skin-to-skin on your body** (your legs or belly are fine if you can't get access to your chest) and cover him with a blanket, shirt, or jacket. (You also might want to note the time. Ya know, for the birth certificate.)

- **If he doesn't breathe or cry right away, don't panic**—he's still receiving oxygen from the umbilical cord. Vigorously dry him off (wiping his nose and mouth) to help stimulate breathing.

- **A gush of blood and fluid will follow his birth,** but it'll seem like more (volume-wise) than it actually is; part of this "gush" is just amniotic fluid.

- **It may take anywhere from 5 to 30 minutes to expel the placenta.** By then, emergency services should have joined you. In the meantime, do not pull on or cut the cord.

- **Make your way to the hospital by ambulance** (so that everyone can be checked out by a doctor) and congratulate yourself on one heck of a memorable birth story!

WHAT IF MY BABY IS BREECH?

So you've tried moxibustion acupuncture and visited a Webster-certified chiropractor. You've had an external cephalic version and painstakingly done your pelvic exercises. But now your due date is merely days away, and your baby is *still* positioned butt-first. What to do?

Well, Mama, you've got a few options.

Option A is to accept the situation for what it is, grieve if necessary, and deliver via gentle Cesarean.

Option B is to find a provider who's got some experience attending vaginal breech births.

True, most obstetricians are no longer trained in the procedure; the increased risks of a vaginal breech delivery, combined with what's commonly referred to as medico-legal pressure (in other words, the threat of a malpractice lawsuit) have made C-sections the go-to method of delivery in the vast majority of breech cases. However, recent research has shown that vaginal breech births are no riskier than planned C-sections when certain conditions are met. In fact, the American College of Obstetricians and Gynecologists reversed its stance on vaginal breech births back in 2006, declaring them a "reasonable" option in the hands of an experienced provider. (Previously, the college recommended C-sections for *all* breech babies.)

According to the American Pregnancy Association, you should meet the following criteria in order to safely attempt a vaginal breech delivery:

- You're at least 37 weeks along.

- Baby is in the frank breech presentation. (Some providers may green-light a complete breech baby for a vaginal delivery, too, as this is the next most favorable position.)

- Baby shows no signs of distress when his heart rate is closely monitored.

- Baby is not too big to pass safely through the birth canal. (Generally speaking, baby should be no bigger than 4,000 grams, or 8 pounds, 13 ounces.)

- Anesthesia is readily available and a Cesarean delivery possible on short notice.

♡ Labor is spontaneous and progresses steadily.

If you choose to move forward with a vaginal delivery attempt, know that your odds will improve significantly if you've got a skilled provider who takes a "hands-off" approach. Mamas who've had one previous vaginal delivery may have a higher chance of success than first-timers.

If you're opting for a C-section, discuss with your provider the potential benefits of delaying the surgery until the onset of spontaneous labor (remember, any amount of labor is beneficial for baby). And although unlikely, it is possible that a breech baby will flip to a head-down position past the 39th week.

WHAT IF I HAVE BACK LABOR?

So, what exactly is back labor? Well, it's pretty much self-explanatory: it's when the full force of labor seems to concentrate in the lower back, directly above the sacrum. And according to the American Pregnancy Association, it's often accompanied by irregular contractions, a labor that's slow to progress, and a prolonged pushing stage.

Sounds an awful like my first birth, doesn't it?

That's because the most common cause of back labor is the position of the baby. More specifically, the "occiput posterior" position—exactly the position my son was in, incidentally—causes the hardest part of baby's skull to put pressure squarely on mama's tailbone. I'm not going to lie to you: this does not feel good. It's not unbearable, it's just really, really uncomfortable.

So how do we fix it?

First things first.
If you think you're experiencing back labor, you'll want to get up and get moving.

Lying on your back only encourages baby's full weight to rest on your spine. (If you

must lie down, try lying on your side.) Walking around, squatting, lunging, or dropping down onto your hands and knees and doing some pelvic rocks, on the other hand, can encourage baby to rotate to a more favorable position.

As for pain relief, counterpressure works wonders. Have your partner, doula, or labor support person use that tennis ball massager we talked about in Week 34, or apply pressure to the points located on either side of your spine. Or try leaning forward in the shower and directing the flow of hot water directly onto your

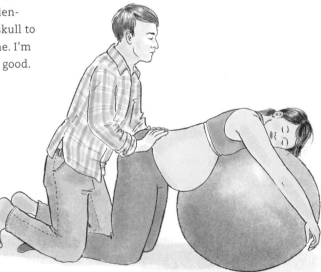

back. You can also soothe your back muscles by using a heated rice sock. (Basically, this is just a DIY hot water bottle: pour some uncooked rice into a tube sock, tie a knot at the top, and heat to the desired temperature in a microwave.) Finally, rebozo sifting (see page 423) can help rotate a posterior baby.

WHAT IF MY LABOR STALLS?

Back in Week 29 (when we were talking about the Cascade of Interventions), I mentioned that the number one cause of unplanned Cesarean in first-time mamas is a labor that stalls or progresses "too slowly." I also mentioned that the standard physicians use to determine how long a "normal" labor should last is *seriously* outdated.

That standard is called the Friedman's Curve. It was invented back in 1955, when a Dr. Emanuel Friedman of Columbia University studied the labors of 500 first-time moms, calculated the average length of time it took each woman to dilate each centimeter, and plotted that data on a graph. Based on his analysis, it became clear that labor seemed to speed up significantly once a woman had dilated to 4 centimeters; in fact, it's from Friedman's research that ob-gyns derived terms like "early" and "active" labor. And though his

---

NOM OF THE WEEK

Red Raspberry Leaf Tea
LABOR DAY EDITION

I've sung the praises of red raspberry leaf tea for months, and now it's time to share with you the formula for my super-strong, extra-concentrated Labor Day Tea, a recipe that is near and dear to my heart; Paloma arrived the day after I started drinking it. Seriously, this is some powerful stuff. You'll want to get the go-ahead from your midwife or doctor first—you don't want to overstimulate the uterus before baby is ready to make her grand entrance—but you'll probably get the all-clear to start drinking the week of your due date. (Drinking the *tea*, that is. It's not time to crack open the wine quite yet.)

To make: add 1½ cups loose red raspberry leaf tea to 4 cups filtered water. Bring to a boil, then reduce the heat, cover, and let simmer for 20 to 30 minutes. Strain, add a natural sweetener if you like, and sip throughout the day.

Oh, and put your midwife on speed-dial.

findings are now sixty-plus years old, they're still considered the obstetrical gold standard. Today, women who don't dilate according to Friedman's schedule—about 1 centimeter per hour—may receive a diagnosis of "failure to progress" and be prepped for an emergency C-section. (Generally, all unplanned C-sections are deemed "emergencies," even if your situation is not in any way life-threatening.)

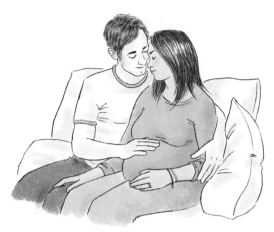

The problem, of course, is that birth in the 1950s bears little resemblance to birth in the new millennium. After all, this was the era of twilight sleep—more than 95 percent of the women in Friedman's study were under some form of sedation. They were also younger (their average age was twenty) and thinner, and their babies were smaller. They were more likely to have a forceps-assisted delivery but less likely to have their labor augmented with Pitocin. Our ideas about what constitutes a "normal" labor in this day and age, in other words, are just plain wrong.

Which is exactly why the American College of Obstetricians and Gynecologists and the Society for Maternal-Fetal Medicine released new guidelines in 2014, redefining the start of active labor as dilation to 6 centimeters (rather than 4) and urging doctors to allow women to labor longer, assuming the baby is not in distress. According to the new standards, first-time mamas should also be allowed to push for at least three hours, longer if they've had an epidural.

These changes, however, constitute a major philosophical shift and take time to implement. Your doctor may still adhere to the old standards. So how can you lessen your chance for an unnecessary Cesarean?

First, remember that it's imperative to stay home as long as is safely possible. (Again, this is where doulas can be such a help!) One of the main reasons first-timers wind up with C-sections is because their labor progressed "too slowly"—even though the standard we use to measure "normal" labors is way outdated. The less time you spend on the hospital's clock, the less you'll be pressured to give birth within some arbitrary time frame.

Once you are admitted, you'll want to create as calming and relaxing an environment as possible. Turning the lights down, listening to some soothing music, diffusing your favorite essential oil, practicing your affirmations, and drowning out the distractions around you can help create a sense of safety, which can reduce your output of labor-stalling stress hormones.

If at some point, your labor does stop progressing, turn to natural remedies to augment your contractions—nipple stimulation and homeopathic remedies are a good place to start.

WHAT IF MY VAGINA . . . *TEARS*?!

I'm not sure if there's anything that sounds worse than having a tear in your vagina—it just makes your skin crawl, doesn't it? But there's no getting around it: during birth, the vagina and the perineum (the area between the vagina and anus) have to s-t-r-e-t-c-h, and sometimes that delicate skin just can't stretch quite fast enough. Anywhere from 40 percent to 85 percent of women delivering vaginally will experience some level of tearing, according to the American College of Nurse-Midwives, although the severity can vary widely. In fact, there are four distinct types:

First degree: A first-degree tear is the least severe, involving only the skin, and will require minimal stitches to repair, if any. It should heal completely within a week or two.

Second degree: Second-degree tears are a little more serious, in that they involve the skin and the muscle underneath the skin. They typically require a few stitches to close, and should heal within two to three weeks.

Third degree: A third-degree tear involves the skin, the perineal muscle, and the muscle that surrounds the anus (the anal sphincter).

Fourth degree: By far the most serious, fourth-degree tears include the skin, the perineal muscle, the anal sphincter, and the tissue that lines the rectum. "Severe" tears (either third- or fourth-degree) are far less common—occurring in 2 percent to 4 percent of vaginal births—but they take considerably longer to heal and are associated with higher risk of long-term complications.

Just as we used to give laboring women enemas to prevent pooping in the delivery room (until we figured out that served no real purpose), old-school physicians had a trick up their sleeves to prevent tearing, too: the episiotomy. This procedure, popular back in the 1960s and 1970s, involves making a surgical cut in the perineum. The idea was that if you cut the vagina *before* it tears, it would be easier to stitch up, as well as quicker to heal.

But just like enemas, episiotomies turned out to be not such a great idea. In fact, they can make things much, much worse. Women who are surgically cut are more likely to develop more severe, spontaneous tears. (Yikes!) Episiotomies may also take longer to heal, are associated with more pain, and up your risk of developing complications, including fecal incontinence and discomfort during sex. (Double yikes!) In 2006, the American College of Obstetricians and Gynecologists issued new guidelines urging doctors to restrict their use, and today episiotomies are considerably less common. Unfortunately, plenty of doctors still do them, often for the wrong reasons, and often without prior consent from the patient.

Strange as it may sound, tearing naturally is almost always your better option.

You can certainly refuse an episiotomy, and it's a good idea to chat with your midwife or doctor about his or her episiotomy philosophy now. It should be a red flag if a provider tells you he routinely cuts episiotomies for all deliveries. Just keep in mind that there *are* a few circumstances in which a cut may be necessary: in particular, if the baby is in significant distress and needs to be delivered immediately.

Want to lower your risk of tearing? I wish I could give you a foolproof solution (with a 100 percent money-back guarantee)—but there isn't one. You can continue performing regular perineal massage (see page 361), and opt for a natural birth (epidurals and Pitocin are both associated with a higher risk of tears). But let me get real with you. Tearing was my second biggest fear about birth, right behind having a C-section. And guess what? I ended up with a second-degree laceration. The good news is that I didn't feel it one bit, and it healed up in a snap. In fact, my midwife explained her love and appreciation for the bounce-back-ability of the vagina like this: "Slap it together, put some stitches in it, and it's good as new."

Yep, she really did say that.

And, yes, I found her words to be true.

WHAT IF I NEED A FORCEPS DELIVERY OR VACUUM EXTRACTION?

FROM MIDWIFE *cynthia*

There was once a time, not so long ago, when almost all physicians used instruments to help facilitate the quick descent and delivery of baby's head. Forceps—which look a bit like a giant pair of salad tongs—were the primary tool, although these days we've also got the option of using vacuum extraction. (It's pretty much what it sounds like, by the way: a little vacuum suction cup is attached to baby's head to help him out.) In my practice, it's rare that we'd need either. Use is generally restricted to situations where the baby's head is visible at the perineum, but prompt delivery is necessary (for instance, if the baby's heart beat is dangerously low for a long time). In these cases, I am fortunate to work with a collaborating physician who is skilled at using both tools.

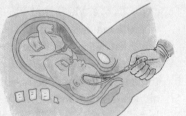

FORCEPS EXTRACTION

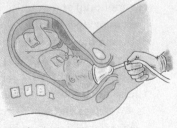

VACUUM EXTRACTION

There are real risks to both the vacuum and forceps: scalp lacerations and certain kinds of brain hemorrhages from a vacuum, for example, or skull fracture and facial nerve damage in the case of forceps. But in *skilled* hands, these tools can make all the difference in how a baby is delivered: vaginally versus Cesarean. Unfortunately, vaginal instrumental deliveries are becoming a bit of a lost art; many physicians just aren't trained to use these tools anymore. That's why it's important to have a sense for your provider's skill set. The safest and best tool is likely the one for which he or she has received the most comprehensive training and the one he or she feels the most comfortable with.

WHAT IF I DON'T LOVE MY BABY?

It's not a fear you'll hear many women admit to publicly, but worrying that you won't fall head-over-heels in love with your baby is surprisingly common. In fact, google "worried I won't love my baby" and watch what happens. Message board after message board, internet forum after internet forum will pop up in the search results, each of them teeming with anxious mamas-to-be who are terrified they'll turn out to be that woman who doesn't bond with her child. These poor women haven't even given birth yet, and they're already convinced they'll turn out to be unloving mothers.

They won't, though. And neither will you. (In fact, just worrying about being a bad mother implies the existence of a pretty robust maternal instinct.)

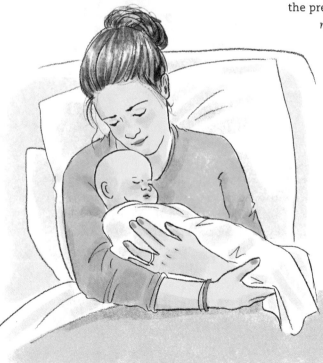

Here's the thing: there's an enormous amount of societal pressure on women to act a certain way—scratch that, to *feel* a certain way—when they're pregnant. After all, you're supposed to jump up and down when you get that positive test (even if the pregnancy wasn't planned), to squeal with delight at the sight of those impossibly cute baby shoes. I mean, this is supposed to be the happiest time of your life, because nothing could possibly be more personally fulfilling than carrying a child because *oh my gosh it's the best thing ever . . . right?*

The truth is that not everyone feels this way—at least not right away, and that's okay. Between the raging hormones, the massive changes to your body, the kooky dreams about giving birth to a toaster, and the unknowns that are part and parcel of all deliveries, and the pressure that comes with trying to do it *au naturel*, it is completely and totally normal to feel overwhelmed by anxiety as opposed to overwhelmed by love.

For the majority of mamas, however, these fears will evaporate the *instant* they set eyes on their baby, and a lot of that will be the hormones talking. One of the greatest benefits of a natural childbirth is that you'll get a massive surge of endorphins (the hormone that triggers euphoria) and produce higher levels of oxytocin in the minutes, hours, and days after birth. (We know that women who are given synthetic oxytocin—a.k.a. Pitocin—during labor, for example, secrete less of the real stuff when they begin breastfeeding.)

But here's something else you won't hear many mamas admit to: for some women, that all-encompassing, I-would-die-for-you kind of love just doesn't kick in right away. It may take days (or even a few short weeks) before the floodgates open. And that's fine, too.

Postpartum depression—which affects up to 1 in 7 new mamas—can also make bonding with baby difficult, but we'll talk more about that in the Special Delivery section, which is coming up soon.

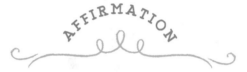

AFFIRMATION

I discipline my mind to focus on love. I breathe in and out, riding each contraction like a wave. I am enjoying each moment as it comes.

mama-do list

- If you haven't already, now's the time to make childcare arrangements for the big day—that's assuming you've already got a kiddo or two, of course, and you're not planning on bringing them along to watch the delivery. If you have fur babies, they'll need care while you're at the hospital or birth center, too!

- Don't forget to keep eating your six dates a day. If you haven't started yet, or you've forgotten, no problem—just start now.

- Quell your fears by reading some positive and empowering birth stories from fellow natural mamas; you can scroll through literally thousands over at mama natural.com.

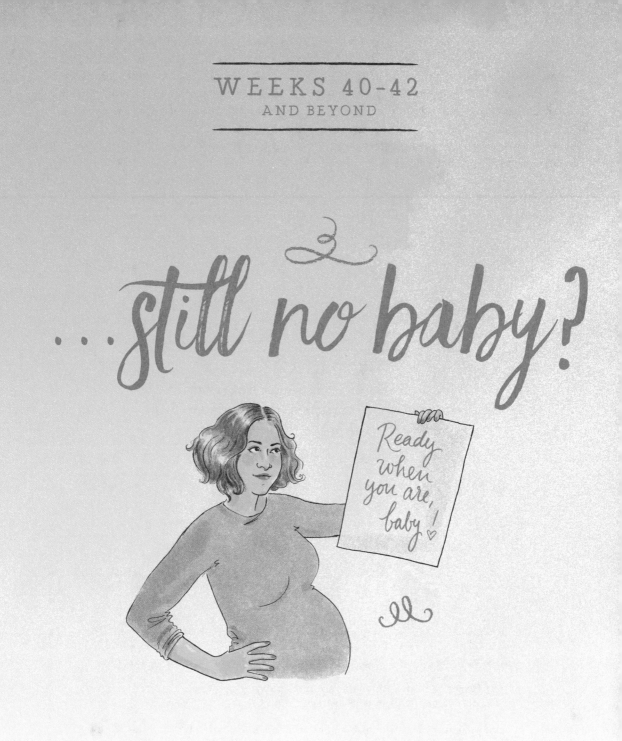

...still no baby?

WHAT'S UP WITH *baby*?

You made it! You've reached the official (if not the actual) end of your pregnancy, Mama! What a wild ride it's been! Baby's really just been marinating in her own juices these last few days, so her official stats—7 or 8-ish pounds (or more) and 19 to 22 inches—should be about the same as they were at 39 weeks. (Even babies that go "post-term" won't necessarily gain an enormous amount of weight. Post-term babes *are* more likely to be classified as "macrosomic"—the technical term for a bigger-than-average baby—but macrosomia begins at just 8 pounds, 14 ounces.) Speaking of juices, the amniotic fluid has been getting a lot of new and interesting flavors lately. Baby, you see, has been busy shedding her coat of lanugo for ten long weeks, but now she's shedding her waxy, cheesy coating of vernix, too. That shed material goes into the fluid, which in turn goes into the baby, which in turn will go into a diaper—as meconium. The longer she marinates, the less likely she is to have any remaining lanugo or vernix at birth.

WHAT'S UP WITH *mama*?

I've always found it strange that many baby books and pregnancy apps end right at 40 weeks. Sure, 40 weeks is the *average* length of a pregnancy—but there's no guarantee that your bun will be fully baked (and ready to come out of the oven) by then. You've only got a 1-in-20 shot of delivering on your actual due date. You've only got a 60 percent chance of going into labor within a *week* of that due date. In fact, "due date" isn't really the greatest term for what's going on here. (If you ask me, "guess date" is more like it!) So as frustrating as it may be to wait, you should relax, take a deep breath and know that baby will come in, well, *due* time.

For some reason (perhaps the improbable size of my growing belly) my husband was convinced that I would deliver our son early, and by the final weeks of my pregnancy he had me pretty much convinced, too. I spent weeks 38 and 39, in particular, on high alert. Every poke in the ribs or potty break seemed like a sure sign that our son's birthday was imminent. But the days continued to tick by on the calendar, my due date drew closer and closer and closer . . . and, alas, nuthin' doin'. As for the office pool, everyone's wagered dates came and went, *sans* baby.

Looking back on it now, I'm not really sure why we were in such a rush. My son ended up entering the world one day *before* his official due date. A dear friend of mine, on the other hand, ended up carrying her first child all the way to 44 weeks. (She went on to have four more babies and—guess what?—every single one of them was born sometime during that 44th week, too.)

Turns out, the length of an average pregnancy isn't as set in stone as we once thought.

In fact, it appears to vary pretty widely. A small study by the U.S. National Institute of Environmental Health Services suggests it may vary by as much as five whole weeks. And there are all sorts of reasons why a mama-to-be might go well beyond her due date.

Genetics, for example, appears to be a factor. Hormonal issues and obesity seem to play a role. First-time mamas are also more likely to carry longer. But the number one cause of post-term pregnancy doesn't have anything to do with your genetics, the health of your baby, or the number of babies you've had.

The number one cause of post-term birth is inaccurate dating. That is, having been assigned the *wrong* due date.

And that's kind of a problem, because mamas who veer too far outside the 40-week window are all candidates for labor induction.

A BRIEF HISTORY OF INDUCTION

Over the last few months, we've talked about the ancient origins of the Cesarean section, the long and winding (and surprisingly political!) history of pain relief during labor, even centuries-old methods of turning a breech baby. So it really shouldn't be a shock to learn that induction—that is, inducing contractions when labor refuses to start on its own—isn't exactly a modern procedure, either.

Hippocrates (commonly regarded as the father of modern medicine, though he died way back in 370 BC) recommended nipple stimulation and mechanical dilation of the cervix. A Roman-era physician, Soranus of Ephesus, was writing about the artificial rupture of membranes (a.k.a. having your water broken) by the second century AD. Doctors in the early 1900s were already experimenting with various forms of hormonal and medicinal induction, in particular injections of quinine and pituitary extract (a kind of precursor to synthetic oxytocin).

And the reason for all these inductions? Back in the day, it was almost always the health of the mother. Pregnancy-related conditions including preeclampsia, gestational diabetes, extreme swelling, bleeding, and infection were—and still are—good reasons to get a baby delivered sooner rather than later. It's only recently that doctors began discovering the potential dangers of going *post*-term (i.e., longer than 42 weeks), even in cases when mama seemed to be tolerating the pregnancy well.

The major ones are fetal distress and stillbirth; research indicates that the risks of both begin to rise after 41 weeks. Additional risks include macrosomia (a post-term baby could theoretically grow too big to safely pass through the maternal pelvis); meconium aspiration (post-term babies are more likely to have their first bowel movement while still in utero); and something called postmaturity syndrome, hallmarks of which include dry, thin, peeling skin, overgrown nails, elongated limbs,

---

NOM OF THE WEEK

Spicy Pineapple

This week we've got two old wives' tales combined into one tasty treat. Pineapple is high in an enzyme called bromelain, which is thought to soften and ripen the cervix. Spicy foods, meanwhile, stimulate the bowels (similar to castor oil)—in fact, some mamas swear that Mexican food kicked their labor into gear. So is this sweet snack enough to bring on contractions, then?

Well, probably not. But this little snack combines salt, spicy, and sweet flavors, and certainly *tastes* delicious. Plus, it's a nice "recipe" to have on hand near the end of pregnancy, when cooking elaborate meals is no longer appealing.

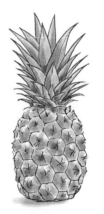

INGREDIENTS

1 organic pineapple

Cayenne pepper to taste

Sea salt to taste

To make, simply core and chop or slice your pineapple, then sprinkle with cayenne pepper and sea salt. Eat with a toothpick or put on a shish kabob stick for a little extra fun. Bon appétit!

and a greenish or yellowish tinge to the skin due to meconium staining.

Given these risks, you can understand why inductions to prevent going post-term haven't just become more common; they've become a standard of obstetrical care. But as induction techniques grew more sophisticated over the years, doctors began to discover something else, too: they afford a certain measure of convenience. None of this waiting on pins and needles for labor to start or driving to the hospital at three in the morning. In the last few decades, it's become possible to *schedule* childbirth.

So guess what's happened? If you said a massive spike in *elective* inductions—inductions that are in no way medically indicated—you'd be right. The rate of induction has more than doubled since 1990; the rate of "early" inductions (those occurring between 37 and 38 weeks) has been on the rise, too.

Unfortunately, these trends have major health consequences.

First, we now know (contrary to previous medical consensus) that weeks 37 and 38 are vitally important to a baby's development; babies born before 39 weeks generally don't fare as well as those who make it full-term—they're more likely to develop

respiratory problems, infections, and low blood sugar, more likely to require admission to the NICU, and more likely to suffer longer-term health problems. In response to the alarming rise of early elective induction, in fact, the American College of Obstetricians and Gynecologists and the Maternal-Fetal Medicine Society actually *changed* the definition of a full-length pregnancy. In the old days (by which I mean, the days before fall 2013) a pregnancy was considered "term" anytime between 37 and 42 weeks. Now, pregnancies are more accurately labeled using the following parameters:

EARLY-TERM
between 37 weeks and 38 weeks, 6 days

FULL-TERM
between 39 weeks and 40 weeks, 6 days

LATE-TERM
between 41 weeks and 41 weeks, 6 days

POST-TERM
42 weeks and beyond

The changes do seem to have helped, by the way—early-term inductions have dropped a bit in the last few years. Plenty of doctors, however, are still happy to induce the moment a mama hits 39 weeks. And that's not always such a good idea, either.

Remember what I said about how the number one cause of post-term pregnancies is inaccurate dating? Modern due dates, you may recall, aren't calculated from the precise moment of conception, but from the first day of your last menstrual period. This dating method is known as Naegele's Rule, and while it can give you a decent estimate of a baby's arrival, it presumes a menstrual cycle that lasts 28 days—that's just not the case for every woman. That means a 42-week-old baby might actually be nearer to 41 weeks. Your 39-week-

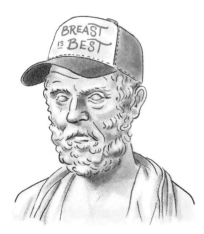

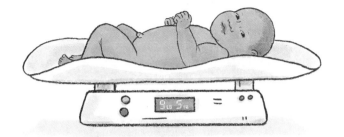

LESS THAN 2% OF U.S. NEWBORNS EXCEED 9 POUNDS, 5 OUNCES.
YET 32% OF WOMEN ARE WARNED THEIR BABIES MAY BE "TOO BIG."

old baby, meanwhile, might actually be closer to early- or preterm, in which case he'd almost certainly benefit from a little more time in the womb.

What about concerns that an overdue baby will become too large to deliver vaginally? It's possible—but not likely.

Less than 2 percent of newborns in the US exceed 9 pounds, 5 ounces. Despite your slim chance of delivering a hefty baby, however, you've got a relatively high chance of being *told* that your baby is "too big." A 2013 survey of new mamas revealed that 1 in 3—or 32 percent—were warned about this very possibility,

but the average weight of their supposedly *enormous* babies at birth turned out to be . . . wait for it . . . less than 8 pounds.

I wasn't kidding when I said ultrasound estimates of fetal weight are notoriously inaccurate.

In the case of stillbirth, it's true that the risk does goes up after a mama clears 41 weeks. It's important to point out, however, that while there is a significant *statistical* increase, the "absolute risk" of stillbirth is still very, very low—less than 1 percent, in fact.

The biggest problem with elective inductions, however? In first-time mamas, they *double* the risk of eventual C-section.

THE PROCESS OF MODERN MEDICAL INDUCTION

While we're stuck with theories as to what triggers spontaneous labor, one thing we *do* know is that a vaginal birth just isn't going to happen until or unless the cervix is ready. Many mamas will begin to dilate and efface in the weeks before birth; but others will not. Instead of thinning and softening, the cervix remains closed and firm. The first stage of induction, then, usually involves an attempt to ripen the cervix—it's called membrane stripping, and your provider might recommend it any time after 39 weeks (if not sooner).

The procedure is simple: during one of your regular prenatal appointments, your provider will insert a finger into the cervix and sweep it around, separating the amniotic sac from the lower uterus. In theory, this may trigger the release of prostaglandins. In reality, there's not a lot of evidence to support the notion. A Cochrane review found that routine sweeping from 38 weeks onward "does not seem to produce clinically important benefits."

In addition to—or instead of—membrane stripping, your provider might want

CALCULATING YOUR BISHOP SCORE

Sometimes letting baby stay is riskier than inducing labor. For example, preeclampsia, intrauterine growth restriction, and decreased placental function are all valid medical reasons to induce. But how do you know if your induction will be successful? And if you're on the fence about induction—if, say, you're 41 weeks and 5 days along and your ob-gyn is knocking on your door with an amniohook—how might you decide if induction is the right choice for you?

Enter the Bishop Score. And, no, I'm not about to enroll you in Catholic school.

The Bishop Score (invented by, yes, a Dr. Bishop back in the mid-1960s) is a simple method of predicting whether the onset of spontaneous labor is likely imminent, and whether induction—if necessary—will prove successful. The score takes into consideration five different components of a vaginal exam, awarding points in each category based on the readiness of the cervix. The higher your score, the greater chance that a medical induction will result in a vaginal delivery (as opposed to a C-section). Scores of 8 or more are associated with a high chance of successful induction. Scores of 5 or below, on the other hand, indicate that labor is not likely to begin on its own anytime soon, and that induction is not likely to be successful.

Here's how the score is calculated based on your most recent vaginal exam:

SCORE

Cervical Position	POSTERIOR 0 points	MID 1 point	ANTERIOR 2 points		
Cervical Consistency	FIRM 0 points	MEDIUM 1 point	SOFT 2 points		
Cervical Effacement	0–30 percent 0 points	31–50 percent 1 point	51–80 percent 2 points	>80 percent 3 points	
Cervical Dilation	0 cm 0 points	1–2 cm 1 point	3–4 cm 2 points	>5cm 3 points	
Fetal Station	-3 0 points	-2 1 point	-1 or 0 2 points	+1 or +2 3 points	

TOTAL SCORE

to try administering topical prostaglandins, a synthetic version of the substance your body produces all on its own (Cervidil is one of the most popular). For some mamas, a single application (delivered via something that looks like a medicated tampon) may be enough to trigger contractions. In rare cases, topical prostaglandins work a little *too* well, overstimulating the uterus (and potentially causing fetal distress). And sometimes not much happens at all.

Assuming your water hasn't broken, artificially rupturing the amniotic sac might be next on the list, and the process is pretty straightforward: your doctor will insert an amniohook deep into the vagina in order to poke a tiny hole in the part of the sac that's protruding through the cervix. This can be uncomfortable—as all vaginal exams tend to be—but it shouldn't be *painful*, since the amniotic sac has no nerve endings. Once your water has been broken, your provider should perform fewer vaginal exams to check your progress in order to lessen the risk of infection.

The final step in the induction process is usually the administration of Pitocin. You'll

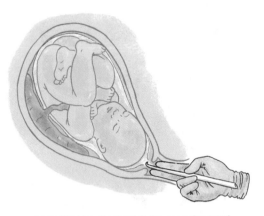

ARTIFICIAL RUPTURE OF MEMBRANES

be started on a low dose, but that dose will be gradually increased until contractions kick in. Of course, you already know the risks: intense, too-close-together contractions and a greater need for pain relief chief among them. In fact, here we are, right smack dab in the middle of the Cascade of Interventions. It's no wonder that inductions extend labor—by an average of three to five hours—and fail so often. As I mentioned earlier, first-time mamas who opt for elective induction double their risk of eventual C-section, according to a study published in the *Journal of Obstetrics & Gynecology*.

NATURAL ALTERNATIVES TO MEDICAL INDUCTION

All of these risks are reason enough to avoid induction—*unless induction is medically indicated*—even if you've gone past your due date. Most women can safely deliver a perfectly healthy baby as late as 42 weeks. (Some will choose to wait even longer; remember my friend, the 44-week mama!) The key is to monitor your and baby's health closely, which is why your midwife or doctor will likely order repeat non-stress tests and/or biophysical profiles if you're headed into late-term territory. (You can always *request* these, by the way.)

But let's be honest. The last few weeks of pregnancy can get really, really uncomfortable.

You're ridiculously huge, you can't sleep, your back hurts, and you're probably desperate to meet your baby. So . . . are you just supposed to sit around, twiddling your thumbs? No way! In fact, unlike the risks associated with medical induction, the following methods of *natural* induction are generally considered safe to start trying once you hit 40 weeks:

THOUGHTS ON NATURAL INDUCTION
FROM MIDWIFE *cynthia*

So, baby's taking a while to make his debut, eh? For first-time mothers, that's not unusual. In fact, there is some research to suggest that first-time mamas commonly go past their due dates—by as many as 10 days. There are definite risks associated with being overdue (in my practice, we generally advise women not to go beyond 42 weeks), but one could argue there are just as many risks associated with premature birth. And as Genevieve mentioned, induction of labor for a baby who is "large for gestational age" is not supported by the evidence. Simply put, women have been growing babies of the same size for decades. Suspicion that a baby is "too large" or that a woman's pelvis is "too small"—in the absence of any other medical conditions—is not a reason to induce any pregnant woman.

If induction does become necessary, there are lots of methods to try—and barring an emergency, you can always opt to try a number of natural methods first. (I usually recommend implementing these methods by 39 weeks as a means to help ripen the cervix.) It's true that most natural techniques are often dismissed as old wives' tales, and many lack strong randomized control trial data, but subjectively many of them have been found to be effective in promoting labor. Medical inductions, on the other hand, are usually only administered in a hospital setting, and the way in which they're administered is usually guided by hospital policy and protocol. My advice is to have a frank discussion with your provider if induction is recommended; understand why you're being induced, and make sure to go over all your options.

♡ **Sex**—a lot of sex. Semen contains prostaglandins, the same hormonelike substance your body emits to bring on contractions, as well as the same active ingredient found in cervical-ripening medications like Cervidil. In fact, it's thought that semen is the biological source with the highest concentration of prostaglandins, which is one reason that sex is an old-school method of natural induction, recommended by doctors and midwives alike. (Other factors that may be at play: orgasm triggers a flood of oxytocin, while the physical aspect of sex may stimulate the uterus.) How effective is sex at inducing labor? From a clinical standpoint, it's hard to say. Studies are extremely limited, and the results of those studies are largely inconclusive. It's also true that sex won't bring on contractions unless your body (and your baby) is ready for birth. However, this is one method that's not only free, but it's a heckuva lot more fun than drinking, say, castor oil—which we'll get to in just a bit. So grab your partner and get it on. (Oh, and according to one experienced mama, third time's the charm.)

♡ **Nipple stimulation.** You already know that nipple stimulation can be an effective way to boost a slow or stalled labor, so it should be no surprise that it can be used to induce labor, too. The most effective way to get an oxytocin boost is to stimulate the whole breast, however, rather than just the nipples. Try performing a slow, rhythmic massage on the breast mound, concentrating on the area behind the areola.

♡ **Evening primrose oil.** This herbal supplement contains prostaglandins and may be taken orally (in capsule form) or applied topically to the vagina and cervix—but it's not without controversy and should definitely be discussed with your midwife or doctor before use. Though studies on the effectiveness of evening primrose oil are limited, there is some indication that oral administration may cause premature rupture of membranes or even lengthen labor.

♡ **Castor oil.** This is another classic method of induction—handed down for generations—as well as another you'll want to discuss with your midwife or doctor. Castor oil is essentially a laxative; it stimulates the bowels to contract, which may stimulate contractions in the uterus. (The usual dose is one tablespoon of castor oil mixed into juice to mask the taste.) The method *does* seem to work; I know plenty of mamas who've had great success with this decades-old remedy. But the potential side effects include pretty

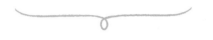

My baby will be born at the perfect time. Instead of counting down the days, I count the moments of being present on this miraculous journey.

terrible diarrhea, which can be uncomfortable at best and lead to dehydration at worst. If the members of your birth team green-light this method, be sure to drink plenty of fluids to rehydrate.

♡ **Pampering and relaxation.** It's important to be calm, relaxed, and psychologically ready for baby—fearful thoughts and anxiety, on the other hand, can trigger adrenaline and other stress hormones that shut down labor. So while these methods may not be backed by hard science, there's plenty of anecdotal evidence to suggest that deep breathing, guided meditation, acupuncture, acupressure, and massage are excellent forms of natural induction. Don't forget to recite your affirmations, too!

mama-do list

● Common homeopathic remedies to induce labor include Pulsatilla, Gelsemium, Caullophyllum, and Cimicifuga. If you're interested in giving homeopathics a go, talk to your midwife or doctor first.

● Get as much rest as possible in these last days or weeks before birth. Take naps. Sleep as much as you can. Watch movies. Stay relaxed.

● Be sure to eat your six dates a day and drink your Labor Day Tea (see page 404).

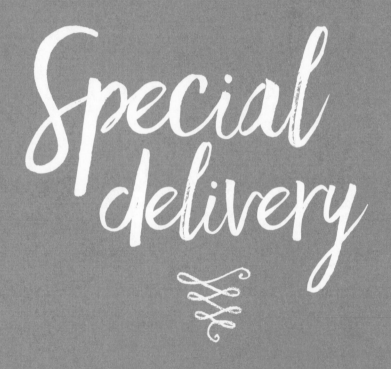

PART FOUR

Special
delivery

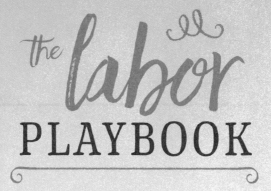

the *labor* PLAYBOOK

YOUR STEP-BY-STEP
(OR SHOULD I SAY, *STAGE-BY-STAGE*)
GUIDE TO A NATURAL CHILDBIRTH.

STAGE ONE: *labor*

PHASE ONE: *early labor*

Over a period of hours, days, or perhaps even weeks, your cervix will gradually begin to efface (thin) and dilate (open). You may notice increasingly frequent (and intense) Braxton Hicks contractions during this process, but it's also possible that you won't feel much of anything at all, especially if this is your first birth. Soon, however, you'll experience your first *real* contraction, followed by another and another and another. Keep in mind that your contractions may be wildly irregular at first—anywhere from 5 to 20 minutes apart—but they'll become progressively stronger, longer, and closer together. Your cervix will continue to dilate, all the way to 6 centimeters.

ADDITIONAL SIGNS OF EARLY LABOR

♡ Intense, menstrual-like cramps

♡ Dull backache

♡ Diarrhea or loose bowel movements

♡ Increased vaginal discharge or loss of the mucus plug

♡ The bloody show

♡ Leaking fluid or breaking of the amniotic sac

POSITIONS TO TRY DURING *early labor*

It's important to preserve your energy, but now's not the time to lie flat on your back. This only compresses the pelvis and encourages a posterior baby to put more pressure against your spine (ouch!). Instead try:

Resting Easy. When you're lying down, rest on your left side, rolling your hip and shoulder downward so that you're as far on top of your belly as is comfortable. Bend the knee of your right leg and rest it on the bed, couch, or floor (using a pillow for support if you need to). This position stretches the muscles in your lower body and allows you to rest without putting pressure on the vena cava. It may also encourage a poorly positioned baby to readjust herself in the womb.

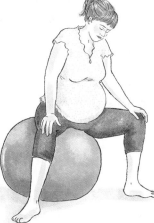

The Birth Ball. Try bouncing atop a birthing ball instead of leaning backward in a comfy chair or recliner. You can also try rotating your hips in a circle, which can relieve lower back pain and keep the pelvis open and aligned. (Some wild-child mamas also like to hula hoop or belly dance to encourage baby to descend!)

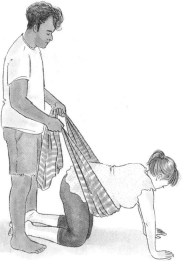

Rebozo Sifting. A rebozo is a traditional garment worn by Spanish American women, as well as a popular tool in the natural birth world. Don't have a rebozo? No problem—an oversized scarf, shawl, or even a baby wrap will do. To do the sift, get down onto all fours. Your partner should wrap the rebozo around your belly, then *gently* pull the loose ends from side to side, jiggling the uterus. This helps to relax the muscles involved in labor and delivery and aids in the rotation and descent of the baby. (Most doulas are well versed in the rebozo technique, too.)

WHAT'S UP WITH BABY?

Baby is beginning his descent through the pelvis—if he hasn't already "dropped" and "engaged," he will soon. Meanwhile, the pressure from his head will help to thin and dilate the cervix. He also may begin rotating in the hours before birth.

WHAT YOU CAN DO

It's common to experience a surge of energy and adrenaline when labor kicks in (baby is finally coming!), but try to stay relaxed—after all, you may be in for a marathon labor. If it's the middle of the night, do your best to get some sleep. If it's midafternoon, make yourself comfortable. At some point over the next few hours, you'll also want to:

♡ Time your contractions periodically, just to see if a pattern is emerging.

♡ Call your doula. Together, you can determine when it's time for her to come and join you.

♡ Stay hydrated—sip some Labor Day Tea and/or coconut water.

♡ Eat something. You'll lose your appetite as labor becomes more intense, so try to get some protein and healthy fats into your system now. You'll need the energy later.

WHAT YOUR PARTNER CAN DO

Early labor is all about staying relaxed and comfortable. Papa can perform some light massage (get out that tennis ball back massager if you need to!), practice timing contractions, whip her up a nutritious meal, or just keep mama company while she naps, reads, or watches movies.

HOW LONG IT LASTS

Early labor is unpredictable; yours could last mere hours, or it could stretch on for days.

WHAT OTHER *natural mamas* SAY

ashton: I knew I was in labor when my water broke: right in the middle of my in-laws' living room on Christmas day!

sabrina: I felt a lot of pressure in my uterus—a little more than when I get my period. When the pressure seemed to increase, I knew something was going on.

claire: My midwives later teased me because I'd been up all night with what I was sure were just gas pains. At my prescheduled appointment the next morning, I kept trying to convince them that I wasn't in labor. They took one look at me and knew that I was. In fact, they strapped me to a monitor to prove to me that these weren't gas pains—they were contractions! I went back home and spent the day resting. About 24 hours later, things got more intense, I lost the mucus plug, and I knew it was time to check in.

PHASE TWO: *active labor*

As you move into active labor, your contractions will become much stronger, much longer, and much closer together. When they're consistently 4 minutes apart, each lasts for a full minute, and hold that pattern for at least an hour, it's generally time to leave for the birth center or hospital. But remember that the 4-1-1 rule is only a guide; some mamas never settle into a pattern that's clear cut. If at any point you have questions about your progress, don't hesitate to call your midwife or doctor.

ADDITIONAL SIGNS OF ACTIVE LABOR

♡ Increased pressure in the pelvis

♡ Intense lower back discomfort

♡ You can no longer talk through contractions

♡ You can no longer be distracted during a contraction; they require your full energy and concentration

♡ Rupture of waters

WHAT'S UP WITH BABY?

Baby is continuing to descend down into the pelvis, putting more and more pressure on the cervix, helping you to dilate an additional 2 or 3 centimeters.

WHAT YOU CAN DO

As your contractions intensify, you'll likely feel them building to a distinct peak—a point at which they're most intense—and then fading away. As your contractions lengthen, the peak will lengthen, too, so it's a great time to employ some of the pain-relief techniques we've talked about: hydrotherapy, deep breathing, homeopathics, acupressure. Do your best to stay relaxed and keep your muscles loose—moaning throughout your contractions can help prevent you from tensing up or holding your breath. You can also try making "horse lips" (a relaxation tactic made popular by renowned midwife and natural birth advocate Ina May Gaskin) by fluttering your lips together while exhaling. This keeps the mouth and jaw loose, which prevents your body from tensing up (and may encourage the opening of your cervix). If you're feeling intense back pain, try taking a warm shower and aiming the water directly on your lower back or getting some counterpressure and massage from partner.

WHAT YOUR PARTNER CAN DO

It's important to create a calming, comfortable space in which to give birth; the more safe and supported mama feels, the less likely she is to start producing stress hormones (which could potentially stall her labor). Partners can dim the lights, keep the door to the room closed, offer fluids from time to time (with a little natural sweetener for an energy boost), play some soothing music, diffuse some essential oils, do some acupressure or massage, and offer *plenty* of encouragement.

HOW LONG IT LASTS

Active labor tends to be much shorter, but much more intense—on average, anywhere from 4 to 8 hours. (It may go even quicker if this isn't your first birth.)

POSITIONS TO TRY DURING *active labor*

Your body will guide you into positions that will help baby rotate and descend, making your contractions more efficient and your labor more comfortable, so go where it takes you. You may find that leaning over a birth ball or getting onto all fours is particularly helpful, but consider giving these moves a try too:

Supported Knee-Chest. This is a great way to potentially reposition an engaged but "stuck" baby. Do not do this if your labor is progressing well and/or baby hasn't engaged. Spread your knees wide, sinking your belly as low as possible, and rest your head and chest on the bed or couch, using pillows for support as needed. Meanwhile, your partner gently pulls back on the ends of the rebozo. Lean your hips into the support he provides.

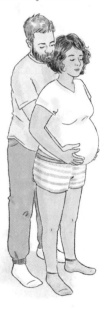

The Abdominal Lift. This move should only be used if you have back labor or baby isn't engaging into pelvis. Wait for a contraction, then direct your partner or doula to gently lift your belly, pulling it up and back toward your spine, as if lifting the baby out of the pelvis. When the contraction ends, direct your support person to gently let go of your abdomen. You can do this move with or without a rebozo.

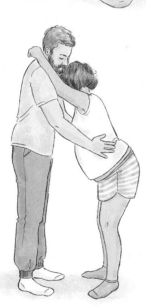

Supported Slow Dancing. Mamas often intuitively sway their hips during contractions; being close to and supported by their partners is comforting, too. Meanwhile, the upright position uses gravity to help baby descend.

PHASE THREE: *transition*

It's almost time to push, Mama, but first we've got to get through the toughest part of labor: transition. During this phase, your contractions will become extremely intense and very close together, occurring roughly every 2 minutes and lasting between 75 and 90 seconds at a time, with very little rest in between. Some women may experience double peaks (in other words, your contraction will build, peak, fade slightly, then peak again before ending). Surging adrenaline may also cause some women to tremble or shake.

ADDITIONAL SIGNS OF TRANSITIONAL LABOR

♡ Nausea or vomiting

♡ You become more vocal (yelling at people during transition is not uncommon).

♡ You may become more discouraged, distressed, or emotional.

♡ You may suddenly request an epidural, a C-section, or other interventions.

♡ You may make irrational statements like "I'm done" or "I'm going home now."

WHAT'S UP WITH BABY?

As the cervix expands those last few centimeters, baby will descend through the pelvic outlet and into the lower part of the vagina. He may also still be rotating, getting into a better position for the pushing stage.

POSITIONS TO TRY IF YOU'VE HAD AN EPIDURAL
FROM MIDWIFE *Cynthia*

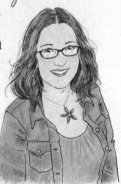

Mamas who've had an epidural often don't have the ability to stand or walk around during labor, but there are still many positions they can utilize to help their babies descend. In fact, many midwives and doulas recommend rotating through four positions every half hour or so: sitting (or semi-reclining), lying on your right side, resting on your hands and knees, lying on your left side. Then repeat. Peanut balls have been shown to shorten labor (and lower the risk of eventual Cesarean), since placing one between your legs while reclining helps to keep the pelvis open.

When it comes time to push, it's actually not necessary for mamas who've had an epidural to deliver flat on their backs. Many hospital beds can be raised to encourage an upright, seated position (allowing gravity to help baby descend). They can also be equipped with squatting bars—mamas who are able to support their own weight (even briefly) can use these bars for stability in order to squat during contractions and birth. Talk to your midwife or doctor about the types of birthing tools that might be available to you on the big day.

POSITIONS TO TRY DURING *transitional labor*

Movement can help bring the baby farther down into the birth canal, enabling transition to pass more quickly, so let your body lead you. Some especially productive positions include:

Lunging or Squatting. Let gravity do some of the work by squatting (on a birthing stool or even—yes!—the toilet) or lunging into a contraction; try lunges on a chair or against a bed, and make sure your partner's nearby for support and balance.

Counterpressure. Climb onto all fours and have your partner apply firm pressure (either with his hands, a warm rice sock, or the tennis ball massager) directly to your sacrum—that's the large, flat bone on the lower back.

The Double Hip Squeeze. While on your hands and knees, have your partner apply firm pressure to the hip bones, forcing them in and up. This pose is excellent for stalled labors, malpositioned babies, and lower back pain, because it mechanically opens the pelvis, making more room for the baby.

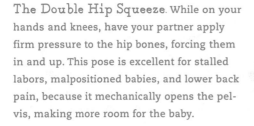

WHAT YOU CAN DO

Transition can be a breaking point. This is the time when some natural mamas may begin to wonder why they didn't just sign up for the drugs—it's common to feel overwhelmed, scared, super fatigued, or just plain freaked out. What's important to remember, however, is that feelings like this are *totally* normal and, actually, a really good sign. (You know the cliché *it's always darkest before the dawn?* Things will only get better from here on out.) Take it one contraction at a time. Focus on your breath and go to your happy place. Getting into a birthing tub can provide some major relief, too.

WHAT YOUR PARTNER CAN DO

Apply counterpressure if mama needs it, fill up the bathtub, offer sips of juice or give her ice chips to munch on in between contractions. Mamas in transition are at their most vulnerable, so help her stay focused and confident— she's almost there. In fact, she's one step closer to holding her baby. Perhaps most important, don't be offended if she tells you to back off (or worse!). Some mamas just don't want to be touched or spoken to at this time. Give her the space she needs but send some prayers or good energy her way.

HOW LONG IT LASTS

As little as 15 minutes to several hours.

STAGE TWO: *time to push*

Ah, sweet relief! The hardest part of labor (for most mamas) is over, and it's time to push this baby out. Luckily, most natural mamas will feel a surge of energy and a powerful urge to bear down, as well as some intense rectal pressure (having a baby sometimes feels a bit like having a very large, very intense bowel movement). During the pushing phase, your contractions will usually space out again, coming every 2 to 5 minutes; meanwhile, because your cervix has completely dilated and effaced, you should be more comfortable. In fact, you may be elated to have reached a more proactive part of labor. Instead of passively letting the contractions wash over you, there's finally something to *do*. Yay!

WHAT'S UP WITH BABY?

As baby descends even farther, the soft bones of his head will mold to the shape of the birth canal and gently stretch mama's vaginal tissue. His head will come out first, followed by his shoulders and the rest of his body. Your provider should then place him directly onto your chest for immediate skin-to-skin contact. While he's on your chest, a birth attendant may cover him with a blanket and begin assessing his health and breathing.

WHAT YOU CAN DO

You probably won't need all that much coaching—trust me, you'll likely feel the urge to bear down and *push*—but you do want to rest in between contractions. Be sure to keep drinking fluids and stay focused on your breathing. Intermittent squatting or rocking back and forth while on all fours can help the baby descend even farther. (Keep in mind that epidurals can sometimes interfere with the body's signaling, so if you don't feel the urge to push, your midwife or doctor can help by confirming that your cervix is fully effaced and dilated and guiding you along. Sometimes this process is called "laboring down," and it can help prevent exhaustion and even vaginal tearing.)

WHAT YOUR PARTNER CAN DO

Help mama get into the pushing position that most suits her—using pillows, a squatting stool, or your own body weight for support and balance. Offer her something to drink in between contractions and encourage her with positive statements: *You are doing so awesome. Our beautiful baby is almost here. I am so proud of you.* You might also ask for a hand mirror. Seeing baby in the bottom of the birth canal can be a huge encouragement for some mamas— just make sure to get her permission first!

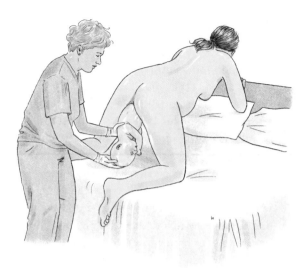

HOW LONG IT LASTS

On average, first-time mamas can expect to push for at least 1 to 2 hours; mamas who've had an epidural, meanwhile, will likely need to push longer (2 to 4 hours, if not more). More experienced mamas may push for only a matter of minutes.

THE RING OF FIRE

Ever heard experienced mamas talk about the "ring of fire"? They're not referring to their love for Johnny Cash songs—as I imagine you knew—but rather a common phenomenon that occurs in the moments before birth: As your baby crowns and emerges through the vaginal opening, you may feel an intense dryness and stretching that literally burns—hence the name. But just as a candle's flame can be put out in a mere instant, the pain dissipates quickly. And by then, most mamas are so overjoyed to be delivering their babies—finally!— that the burning sensation is *almost* welcome.

POSITIONS TO TRY *while pushing*

Some mamas will be most comfortable on their hands and knees, but it's important to push in the position that feels right to you. Try:

Squatting. Using a squatting bar or stool, your partner, and/or a rebozo, try sinking deep into the squat and curling your upper body over your belly to push out the baby. Be sure to rest in between surges, as squatting for *long* periods can promote swelling.

Supported Semi-Seating. Pull your knees to your chest, using your partner, a pile of pillows, or an elevated hospital bed to support your back.

Side Lying. A great option for mamas who've had a very long (very exhausting) labor: Bend your knees, and pull the knee of your upper leg in toward your chest.

WHAT YOU CAN EXPECT DURING LABOR

FROM MIDWIFE *cynthia*

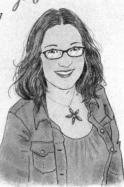

The amazing and miraculous changes that occur in a woman's body during labor astound me, even to this day. In fact, I've always felt lucky to be invited into someone's birth space. There is a palpable aura that surrounds a laboring mama—most providers, nurses, and doulas I've spoken with have felt it, too. It causes those present to rock and sway rhythmically in time with contractions. It casts a warm, fuzzy haze over everyone in the room.

But beyond that, every birth I've ever witnessed has been utterly unique and different. I've attended a birth with a dozen of mama's family members, all of whom danced and celebrated and cheered (loudly!) during the pushing phase. I've attended an intimate birth with a strict no-noise rule, which everyone observed until the baby emerged and the father whispered the first words, a prayer, directly into the newborn's ear.

In total, the births I've witnessed actually have had more differences than similarities, and it's impossible to know exactly how long a labor will last, how a mama might cope or what she will and won't like during the birth process.

Some women have very long labors; some only last a few hours. Some mamas may vomit or have diarrhea, some not at all. Some women love certain positions; others loathe them. And from a provider's standpoint, I choose not to sweat the small stuff. My job is to ensure mama's health and baby's safe passage, so I don't care if you want to labor without your clothes on; I don't mind if you want to make a lot of noise or scream the whole way through. Ultimately, you birth the baby the way *you* want to. I may give suggestions from time to time, but unless there's some major medical concern, I don't necessarily expect a mama to do exactly what I say. My philosophy has always been to be patient and to give her the space to do what feels natural.

megan: I delivered my baby on all fours. I got on top of the bed on my hands and knees and just didn't want to move. I liked being able to have my head in the pillow. I'm kind of shy and private, so I think that helped me to just feel like I was in my own space.

mariska: I gave birth on a birthing stool. Gravity helped a lot! I had a sense of control, and I felt so much stronger on the birthing stool than lying on a bed. I really felt each contraction pushing the baby out, so it felt like the most natural position to give birth in.

kjelse: As soon as I hit transition, I went to all fours on the bed. I wanted to give birth in the water, so when a break between contractions came, my husband and midwife helped me into the tub, where I ended up giving birth in a position that was part all fours and part squat. I just followed my instinct in how to move.

laci: I had a home water birth, so I expected to deliver in a squat or on my hands and knees. I did move around into various positions during the contractions, but when it came time to push, I felt like I needed to lie back against the side of the pool, which surprised me. Your body tells you exactly what it needs to help the baby out!

DON'T CUT THAT CORD!

All throughout your pregnancy, baby's lungs have been filled with amniotic fluid. Of course, it's impossible to breathe underwater, so his only source of oxygen has been you—oxygen from your blood transfers to his blood inside the placenta and then travels to his body via the umbilical cord.

At the moment of birth, however, everything changes.

As baby takes those first, gasping cries, the fluid will begin draining from his lungs, and the alveoli (those little grape-like sacs) will begin filling with air. Meanwhile, blood from his heart will start flowing to the lungs in order to take up oxygen. It's a dramatic transition, all right, and there's not a lot of margin for error. But that's why there's a nice little insurance policy. During the first few minutes after birth, baby will receive oxygen from not one, but *two* sources: his newly functioning lungs *and* the placenta, assuming the umbilical cord is still attached and still pulsating. When the transition to the outside world is complete—in other words, once baby's breathing has regulated—the flow of blood through the umbilical cord will stop all on its own.

You might wonder, then, why it's common practice to clamp and cut the umbilical cord mere *seconds* after baby makes his debut. But in the old days, there were actually quite a few reasons.

Back in the 1950s, for example—a.k.a. the era of twilight sleep—the drugs mamas were given were often intense enough to cause respiratory distress in newborns, and it wasn't uncommon for an infant to need immediate resuscitation. The rise of the Cesarean also likely played a role in early clamping; after all, it's easier (for the doctor, at least) to clamp and cut the cord, remove the baby from the surgical venue, and continue along with the procedure. The *major* benefit to early clamping, however, is that it was thought to speed delivery of the placenta, reducing the risk of postpartum hemorrhage.

Turns out that last part, however, just isn't true: research has shown there is no correlation between maternal hemorrhage and cutting of the umbilical cord. We also now know there are numerous reasons to delay cord clamping.

For one thing, waiting a few minutes to cut the cord boosts a newborn's iron stores—by as much as 30 percent (!) more iron-rich blood is transferred to the baby—significantly lowering his risk of anemia. He'll also get a bigger influx of stem cells and maternal antibodies, and have a lower risk of respiratory distress. In premature babies, delayed cord clamping is associated with a reduction in hemorrhages and reduces the need for eventual blood transfusion. A 2015 study published in *JAMA Pediatrics* indicates that delayed cord clamping may be associated with improved fine motor and social skills *years* down the line. The benefits are so profound, in fact, that the World Health Organization now recommends "late cord clamping"—performed between 1 and 3 minutes after birth—unless a baby needs

$\longrightarrow$

immediate resuscitation. (Curiously, the American College of Obstetricians and Gynecologists has not yet updated its guidelines, although it does recommend a delay of 30 to 60 seconds in preterm babies.)

If you'd like to opt for delayed cord clamping, you'll need to include this in your birth plan and discuss your wishes with your doctor or midwife and doula. How long should you wait? That's up to you.

Many natural mamas will choose to delay clamping until the cord stops pulsating, or for at least 3 to 5 minutes, which is about how long it takes for baby to receive a full transfusion. Others may choose to wait until the placenta has been delivered. One important thing to keep in mind: you may not be able to delay cord clamping (or may not be able to delay it for *long*) if you're planning to donate or bank your baby's cord blood. There is currently no medical consensus on delayed clamping as it relates to cord blood retrieval, but the more blood that flows into your baby, the less blood is available for collection and storage. You'll need to decide which of these is most important to you—either baby receives those extra stem cells now or you collect and pay to store them.

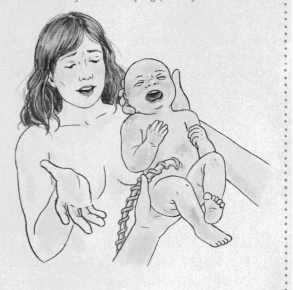

STAGE THREE: *meeting your baby*

(OH, AND DELIVERING THE PLACENTA, TOO)

All that waiting and worrying and wondering over the past nine or ten months and then—poof!—just like that, your sweet baby is here. These next few minutes will be positively magical. (I call it "new baby bliss.") But even though you've made it through delivery, your job isn't *quite* over yet. In fact, your uterus is still contracting—although you may not even notice, since you'll be basking in the afterglow of birth. Some mamas, however, will experience some mild cramping and rectal pressure when the placenta detaches from the uterine wall and is ready to come out.

WHAT'S UP WITH BABY?

Barring any medical complications, baby should be lying skin-to-skin on your chest. He's likely taking in the world around him, curling his hand around your finger, and may even be showing signs that he's ready to breastfeed. But here's something you won't often hear mamas admit to or discuss: adorable and pre-

WHAT OTHER *natural mamas* SAY

rhiannon: Birth is indescribable. I felt this little being leave my body and all of a sudden the person I had dreamed of and wondered about for nine months was cuddled up on me, breathing, blinking, and reacting to my touch!

kathleen: I cry just thinking about it. I gave birth on a stool in the tub. In one smooth motion, I pushed and my midwife lifted him to my chest. I was crying and laughing and kissing my husband and overcome with emotions—so much so that we forgot to check if it was a boy or a girl! It wasn't until a nurse asked that we remembered to look.

tenell: Words could never describe the magnitude of that life-changing moment. Intense love—the most intense love you have ever felt, times a million. The exhilaration. The adrenaline. The overwhelming sense of accomplishment. The joy. The birth of our son and daughter have been, hands down, the moments I will always cherish most.

cious as they are, brand-new babies sometimes look a little worse for wear, especially after a vaginal birth. They've been through quite an ordeal, after all. So don't be surprised if his head is a bit cone-shaped, if he's got hair in all the "wrong" places (like his back and upper arms instead of his head), if he's a little bloated and puffy (especially if you received IV fluids during labor), or if his skin is blotchy or bruised. All of this is very common in newborns, and generally clear up on their own in a matter of days or weeks.

WHAT YOU CAN DO

Skin-to-skin contact helps boost oxytocin production, which accelerates delivery of the placenta (thus helping the uterus shrink back to its usual size and minimizing bleeding). To speed the process along, your provider may knead or massage your abdomen and will likely ask you to push while gently tugging on the umbilical cord. (Some mamas may benefit from a small hit of Pitocin to encour-

age contractions. As an alternative, you can try rubbing a very small amount of clary sage essential oil—mixed with coconut oil—directly onto your belly.) Once the placenta has been delivered, your midwife or doctor will inspect it to make sure it's fully intact; you don't want any residual pieces of placenta hanging around inside your uterus, as this can cause complications. If you're planning to take your placenta home, now's the time to have your partner or doula get out that plastic bag or cooler, as the organ needs to be put on ice. Finally, your provider will stitch up any tears.

WHAT YOUR PARTNER CAN DO

Take some photos, offer skin-to-skin contact if mama's busy delivering the placenta, and be ready to navigate newborn tests and screenings—more on that in a bit.

HOW LONG IT LASTS

On average, anywhere from 5 to 20 minutes.

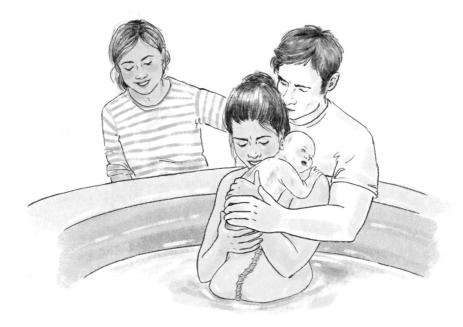

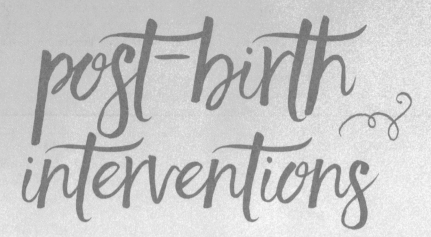

post-birth interventions

NEWBORN TESTS AND SCREENINGS

Natural mamas are often so fixated on pregnancy and avoiding unnecessary interventions during birth that they often forget they'll be faced with a ton of choices *after* birth, too. Here's a look at the routine tests, interventions, and screenings you can expect between the moment baby arrives and the moment you both head home from the birth center or hospital. Review the list now, and discuss your preferences with your healthcare provider *before* those contractions kick in—you don't want to be making important decisions about baby's well-being without having done your research!

THE APGAR

Immediately after birth, your provider should place baby directly onto your chest and abdomen for skin-to-skin contact. Newborns can't regulate their own body temperature well, but the close contact with mama will keep him warm, not to mention lower his output of stress hormones, flood him (and you!) with oxytocin, and help with the initiation of breastfeeding. A nurse may dry baby off a little and cover him with a blanket. While you're bonding, a nurse will also perform a standard assessment of baby's health, called the APGAR.

The APGAR—named after Virginia Apgar, an anesthesiologist who invented the protocol back in the early 1950s—is a quick way to determine if a newborn needs any kind of emergency medical care. APGAR also stands for the five factors that are scored on a scale of 0 to 2, for a total possible score of 10:

- ♡ **Appearance** (Is baby pink, or bluish-gray, indicating poor circulation?)
- ♡ **Pulse** (Is it strong and fast or slow and sluggish?)
- ♡ **Grimace response** (a.k.a. reflexes)
- ♡ **Activity** (Is he kicking and moving his arms, or is he "floppy"?)
- ♡ **Respiration** (Is his breathing erratic, or does he have a good, healthy cry?)

APGAR scores of 7 and above are indicators of good overall health (keep in mind that scores of a "perfect 10" are very rare). Scores of 3 or below at the 1-minute mark indicate the need for emergency medical intervention, including but not limited to resuscitation. Five minutes after birth, the APGAR is repeated and recalculated. Low-scoring babies who have failed to improve may require very close monitoring or additional intervention.

WHAT ARE MY NATURAL OPTIONS?

Barring a medical emergency, the APGAR can (and should) be performed while baby lies on your chest—when a newborn is stable, there's no medical reason to separate him from his mother or move him to an incubator or radiant warmer. In fact, even babies who need a *little* bit of help with their breathing (like, say, additional suction) tend to do better when they're allowed to stay with mama and the umbilical cord remains attached and unclamped. You'll want to indicate your desire for immediate skin-to-skin contact (also called "kangaroo care") on your birth plan, as well as discuss your wishes with your midwife or doctor. Because, unfortunately, the standard practice used to be (and in some cases, still is) to remove baby to a warmer, wipe him down, weigh him, footprint him, swaddle him, and present him back to mama; sometimes for mere moments before whisking him away to the nursery for additional observation.

In the event that mama can't provide skin-to-skin contact (if, say, she's under general anesthesia), papa should be allowed to step in.

Additional routine procedures—weighing the baby, footprinting, etc.—can be delayed for an hour or so, until mama has bonded and/or initiated breastfeeding. Keep in mind that you *may* need to hand baby off while delivering the placenta; after my daughter's birth, for example, I needed to get out of bed, assume a standing position, and really bear down. However, this is pretty rare.

ANTIBIOTIC EYE OINTMENT

In the days when nurses were accustomed to evaluating baby on a radiant warmer away from his mother, they were busy administering some other post-birth interventions, too. One of those was the application of eyedrops or ointment, which guards against STI-related eye infections in newborns, some of which have been known to cause blindness. Standard treatment used to be silver nitrate (which was super-irritating and could, ironically, *cause* infections). These days, babies are given a gentler, milder antibiotic—usually erythromycin.

And I know what you're thinking—I was tested for STIs including syphilis, gonorrhea, and chlamydia during pregnancy (during the first *and* third trimesters), so baby only needs this if I've tested positive, right? Wrong. All babies—even C-section babies—are given the ointment, regardless of a mother's STI test results. Partly, this is because you could theoretically be infected with certain STIs and have no symptoms, and partly it's because babies can *sometimes* get a mild case of conjunctivitis from exposure to healthy bacteria in the vagina. The treatment is not 100 percent effective, however, nor is it standard procedure in many countries outside the Unites States, including the UK.

WHAT ARE MY NATURAL OPTIONS?

Who wants a bunch of goop in their eyes right after birth? Doesn't sound pleasant to me! Some even believe that erythromycin can make a newborn's already poor vision worse (and blurrier), which could theoretically interfere with her ability to bond and breastfeed. For this reason, some natural mamas choose to delay the application of eye ointment for an hour or two, or until they've been able to initiate breastfeeding. Of course, other mamas may prefer not to give baby unnecessary antibiotics *at all*, and provided you've tested negative for any and all STIs and were celibate during pregnancy or in a committed, monogamous relationship, you should be able to safely decline this intervention. Know that most states are required by law to administer antibiotic eye ointment. Some hospitals and birth centers will let you decline without much fuss (you'll likely have to sign a medical waiver), but some have been known to call Child Protective Services (or threaten to call, as an intimidation tactic). Discuss your wishes with your healthcare provider well in advance, and indicate them on your birth plan.

THE VITAMIN K SHOT

Adults get vitamin K from two main sources: their diet (leafy green veggies are a great source) and bacteria in the gut and intestines. Newborns, however—whose microbiomes are

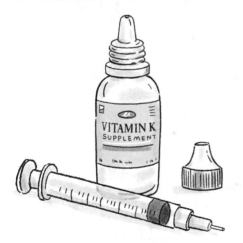

still being colonized and who don't exactly eat a lot of spinach and kale—usually have some level of vitamin K deficiency, and that's a problem. Vitamin K is crucial for blood clotting, and lack of this important nutrient can lead to spontaneous and severe internal bleeding. The condition is called vitamin K deficiency bleeding (VKDB) or hemorrhagic disease of the newborn (HDN), and though rare, it is *very* serious. Early-onset VKDB develops within the first 24 hours; classic VKDB between 1 and 7 days postpartum; and late-onset within 2 weeks and 6 months after birth. To protect against VKDB, the American Academy of Pediatrics has recommended a vitamin K shot—an intramuscular injection, administered into baby's thigh in the hours after birth—since the 1960s.

WHAT ARE MY NATURAL OPTIONS?

In the natural world, there are really two main concerns floating around about the vitamin K shot. The first is that it's a *mega-dose* (although, it's important to point out, side effects associated with the shot are so rare they're virtually unheard of). The second is that the shot contains a synthetic version of vitamin K and some not so great ingredients and preservatives. In the event that you're perusing the internet, concerns that the vitamin K shot might increase baby's risk of leukemia have been completely disproven.

There *are* alternatives to intramuscular vitamin K:

♡ You can ask if your birth center or hospital offers a preservative-free version of the shot (which does still contain some less than desirable agents).

♡ You may inquire about oral vitamin K drops for your child. (There are a few different oral vitamin K regimens. Some suggest three doses, administered at birth, one week, and one month. The Danish regimen, meanwhile, involves administering drops weekly for the first three months.) Studies *have* shown the oral version to be effective in preventing some instances of VKDB, though not nearly as effective as the shot. You should also know that there isn't an FDA-approved version of oral vitamin K available in the United States. Some midwives may provide oral vitamin K, or it can be purchased online. Drops sold via the internet, however, are sold as supplements, and are therefore not regulated by the FDA.

♡ Or, you can decline the shot, just as you may decline any intervention, but be sure that you fully understand the risks. It's important to point out, too, that many states mandate the administration of vitamin K. Some (New York, in particular) do not allow you to decline the shot via waiver or religious exemption.

Full disclosure: I declined the vitamin K shot with each of my children, but if I had to do it all over again, I'd almost certainly change my mind. (I'd likely opt for the drops.) While I love to avoid anything "unnatural," I believe this is a situation where the rewards outweigh the risks of the injection. Interesting to note: in the last few years, we've started to see a small surge in cases of VKDB, specifically in babies whose parents declined the intervention. The effects of vitamin K deficiency bleeding can be catastrophic; late-onset VKDB, in particular, is often fatal. You should not decline the shot until or unless you've had a very detailed discussion with your healthcare provider. And at an absolute minimum, you might consider taking a vitamin K supplement in the weeks and months after birth. (There is some extremely limited evidence to suggest that taking a large daily supplement may raise the level of vitamin K in *breast milk*; however it's not clear how much of this vitamin K a newborn might absorb. There also haven't been any studies on the relationship between maternal supplementation and instances of VKDB.) Finally, know that babies who are exclusively formula-fed have a nearly non-existent risk of VKDB, as infant formula is fortified with high levels of vitamin K.

BABY'S FIRST BATH

Sometime in the hours after baby's birth, he'll very likely be offered a bath by one of the labor and delivery nurses. For years, babies were bathed right away for basic hygienic purposes, as well as for aesthetic reasons— in other words, to wipe off all that gloopy, cheesy residue. In the past few years, however, we've learned much more about the incredible benefits of vernix caseosa. It's loaded with antimicrobial properties that protect against infection; it's an incredible natural moisturizer; it helps regulate baby's temperature; and left intact, leads to more successful breastfeeding.

Even the World Health Organization now recommends delaying baby's first bath for at least 24 hours.

In response to this emerging research, some hospitals have begun delaying baby's first bath by anywhere from 4 to 12 hours; some, however, will still rush to bathe baby.

WHAT ARE MY NATURAL OPTIONS?

Babies are not born "dirty," and you can reasonably delay his first bath by a day or two. (You could even wait as long as a whole week, or until baby has his first diaper, uh, *explosion*.) Until then, a light rubdown or spot check with a towel to remove any amniotic fluid, blood, or meconium is sufficient. You'll want to specify your wishes on your birth plan and discuss them with any provider who attends to baby while in the birth suite. Keep in mind that babies who have not yet been bathed might have a little sticker or sign attached to their bassinette, instructing all hospital or birth center staff to wear gloves when handling him (this prevents exposure to any residual blood or bodily fluids). If, after a 24-hour delay, you opt to bathe baby for the first time while still in the hospital, you may want to use your own personal care products. (Hospitals often use commercial soap, which may contain parabens and/or sodium lauryl or laureth sulfate.) You'll also want to steer clear of talc-based baby powder, as it may be laced with other things, including asbestos. It's also not good for baby's lungs.

THE HEPATITIS B VACCINE

Hepatitis B is an infection of the liver caused by the Hep B virus. Luckily, most people who become infected will be able to fight off the disease, after which they'll have lifetime immunity. Others, however—in particular, children and newborns—may develop a chronic case, which can lead to serious complications, including cirrhosis of the liver and liver cancer.

And, yes, Hepatitis B can even be fatal. In children, the most common form of transmission is from mother to child during birth; this is partly why a newborn Hep B vaccine, administered before you're discharged from the hospital or birth center, has become a standard of care. The CDC recommends additional doses at 1 month and 6 months. Babies born to infected mothers, meanwhile, will also receive a Hepatitis B immune globulin shot, which helps to fight off the virus.

WHAT ARE MY NATURAL OPTIONS?

As we've discussed before, vaccines have become a hot topic of debate in the last few years. The Hep B vaccine is particularly controversial, however, because Hep B is often thought of as an adult disease because it's most commonly acquired in one of two ways: via sex with an infected person or by sharing a dirty needle. Since babies aren't generally having sex or doing drugs, many natural parents wonder why in the world it would be necessary to vaccinate a newborn. But public health advocates have quite a few reasons.

First, even though you were tested for Hepatitis B during your pregnancy, there is a small window during which you might contract the virus and not know it, in which case you could theoretically pass it to your newborn. Second, there is always a (rare) possibility of transmission during a blood transfusion—in the unlikely event that your baby needed one, this might further increase his need for a Hep B vaccine. Third, sex and drugs are *not* the only way the virus is spread. For example, it can be transmitted from child to child. There have been some instances of transmission from child to child in daycares, usually after somehow sharing bodily fluids—and then from sibling to sibling within the home.

Is the risk of transmission high? No.

It is possible? Yes.

And that's the thing: very young children who are infected have a much higher risk of developing a life-threatening complication. The vaccine is also administered this early in an attempt to eliminate asymptomatic carriers and eliminate the virus completely. As with most things in parenting, it really comes down to doing the research and making the best choice for your family.

As an alternative, you may opt to delay administration of the vaccine (by anywhere from a few months to shortly before baby enters daycare or preschool, when his risk of transmission may increase). But if you do get the vaccine, be sure your baby is healthy and stable. (The CDC actually recommends delaying the Hep B vaccine in very premature babies—those weighing less than 2,000 grams, or 4 pounds, 7 ounces—until hospital discharge or as late as one month after birth.) You can also decline the vaccine, just as you may decline any intervention. Know that some doctors and/or hospitals will insist on the vaccine, and some have been known to call Child Protective Services (or threaten to call, as an intimidation tactic). Talk to your healthcare team about what's best for your baby.

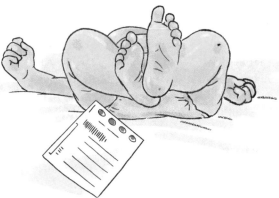

NEWBORN SCREENING PART I: THE HEEL PRICK

Sometime between 24 and 48 hours after birth—not before and not after—baby's heel will be pricked in order to draw a few drops of blood to test for a variety of (rare) genetic, developmental, and metabolic disorders. The procedure is often called—wait for it—the "heel prick test." It may also be referred to as the "PKU," because one of the disorders it screens for is phenylketonuria, an inherited condition that can lead to intellectual disability (or what used to be known as mental retardation).

So, if you already submitted to all those genetic tests and screenings during pregnancy, why is a heel prick necessary? Simple: most of these disorders aren't detectable until birth. And though they're all rare, many of them can be treated if caught early. Galactosemia, for example, is an inherited disorder that prevents baby from breaking down galactose, a simple sugar found in milk—including breast milk. If detected early enough, proper adjustments to baby's diet can be made. If left undetected, galactosemia is fatal.

All fifty states screen for a variety of conditions, although the exact panel of testing will vary from state to state. (If you believe baby has a predisposition to some certain disorder, you can request additional screening.) Because the heel prick is not diagnostic, know that results are not conclusive. A positive result merely indicates the need for more advanced testing. As with all screenings, false positives are also possible.

WHAT ARE MY NATURAL OPTIONS?

The heel prick is one intervention you'll likely choose *not* to decline—there is no immediate intervention associated with the test, no shot to give or medication to take; it's just a blood draw. And though baby may cry (and that is no fun) you can request that the heel prick be performed in your room, so you can cuddle, comfort, and/or nurse baby during or immediately after the procedure.

NEWBORN SCREENING PART II: THE HEARING TEST

Another component of routine newborn screening includes a hearing test, and while that may seem like overkill—I mean, do we really need to test a day-old child's *hearing?*—hearing loss is actually a relatively common birth defect. It's also one you'll want to catch early: undiagnosed hearing loss or deafness can have long-term consequences, including language delays and speech development problems.

There are two types of newborn hearing tests available; based on your individual hospital or birth center's policies, you may be offered one or both:

♡ The otoacoustic emissions (OAE) test determines how baby's *ears* respond to sound. During the test (which may take anywhere from 5 to 10 minutes), a tiny earphone and microphone will be placed in baby's ear and some sounds will be played. When a baby has normal hearing, an echo is reflected back into the ear canal, which is then measured by the microphone. The absence of an echo may indicate hearing loss.

♡ The auditory brainstem response (ABR) evaluates how baby's *brain* responds to sound. During the test, a tiny earphone will be placed in baby's ear; he'll also have some electrodes placed on his head, and some sounds will be played. A lack of consistent response in the brain may indicate a hearing problem.

Babies who "fail" the test may need only a second screening; for example, if baby fails the OAE, he may then undergo the ABR. Babies who fail more than once should be referred to an audiologist for more comprehensive testing. (Keep in mind that it's relatively common for a newborn to fail at least once; the little hairs inside baby's ear can get wet, which can affect the echo. Paloma failed her hearing test the first time. A few hours later we retested her, and she passed with flying colors.)

WHAT ARE MY NATURAL OPTIONS?

Most states in the United States mandate the newborn hearing test. Some, however, do not, in which case you may be *offered* the test, or

you may have to *request* it—and you should. Even babies that seem to respond well to the sound of your voice or to noise in the room can sometimes still have some degree of hearing loss. Luckily, both the OAE and the ABR are completely noninvasive. In fact, they can each be performed while baby sleeps! You and/or your partner can be in the room while the test is being performed, too.

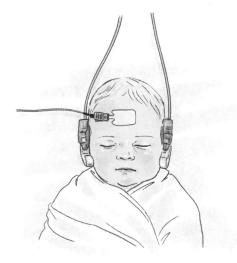

NEWBORN SCREENING PART III: CRITICAL CONGENITAL HEART DISEASE (CCHD)

The newest component of newborn screening is a test for critical congenital heart disease, which is actually a group of heart defects that are all easy to miss during a routine physical exam, but which may become life-threatening—or potentially fatal—if left undetected and untreated. The screen is fast, noninvasive, entirely painless, and completely risk-free; all that's required is a few minutes of your time and a machine called a pulse oximeter.

Say what?

At some point during your labor—or any other time you've been admitted to the hospital—did a nurse ever slide a little clamp onto the end of your index finger? That's the pulse oximeter, and it measures the amount of oxygen circulating in your blood. When testing newborns, the clamp (which is usually more of a soft cuff) is placed on baby's hand or foot in order to get an accurate reading.

WHAT ARE MY NATURAL OPTIONS?

At the time of this writing, not all fifty states have included pulse oximetry in their newborn screening panels, so you may have to ask for it—and I'd encourage you to do so. The test is best performed right around 24 hours after birth. Babies who receive an abnormal result will be rescreened (perhaps several times) before being examined by a pediatrician or specialist and referred for more comprehensive tests.

JAUNDICE

Every day, your body breaks down old red blood cells, a process which creates a waste product called bilirubin, which is then filtered out of the blood by the liver. A newborn's liver, however, is still immature, and often isn't efficient enough to handle the job. The buildup of bilirubin in his system can then cause jaundice. This is a super-common condition—affecting as many as 60 percent of infants—and it's virtually impossible to prevent. Luckily, it's almost always mild, resolves on its own, and has no adverse side effects. (The main symptom of jaundice is a yellowing of the skin and sometimes the whites of the eyes.) In very rare cases, though, abnormally high levels of bilirubin can progress to a condition called kernicterus, which can cause brain damage. For this reason, all babies are monitored for jaundice—either visually, via a blood test, and/or via something called transcutaneous bilirubin measurement (TcB), which involves using a meter to send a quick flash of light through baby's skin to measure bilirubin levels. Newborns with mild jaundice may be offered phototherapy, which involves placing a naked baby under special UV lights.

WHAT ARE MY NATURAL OPTIONS?

Natural mamas may want to forego phototherapy if it's suggested to treat a *mild* case of jaundice or for use as a preventive measure. That's because two companion studies, both published in *Pediatrics* in 2016, have suggested that phototherapy may *slightly* increase the risk of childhood cancer. It's important to point out that these are preliminary studies, and the results are nowhere near conclusive, but you may want to err on the side of caution, just in case.

Alternatively, mild jaundice can easily be treated via two natural remedies: the first is a bit of exposure to natural sunlight, although not *direct* sunlight—too much sun exposure can easily sunburn a baby's delicate skin. Instead, baby may be undressed and placed next to a closed window for 15 minutes at a time, a few times a day. The second method is to increase the frequency of feedings to encourage more frequent bowel movements (which is how the body "dumps" the excess blood cells). Jaundiced, breastfed newborns should generally be fed often—at least every 2 hours or so during the day—until the condition clears up.

CIRCUMCISION

Routine infant circumcision has been the cultural norm in the United States for generations. Many parents don't think twice about circumcising their newborn sons. (I know I didn't give it much thought until I found out I was pregnant with a boy!)

And yet, globally, the practice of circumcision is hardly the norm. Approximately 70 percent of the world's male population is *intact*—that is, with foreskin. And the medical arguments in favor of circumcision appear increasingly dubious.

The fact is, no medical organization worldwide recommends routine infant male circumcision, and yet it is the most common surgical procedure done in the United States.

HOW DID WE GET HERE?

Male circumcision is practiced as a religious rite by some Jews, Muslims, and Christians. In Genesis 17 of the Hebrew Bible, circumcision is viewed as part of the Abrahamic covenant between God and His people.

However, religion played a smaller role in the rise of circumcision in the United States. Some research suggests that the original motivation for circumcision was to temper male sexuality and concerns that the foreskin was "unclean."

British doctor Sir Jonathan Hutchinson was an early proponent of circumcision and had this to say about the foreskin: "It constitutes a harbour for filth, and is a constant source of irritation. It conduces to masturbation and adds to the difficulties of sexual continence. It increases the risk of syphilis in early life, and of cancer in the aged."

In the late 1800s, Dr. Lewis Sayre, a New York–based orthopedic surgeon, started using circumcision as a "cure" for various boyhood ailments. He stated: "I am quite satisfied from recent experience that many of the cases of irritable children, with restless sleep, and bad digestion, which is often attributed to worms, is solely due to the irritation of the nervous system caused by an adherent or constricted prepuce [foreskin]."

Sayre's prominence within the medical profession (he later became the president of the American Medical Association) allowed his message to reach a wide audience. Before long, many physicians advocated universal circumcision as a preventive health measure.

ARE THERE MEDICAL BENEFITS TO CIRCUMCISION?

The medical benefits of circumcision may not be as significant as once thought. For example, the belief that intact boys will get urinary tract infections (UTIs) has been criticized by many doctors and researchers. While there may be a slight increase of UTIs within the first year of life in intact infants, the overall risk is still low. (Interesting to note: Women are eight times more likely to get UTIs compared to men, and yet they manage to treat them with either natural remedies or antibiotics.)

Another rationale for circumcision is that it may help prevent STDs. Some studies in Africa suggest that circumcision reduces the risk of HIV infection in men by approximately 60 percent. But the U.S. Centers for Disease Control and Prevention found that men in the United States were no more or less likely to contract HIV if they were circumcised. Moreover, the HIV/AIDS rate in the U.S. is 2 to 6 times higher than in Northern Europe, where most men are intact.

And while circumcision may decrease a man's risk for genital herpes, in studies the results were statistically insignificant. Furthermore, a meta-analysis of sexually transmitted infections and male circumcision concluded: "Any policy of circumcision for the general population to prevent sexually transmitted infections is not supported by the evidence in the medical literature."

THE FUNCTION OF FORESKIN

As I began researching the topic of circumcision, I was surprised to learn all the functions of the foreskin, which include, among others:

Protection

The glans or head of the penis is intended to be an internal organ, similar to an eyeball under an eyelid. The foreskin serves as a barrier or sleeve that can help keep bacteria, bad microbiota, pollutants, and other harmful substances away from the glans and out of the urinary tract. The foreskin also keeps the penis warm and moist, especially when exposed to cold, dry, or harsh climates.

Lubrication

The foreskin's inner mucosal layer keeps the glans of the penis moist. This can help prevent the penis from chaffing, which is common in circumcised men. With this built-in natural lubricant, intact men generally don't need sexual lubricant. Women may also benefit, with less vaginal dryness, especially in later adulthood.

Sensitivity

The foreskin is as sensitive as the palm of your hand or the lips of your mouth. The foreskin features between 10,000 and 20,000 (some say up to 70,000!) specialized nerve endings—this is a greater density and variety of nerve endings than on any other part of the penis. Studies of men who were circumcised later in life reported less sexual sensitivity and satisfaction without their foreskins.

RISKS OF CIRCUMCISION

The act of circumcision is not without risk. Side effects may include bleeding, infection, and pain when insufficient anesthetic is used (which is unfortunately quite often the case). Less common side effects include excessive foreskin removal, meatitis (inflamed urethral opening), meatal stenosis (narrowing of the urethral opening), and inclusion cysts along the edge of the circumcision scar.

WHAT OTHER COUNTRIES SAY ABOUT CIRCUMCISION

CANADIAN PAEDIATRIC SOCIETY

The procedure often raises ethical and legal considerations, in part because it has lifelong consequences and is performed on a child who cannot give consent. The CPS does not recommend the routine circumcision of every newborn male.

BRITISH MEDICAL ASSOCIATION (BMA)

The medical benefits previously claimed, however, have not been convincingly proven, and it is now widely accepted, including by the BMA, that this surgical procedure has medical and psychological risks.

ROYAL DUTCH MEDICAL ASSOCIATION (KNMG)

KNMG regards the non-therapeutic circumcision of male minors as a violation of physical integrity, a constitutional right that protects individuals against unwanted internal or external physical modifications.

SWEDISH MEDICAL ASSOCIATION

The Swedish Medical Association's Code of Ethics and Liability Council now stands unanimously behind a statement about ending male circumcision without prior consent. It should be done when the boy is no less than 12 or 13 years of age.

WHAT IF CIRCUMCISION IS PART OF MY RELIGION?

That is between you, your faith, and your God. For Jewish parents looking for alternatives, you might want to consider a *brit shalom,* which is a rabbinical blessing ceremony that does not include circumcision. Bottom line: It's important to do what's right for you and your family in the context of your own religious tradition.

WHAT ARE MY NATURAL OPTIONS?

Your most natural option is, of course, to leave your son intact. You may be interested to know that approximately 50 percent of male newborns in the United States are left intact these days. On the fence? Keep doing your research with your partner.

Intact? Don't retract!

Caring for an intact penis is easy: Do absolutely nothing. When you bathe your child, just let the warm water take care of cleansing his penis. You don't have to add soap. More important, never force back (or retract) the foreskin, as this can cause serious problems. (Be sure your pediatrician doesn't do this either!) The foreskin will naturally retract from the penis as your child gets older.

bonding and recovery

THE FIRST 48 HOURS WITH BABY... AND BEYOND!

Yay! All the action and commotion of birth has subsided, and now it's just you, baby, and close family. These first few days are the perfect time to get started with skin-to-skin contact, breastfeeding, babywearing, and more.

BREASTFEEDING AND KANGAROO CARE

In the spring of 2010, an Australian woman went into labor with twins, a boy and a girl, 13 weeks prematurely. Her daughter, the second born of the tiny twosome, let out a good healthy cry and quickly stabilized, despite her size. The boy, however, wasn't breathing. Doctors, nurses, and a whole team of medical professionals attempted to resuscitate the newborn for nearly half an hour, but it was no use. The baby, named Jamie, was pronounced dead. And the mama, overcome with grief, asked to hold her son for a few moments to say her good-byes. She unswaddled him, placed him directly onto her chest, and instructed her husband to remove his shirt and climb into bed. Instinctually, she just wanted to keep her son warm.

And it was likely that instinct that saved her son's life.

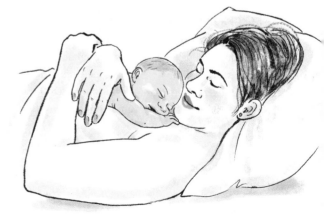

After 5 minutes or so, Jamie gasped. A short while later, he moved. Doctors were convinced these tiny flinches and twitches were just reflexes and warned the mother not to get her hopes up. But then, two hours after his traumatic birth, still lying in the arms of his mother, Jamie opened his eyes. The doctors couldn't deny it anymore—the baby was *alive*. And today, he's a healthy, active, normal child. In fact, he's thriving.

This is the power of skin-to-skin contact, also called kangaroo care. And as you can see, it goes far beyond snuggling. When a newborn is removed from his mother, he begins to show signs of distress. When placed on his mother's chest, however, he is comforted. Babies who receive immediate skin-to-skin contact cry less and emit fewer stress hormones. As I've mentioned again and again, kangaroo care helps regulate an infant's body temperature. (Amazingly, your chest will heat up to warm a cold baby, and cool down when baby's too warm—the phenomenon is called thermal synchrony.) Mother and child will synchronize their breathing and heartbeats, too. The close contact triggers a flood of oxytocin, allowing for better bonding, essentially cementing or hardwiring the maternal (and paternal!) instinct. We also know that kangaroo care is associated with better breastfeeding. In fact, it's *baby* that usually prompts the first feeding. Despite all these measurable benefits, however, only about 40 percent of hospitals implement skin-to-skin care after uncomplicated vaginal births as a matter of routine, according to the CDC.

GETTING STARTED

When placed skin-to-skin (covered by a blanket but *not* swaddled) on mama's chest, healthy babies react in much the same way: they cry, which helps the lungs expand and drain amniotic fluid, and then become calm and alert. If placed tummy to tummy, below and between the breasts, they'll gradually begin to kick and crawl toward the nipple. (The phenomenon is appropriately called the "breast crawl".) If placed alongside mama's belly (in a cradle hold), they'll begin to "root"—that is, instinctively turn their heads and open their mouths. When baby finds the nipple, he may lick, touch, or massage the breast before latching all on his own. The entire process may take an hour or so, with lots of breaks for resting—birth is *exhausting!*—but it's primal and instinctual. So long as baby's healthy, there's no need to rush him, to force that initial feeding, or to separate him from his mother for weighing or footprinting or tests. All that can wait.

HOW HUNGRY IS MY BABY?

In the first hour or so after birth, not very. A one-day-old baby's stomach is about the size of a gum ball, and during his first few feedings, he'll only be getting a tiny amount of colostrum. This pre-milk is the perfect blend of protein, nutrients, and maternal antibodies to support his new life on land—in other words, it's the exact right amount and just what baby needs. Over the next few days, his stomach will grow, and by the time he's ready to eat more in a single sitting—guess what? Your milk will have come in.

HOW OFTEN SHOULD I NURSE?

Because baby's stomach is so small, he doesn't need to eat *much*, but he does need to eat *often*—at least every 2 hours over the course of the first week (with no more than a 4-hour stretch over a 24-hour period). Brand-new babies, however, are usually very sleepy—seriously, being born is exhausting!—so you may need to wake her up in order to nurse. Baby should be allowed unlimited time at the breast

THE STAGES OF BREAST MILK

✤ Colostrum, a nutrient-dense "pre-milk," is baby's first food. It's high in protein and antibodies, which help to seal baby's gut and boost his immunity.

✤ Between two and five days postpartum, your colostrum will turn whiter in color as it changes to *transitional milk*, which is lower in protein and higher in natural sugar and fat. This helps baby pack on those adorable rolls.

✤ Roughly two weeks postpartum, your *mature milk* will come in, which is a balance of foremilk (higher in water and carbs for quick energy and hydration) and hindmilk (rich in satiating and calorie-dense fat).

Keep in mind that your breast milk is a dynamic food—it will *continue* to evolve to meet the needs of your growing child. See? Mamas really do have superpowers!

A NEWBORN'S STOMACH

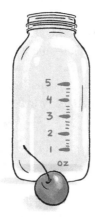

DAY ONE
SIZE OF
A CHERRY

1–1.5 TEASPOONS

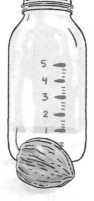

DAY THREE
SIZE OF
A WALNUT

0.75–1 OZ

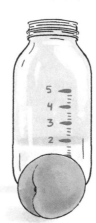

ONE WEEK
SIZE OF
AN APRICOT

1.5–2 OZ

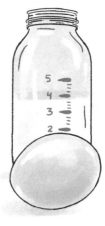

ONE MONTH
SIZE OF
A LARGE EGG

2.5–5 OZ

as long as she's actively sucking. After a feeding, she'll typically go back to sleep.

WHAT IF BABY ISN'T GETTING *ENOUGH* FOOD?

Highly unlikely, provided you're feeding often enough. (This is one of the many advantages to "rooming-in," rather than sending baby to sleep in the nursery.) Still, not producing enough milk or not getting baby enough food is the number one breastfeeding-related concern for new mamas, as well as one of the main reasons so many women rush to supplement—that is, to boost baby's intake with a bit of formula.

There are quite a few reasons you'll want to avoid this, if possible.

First, constant suckling at the breast triggers the release of prolactin, the hormone responsible for milk-making. Skipping feedings can lead to diminished milk supply—and then you really could have a problem.

Second, the introduction of a bottle this early can lead to nipple confusion. Since an artificial nipple doesn't require the same jaw and tongue coordination, baby may begin to prefer the bottle over the breast. Even more significant, the flow of the bottle is much faster than the flow of milk from the breast, so a baby can quickly develop a flow preference. Fast-flow bottles (in particular the kind most hospitals use) also mean baby will have a harder time *stopping* when satisfied.

Third, *all* babies lose a bit of weight in the first few days after birth. Partly, this is just water weight. (Remember, baby has been floating in a sea of amniotic fluid for nine long months. Studies indicate that IV fluids given during labor may artificially inflate baby's birth weight, too.) Baby is also still learning to feed, ingesting a tiny amount of colostrum, and sleeping a bunch. So long as baby loses

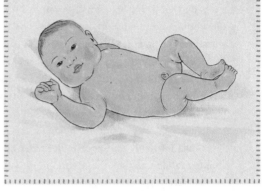

The benefits of mama-baby bonding immediately after birth are so profound that this special time is often referred to as the "Golden Hour." Shoot for as few interruptions and interventions as possible until you've snuggled and initiated breastfeeding.

no more than 10 percent of his body weight, and isn't showing signs of lethargy or unusual fussiness, there should be no reason to supplement.

If you send baby to the nursery at some point—say, for a newborn screening—make sure you've indicated your preference for exclusive breastfeeding, to the midwife, doctor, and nurses on staff. Otherwise, hospital personnel may assume they've got the green light to bottle-feed.

WHAT IF I'VE HAD A CESAREAN?

If you've opted for a gentle Cesarean, you should be able to have immediate skin-to-skin contact with baby and initiate breastfeeding. If for some reason you need to be fully sedated, however, or if you require medical attention after the birth, Papa can (and should be allowed to) stand in for you. Men can't breastfeed, of course, but they can absolutely provide

BEWARE THE SECOND NIGHT:
BREASTFEEDING TIPS

FROM NURSE/DOULA (AND IBCLC) *maura*

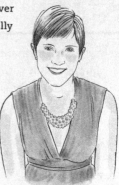

The first 24 hours with a new baby are blissful. Mamas tend to be over the moon, of course, but after the intensity of labor, babies are usually content to sleep most of the day and night away.

The *second* night after birth, however, is a whole different story. By then, your baby has figured out that she's no longer in the womb, and this bright, loud, busy world can be a bit over-stimulating. The smell of your breasts and the sound of your heartbeat are home, so she'll crave warmth and snuggles, and as soon as you finish nursing and put her down for a nap, she'll wake up, begging to nurse again. Over and over, you'll find that baby will nurse for just a short time, fall asleep, and protest loudly as soon as you put her down.

Since it's likely that your milk hasn't come in yet, most new mamas worry that baby is simply *starving*. In fact, the second night is when many women—even those who'd planned to exclusively breastfeed—decide to offer formula supplementation. In reality, though, your colostrum provides the perfect amount of nourishment. Supplementation, on the other hand, can affect your body's long-term milk supply, as well as interfere with a baby's natural desire for the breast over artificial nipples and pacifiers.

So, how to make it through the dreaded second night? A few tips:

- Babies slip into a light sleep (from which they are easily wakened) first, so after she's finished nursing, keep her skin-to-skin—no burping necessary—until she seems to have entered a deeper sleep. You can then transfer her to a bassinet or bed.

- Your baby's hands can provide comfort, so don't cover them up with mittens. Instead, let her use her hands and fingers to touch and massage your breasts; this further stimulates the production of prolactin.

- Keeping an eye on baby's output can offer you reassurance that she's getting enough to eat. During the second 24 hours after birth, you should expect two wet and two dirty diapers.

- Remember, this is just a phase—it won't last forever. Make sure you've got some help lined up for the following day so you can rest and recover.

some of the same benefits to baby, including blood sugar stabilization and temperature regulation. Papa can take his shirt off or just unbutton his shirt—whatever he's most comfortable with.

WHAT IF MY BABY NEEDS TIME IN THE NICU?

There are all kinds of reasons a baby may need to spend a little time in the neonatal intensive care unit. He might stay only a few hours, for example, if he needs extra help with his breathing. Or he might stay for a matter of weeks if, say, he's extremely premature. Virtually all NICU babies, however, do better when they're allowed skin-to-skin contact. In fact, the benefits of kangaroo care are often *more* pronounced for babies who are struggling. Studies show that even short sessions—no less than an hour at a time, to prevent distressing the baby—are associated with improved growth and weight gain, fewer infections, better sleep, and less crying. Kangaroo care decreases maternal stress levels, too, which is important (a stressed-out, worried mama may have a harder time bonding). When it comes to breastfeeding, a NICU baby may not yet have the strength to suckle at the breast, but he may be able to take your milk via feeding tube. (Regardless, you'll want to pump regularly in order to keep up your milk supply until it's time to go home.) Talk to your healthcare provider about ways you might maximize breastfeeding and skin-to-skin contact while baby is growing and getting stronger. Many NICUs have their own independent lactation consultants— ask if yours does, too. Finally, don't be afraid to talk to other NICU mamas, as they can offer a wealth of guidance, strength, and support.

> ### HOW MUCH IS ENOUGH?
>
> Monitoring baby's daily "output" can confirm that she's getting plenty to eat.
>
> **Day 1:** Expect at least one wet diaper ("wet" equates to about 3 tablespoons of urine)
>
> **Day 4:** Six wet diapers and at least 3-4 poopy diapers daily
>
> **Day 14:** Baby has returned to her original birth weight (or gained weight)

WHAT'S UP IN THE DAYS AND WEEKS AHEAD

If your birth center or hospital has a lactation consultant on staff, she might swing by to see you sometime in the first 24 hours or so after birth. You can also, of course, request to be seen—and you should! (Know that not all hospitals have lactation consultants available on off hours and weekends.) But in the absence of an IBCLC, definitely seek breastfeeding assistance from your midwife and nurses. After that initial feeding, it's important to make sure you've got the latch right and you're able to breastfeed without any pain. (A little soreness or tenderness, sure, but not *pain*.) Getting help now can go a *looong* way toward establishing a successful relationship. You can also go ahead and set up an in-home consultation for shortly after you're discharged.

Even when you're not breastfeeding, though, you'll still want to get in plenty of skin-to-skin time with baby.

YOU GOTTA KNOW ~~WHEN~~ HOW TO HOLD 'EM

In the immediate days postpartum, you may be comfortable nursing in only one or two positions—after all, it takes awhile to get the hang of breastfeeding. Once you and baby have gotten a little more comfortable, though, it's a good idea to occasionally switch things up. Rotating positions alters the orientation of baby's latch and the placement of his chin on the breast and nipple, which can come in handy if you're feeling any soreness. So without further ado, here's a look at the top five most popular holds, plus a bonus for mamas who've got a double blessing:

Laid-back (or Biological) Breastfeeding

This position can be a lifesaver in the first week or so after birth, the period when baby is still mastering the latch and you're still fatigued and recovering. It's also a huge help for mamas who are struggling with a fast

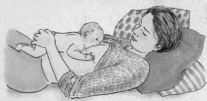

LAID-BACK BREASTFEEDING

letdown; when baby's head is upright, the milk has to flow *against* gravity, which can help slow the flow. Try reclining in bed or a comfy chair—but prop yourself up with pillows, so you're resting at about a 45-degree angle—and place baby tummy to tummy, between the breasts. He will likely move to the nipple on his own, but you can help him if need be.

The Cradle

The most classic of all breastfeeding positions, the cradle involves resting baby in the cradle of your arm, supporting his head, neck, spine, and bottom with your forearm. (Support your forearm, though, with a pillow or the armrest of a chair—even babies this small get heavy faster than you'd think!) In this position, baby's entire body should be turned to face you. In other words, his head shouldn't be turned to the side. Keep in mind that the cradle can be tricky for babies who are still learning to latch, though, so you may want to stick with the cross-cradle for the first month or so.

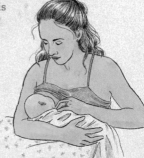

THE CRADLE

→

The Cross-Cradle

In this variation on the classic, mama supports baby with her *opposite* arm—so if he's feeding on the right breast, you'll use your left arm to gently hold his neck and shoulders. With your free hand, you can lift or lower the breast slightly to help baby latch on. One important tip: you should always bring baby up to meet the boob, not bring the boob down to meet baby. (Doing so makes for a bad latch and poor posture.)

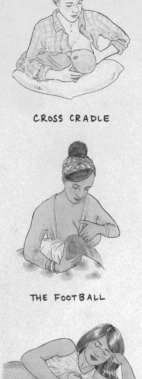

CROSS CRADLE

The Football

For mamas recovering from a Cesarean, this position can provide some much-needed relief—no need to put any pressure or weight on your abdomen. Using a pillow for support, lay baby next to you and tuck him under your arm, as if holding—yup—a football. (Not a sporty mama? Think of this position like holding a purse.) If baby's feeding on the right breast, you'll use your right hand to support his head and neck. Just be sure not to force his head *up* to the breast. His nose should be level with your nipple before he latches on.

THE FOOTBALL

Side-Lying

Breastfeed without having to get out of bed! This one is great for sleep-deprived mamas. Just lie side-by-side with baby, tummy to tummy, and pull him close. You can support his head with your hand. Know that this position may take some practice for newborns.

SIDE-LYING

The Tandem

Or, as I like to call it, the double football. Mamas of twins—or mamas of a newborn and a toddler—may opt to tandem breastfeed. And, yes, it *can* be done! Nursing two at a time not only cuts down on your workload, it makes for great bonding between siblings. If you've got twins, try supporting both babies on either side of a nursing pillow. If you've got a toddler, he can curl up next to you in a semi-sitting position while you cradle the baby.

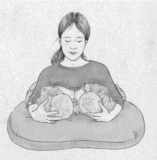

THE TANDEM

BABYWEARING 101

Babywearing—the practice of wearing baby in a sling, wrap, cloth, or carrier—has come back into vogue in the last few years, and one of the greatest benefits for mamas is convenience: You can provide skin-to-skin contact and cuddles while remaining totally hands-free. And trust me, this is *huge*. You'll be able to make phone calls, fold laundry, prep dinner, or just go for a walk (and you'll burn extra calories thanks to baby's added weight!). Babywearing also supports breastfeeding due to baby's close proximity to the boobs. Studies suggest that consistently carried babies aren't as fussy and cry less often. (Sign me up!)

❧ Once positioned in the carrier, make sure baby's airway is unobstructed. You should never have to move or adjust fabric in order to see his face, nor should his forehead be pressed flat against your chest (you can gently move baby's head so that his ear rests against your chest instead). Keep an eye on his chin, too: it should never rest on his chest, but rather be tilted upward.

❧ Baby should stay in an upright position, and her knees should always be higher than her bottom. (Newborns can be worn in a cradle position, so long as their faces are high and clearly visible.) Avoid forward-facing carriers or carriers that encourage baby's legs to dangle, as they don't support proper positioning and can lead to hip dysplasia.

❧ Whether new or gently used, inspect your carrier periodically for signs of wear and tear.

❧ Know that practice makes perfect. When testing carriers (or new ways of carrying), position yourself over a soft surface until you're confident with the method and/or use a spotter.

You might also consider joining a local babywearing group—you'll get tips, tricks, and support, as well as a chance to try out different carriers *before* you shell out the cash. Visit babywearingInternational.org to find one near you.

SAFE BABYWEARING

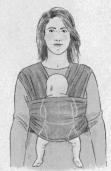
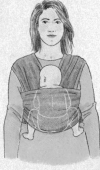

BAD   GOOD

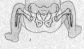

THE MIGHTY SWADDLE

Swaddling is an ancient practice seen all over the world. It's also a standard in hospital maternity wards—ever noticed how all those babies are tightly wrapped in their blankets, like little burritos? Partly this is because swaddling mimics the cozy comfort of being in the womb. And partly it's because a tight wrap can suppress baby's Moro reflex. Just as babies instinctually "root" for the nipple, they also startle easily—at loud noises, sudden movement, or the sensation of falling. This is an involuntary protective mechanism, and it'll disappear around month six. But until then? Babies can easily startle themselves awake. Research shows that swaddled babies cry less and sleep longer, so you'll want to master this technique!

Keep in mind that a swaddled baby should *always* be able to bend his knees and move his legs and hips freely inside the blanket. He's spent the last nine months curled up in the fetal position; sudden straightening of the legs (by, say, a too-tight swaddle) can pull his immature hips from the socket, and lead to a condition called hip dysplasia.

It's also important to point out that babies should *not* be swaddled if you're planning on bedsharing. While most babies seem to love swaddling, a few of them—for whatever reason—just don't. If your little one doesn't take to the swaddle, don't force it. You may want to try a small sleep sack instead.

HOW TO SWADDLE YOUR BABY

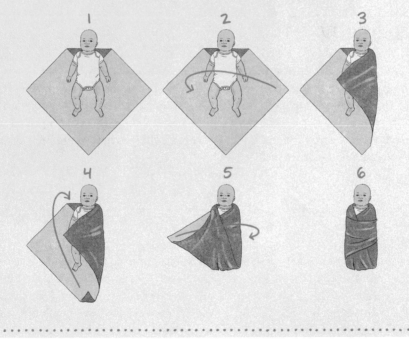

1
2
3
4
5
6

In fact, you can combine the two—skin-to-skin bonding and breastfeeding—with something called laid-back breastfeeding (or the biological breastfeeding position). Try reclining in bed, supporting your back with a heap of pillows, and placing baby between your breasts, covered with a light blanket to keep her back warm. In this position, she can nurse on-demand. If you're feeling modest, try wearing a button-down blouse. It can be opened when you're snuggling, but you'll still have your back, arms, and sides covered.

Know that kangaroo care shouldn't stop when you bring baby home, either. Babies crave this continued closeness for at least the first three months—or what's often referred to as the *fourth* trimester. (If you weren't able to provide much skin-to-skin contact in the hospital, it's not too late!) A baby carrier like a Moby Wrap makes this super-simple; just place baby in the carrier against your bare chest, wearing a diaper only. If and when she wants to nurse,

> Hundreds, if not thousands, of distinct bioactive molecules are found in mother's milk, which protect against infection and inflammation. These molecules also bolster the immune system, contribute to organ maturation, and help establish a healthy microbiome. Breast truly is best!

you can take her out or nurse her right in the carrier.

Finally, make sure papa or your partner is getting plenty of snuggle time in the first few weeks and months, too. Dads also get a boost of oxytocin when providing kangaroo care. Better bonding will take some of the pressure off you, too—you won't be the only one who's able to soothe and comfort a cranky baby.

REST AND RECOVERY

Baby is really, finally, here. You've spent hours gazing into her beautiful eyes. You've managed to navigate that first feeding. You might have even changed a diaper or two. But now baby's drifted off into a deep, post-birth sleep, which means it's time, Mama, to take care of *you*.

GETTING STARTED

As much as is humanly possible over these next few days, try to get some rest and some sleep. Yes, birth is exciting. It's natural to want to call everyone you've ever known, to post a thousand pictures on Facebook, to socialize with visiting friends and family. Your body's been through the wringer, though, and you're gonna be up every 2 to 3 hours throughout

the night to breastfeed. So—I can't stress this enough—do your best to sleep when the baby sleeps. Snooze when baby's snoozing. Nap when baby's napping. Here's a peek at how recovery will go when you're up and about:

OH, SO *THIS* IS THE POSTPARTUM BLEEDING WE'VE BEEN TALKING ABOUT?

The first time you stand up after delivering baby, you may feel a rush of blood coming from between your legs. That's right—you do all this work creating and growing and birthing a baby, and then get rewarded with what amounts to a big, fat menstrual period. (Although, you do get a *baby* out of the deal, too, of course.) Lochia is the technical term for this bloody, mucus-y discharge (which may contain clotty chunks of shed uterine lining), and *all new mamas* experience it—even those who've delivered via C-section. The bleeding comes from what amounts to a "wound" on the uterine wall, the spot where your placenta detached itself. You may notice the bleeding seems to intensify immediately after breastfeeding; this is because oxytocin signals the uterus to con-tract, squeezing out all that excess blood and tissue and, actually, *speeding* healing. Lochia may last anywhere from 1 to 6 weeks before gradually tapering off—during those last few weeks, you won't need to wear more than a panty-liner. In the meantime, though, you'll have your choice of strange new undergarments: mesh panties, regular (oversized) panties and a giant maxi pad, or a disposable panty-maxi pad combo.

WHAT OTHER *natural mamas* SAY

kimberly: After the birth of my first baby, I was a little worried because I didn't know what I was doing. After the next four? I was like, Get me outta here so I can sleep!

irene: Our third child was born at home. The midwives stayed for about two hours after delivery, and then my husband and I were able to take a long nap while baby enjoyed that long after-birth sleep. Words truly can't describe how peaceful and comforting that experience was! No strangers to bother us, no machines, no cords, no noises, no visitors. Just a heavenly peace.

barbara: We stayed in the hospital for forty-eight hours. I was excited to get home, but I was nervous, since I had no idea what to expect from a newborn. I remember coming home and staring at her, waiting for her to do something so we could then do something for her.

allison: We stayed in the hospital for three days because I wasn't confident with breastfeeding. But the most intense emotion I felt was actually a little bit of sadness—the first part of the experience was over. I wanted to soak it all up, and I wasn't ready for it to be over yet!

sara: After forty-eight hours in the hospital, I felt ready to go home. I wanted to be in my own house with my newborn and start the real-world experience of being a mother. They do so much for you in the hospital, it's not quite "real" until you go home.

WHAT YOU NEED TO KNOW
ABOUT POSTPARTUM DEPRESSION
FROM MIDWIFE *Cynthia*

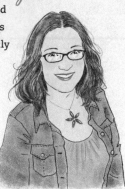

While there's something to be said for that initial burst of joy and excitement following delivery, once the reality of parenthood sets in, many mamas struggle. The sleep deprivation (yes, babies really *do* need to be fed every two to three hours), the physical aspect of recovery, and the hormonal fluctuations can create a kind of perfect storm, setting the stage for the onset of postpartum mood disorders. During the first two weeks after birth, lots of new moms will experience a mild case of the "baby blues"— they may cry or weep or feel a roller coaster of emotions. Beyond six weeks postpartum, however, lingering symptoms are a sign that it's time to seek help.

Based on my own experience as a midwife, it's my opinion that postpartum mood disorders are underreported. There's a social stigma in our society surrounding mental health disorders, and when families speak openly with me about mental health issues, they often describe feeling isolated and alone. Feelings of inadequacy, impaired bonding, or increased irritability seem to predominate what usually is a happy time. For many of these families, having a support system in place (whether that's immediate family or a squad of mom friends) can make all the difference. I'm a true believer in the idea that it takes a village to raise a child. Historically, families lived in tribes; both blood- and non-blood relatives looked out for one another. But this isn't so commonplace anymore. Families don't always live in close proximity; rarely are there multiple generations sharing a home. Some new mamas are single parents, trying to figure out a way to go it alone. For all these reasons, I do my best as a provider to address risk factors for postpartum mood disorders *during* pregnancy and not wait until it's time to bring the baby home.

Women with a history of depression or anxiety disorders are at an increased risk for postpartum depression and postpartum anxiety, respectively. Women with a history of untreated bipolar disorder are at a higher risk of developing the most severe of postpartum mood disorders: postpartum psychosis. It may be easier said than done, but if you're struggling to cope the first step is to reach out and call your provider. Utilize the paging or on-call system if you need to talk and it's after business hours. If you feel that you're a danger to yourself or those around you, call 911 or head to an emergency room. You should not be alone. Call a friend. Call a trusted family member. If you have the means, hire a postpartum doula—that's right, doulas aren't just for labor support. Some women may need antidepressant or antianxiety medications to help regulate their mood and improve their symptoms. You can discuss the safety of these medications while breastfeeding with your provider, as some are considered low-risk. Following your six-week checkup, resume exercise and activity if you've been physically cleared. For many women, getting out of the house, socializing with friends, or meeting other new mamas can help them feel less isolated. For others, going back to work and interacting with other adults will boost their mood. Enlist help with chores, preparing meals, and running errands. Make time for yourself, as well as one-on-one time with your partner. And don't hesitate to contact any of these hotlines:

Postpartum Support International
Phone: 800-944-4PPD

Postpartum Education for Parents
Phone: 800-564-3888

National Suicide Prevention Hotline
Phone: 800-273-8255

What's Not Normal (or, When to Call Your Midwife or Doctor): Needing to change your maternity pad more than once an hour, for more than an hour or two, foul-smelling discharge, or clots bigger than a golf ball. The intensity of the flow can also be an indicator that it's time to slow down. I found that I bled more on days when I was on my feet a lot, or if I went walking for too long in the early days postpartum. I saw this as a gentle reminder to relax and give my body the time it needed to fully heal.

WHY AM I SWEATING SO MUCH?

Here's another, well, interesting thing about having a baby: You're not only recovering, and resting, and *bleeding*, you'll also be sweating more than a marathon runner, even when you're barely moving a muscle. Your pits might be stinkier than usual, too. (Great!)

Although breaking out into a cold sweat isn't much fun, there are a few reasons for the postpartum flood. First, remember all that extra fluid you were carrying around during your pregnancy? Well, it's got to go somewhere. (Expect a frequent urge to urinate—a sensation you're no doubt familiar with by now.) The wild hormonal surges that occur after birth also play a role in this excessive sweatiness. Too much sweating, however, can leave you dehydrated, so don't skimp on the fluids. You'll need plenty, anyway, to support breastfeeding.

What's Not Normal (or, When to Call Your Midwife or Doctor): Fever or extreme chills.

WHY AM I SO GASSY?

Oh, Mama. Nobody tells you about any of this stuff *before* you get pregnant, do they? Flatulence is another super-common side effect of having a baby, and it's triggered by a number of factors. First off, your intestines and digestive organs have been squished for the last several months and are just now starting to relax and settle into their usual position—let them toot a little in celebration! Constipation is another factor, as it's quite common in the days and weeks postpartum (oh, don't worry—we'll get to *that*). The physical act of birthing a child also puts a ton of pressure on the pelvic floor muscles, rectum, and anus. When these muscles are weakened, it's easier for gas to just sort of, ya know, slip right out. You may even notice some air whooshing out of your vagina, too.

What's Not Normal (or, When to Call Your Midwife or Doctor): Unfortunately, the smell is normal. Serious pain or discomfort, however, is not.

I'VE GOT STITCHES *DOWN THERE*— NOW WHAT?

Whether you had a vaginal delivery with no tearing or an episiotomy that had to be sutured, your vagina and perineum are going to be pretty sore for at least a few days if not a week. To soothe basic aches and pains, try taking regular warm sitz baths or spritzing your bits with Motherlove Sitz Bath Spray. (If you followed my packing guidelines, it should already be in your go-bag. Hooray!) Sitting on a pillow can take pressure off the affected area, as can lying on your side or applying ice.

When it comes to cleaning and caring for perineal stitches, well, that's a little more complicated. Luckily, your midwife and nurses should give you detailed instructions on everything from dressing to bathing, as well as regularly monitor your lady parts for signs of infection in the days before you head home. You'll be asked to change the pad you're wearing frequently, as well as given a periwash bottle (a.k.a. a fancy squeeze bottle). Since urine is acidic, it can be extremely irritating against raw, sensitive skin. Aiming the periwash bottle at your perineum while you pee, however, can relieve any burning. Finally, you'll want to pat yourself dry—no rubbing for at least a few days. Mild tears usually heal in about a week.

What's Not Normal (or, When to Call Your Midwife or Doctor): Swelling, extreme pain, redness, or foul odor, all of which can be signs of infection.

WHY AM I AFRAID TO POOP?

Just as flatulence is common in the days and weeks after birth, so too is constipation, for

JUST FOR DADS: DON'T BE A SILENT PARTNER

No one knows your partner better than you, so if mama seems unusually emotional, depressed, or just not like herself for weeks and weeks after the birth, talk to her. Encourage her to communicate with you about her feelings. Help her find time for things she especially loves, such as going for walks or seeing a movie. Make sure you're providing lots of support not only with baby but also around the house (enlist some outside help if need be). And if necessary, help her seek out professional support and guidance. Postpartum depression can be incredibly isolating, so do your best to make sure Mama knows she is not alone.

much the same reason: the trauma of delivery weakens the muscles of the pelvic floor and rectum, and can knock your digestive system a little out of whack. The biggest issue regarding the first post-birth bowel movement, however, is typically fear. After pushing out a baby, the last thing many mamas want to do is bear down. Lots of women feel as though their insides might fall right out of their body and into the toilet (they won't), since the internal organs are settled back into their usual positions. Others may be terrified they'll reopen their incision or split their stitches (that won't happen, either). The longer it takes to get past that first trip to the bathroom—and the more your anxiety builds—the worse constipation gets, so here's what you want to do to keep things moving from the very beginning:

♡ Drink plenty of fluids. Lots of liquids will help soften your stools.

♡ Start boosting your intake of magnesium immediately after birth (with your doctor or midwife's approval, of course). Many hospitals and birth centers will offer you a stool softener. Personally, I prefer to take Natural Calm magnesium supplement since it's non-irritating. And I really can't stress this enough: Take *something* to soften and/or encourage bowel movements right away to ensure you won't have any bathroom issues.

♡ Eat 2 pears a day. You'll want to eat plenty of fiber: whole grains, beans and legumes, nuts, and fresh fruits and veggies are all good options. Pears, in particular, are known for their laxative effect.

What's Not Normal (or, When to Call Your Midwife or Doctor): Painful bloating or bloody stools.

WHAT ABOUT RECOVERING FROM A C-SECTION?

For the first 24 hours or so following a Cesarean, your incision will be covered by a sterile bandage. You may be given an ice pack to help reduce swelling, an array of pain medication, and will need to stay in bed for anywhere from 4 to 24 hours. Soon, though, you'll be ready to sit up, and then to stand up (with help, of course), but you'll need to take it easy. During your hospital stay (three to four days on average, for a C-section) your nurses will monitor the incision site and change the dressing. They'll also give you plenty of instructions before heading home. You'll be advised to keep the area clean and dry, to avoid scrubbing or rubbing in the shower (just let soapy water wash over it), and to keep a maxi pad over the wound for the first week or two to absorb sweat and drainage.

What's Not Normal (or, When to Call Your Midwife or Doctor): Fever, increasing pain, or redness, swelling, or oozing at the site of the incision.

WHAT'S UP IN THE DAYS AND WEEKS AHEAD

Exactly how long you stay at the birth center or hospital will depend, of course, on quite a few factors: the circumstances of your delivery, the specifics of your insurance coverage, and your own personal preferences, to name but a few. No matter how long your stay, though, you won't be leaving empty-handed: Your nurses will give you *plenty* of info and accessories (baby blankets, maxi pads, and the like). They'll make sure you're comfortable changing a diaper, know what kinds of signs and symptoms to watch for (like the onset of jaundice) and how to take care of baby's umbilical cord—most will even make sure you've correctly loaded baby into his car seat.

When it finally comes to taking baby home, though, you may start to feel a little sweaty and anxious. But, Mama? That's *normal.* Every new mother doubts her abilities from time to time, and feels overwhelmed. Over the next few days, weeks, and months, you and baby will learn together, as well as learn from each other. In the meantime, your first appointment with the pediatrician should be just around the corner, and four to six weeks from now (or perhaps a bit sooner, if you've had a C-section) you'll head in for your postpartum checkup. Your midwife or doctor will take a peek at your vagina, perineum, and incision scar (assuming you have one), as well as palpate your uterus. She'll examine your breasts, take note of your weight, and monitor your blood pressure. She'll also be ready to answer any and all of your questions—so bring a list.

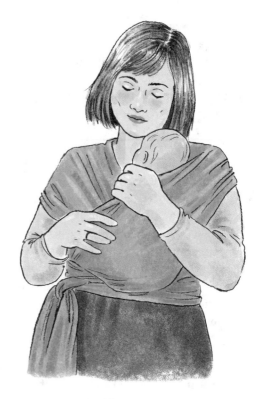

NATURAL REMEDIES FOR THE BABY BLUES AND POSTPARTUM DEPRESSION

Crunchy mamas who are struggling to cope with the adjustment to parenthood may want to try some natural remedies to boost and regulate their mood—and that's fine. You can experiment with the following methods *before* trying medication, or give them a go in addition to medication prescribed by your doctor. Remember, though, that postpartum depression is something you don't want to mess around with; if you're feeling blue, you'll still want to be closely monitored by your midwife or doctor even if you're going the all-natural route.

Increase Your Omega-3 Intake (especially DHA and EPA from fatty fish). A growing body of research suggests that omega-3 fatty acids are useful in regulating mood, so it's interesting to point out that brand-new mamas often have omega-3 *depletion*. During pregnancy, your body shuttled most of its DHA to baby's developing brain. Even if you weren't comfortable taking cod liver oil during pregnancy, it's a great source of omega-3s now that you've given birth. You can also aim to eat oily fish, such as sardines and salmon, two to three times a week.

Boost Your B Vitamins. These energy and mood nutrients tend to plummet postpartum, too (particularly folate and vitamin B_{12}). Talk to your midwife or doctor about taking a supplement, and look for methylated forms if you have the MTHFR mutation. You can also eat nutritional yeast flakes or liver, which are both high in B vitamins.

Get Moving. Believe it or not, studies have suggested that daily exercise can be just as effective as antidepressants. Unfortunately, it can be difficult for a depressed mama to find the motivation to break a sweat. Consider enlisting a buddy to join you for a daily walk. If childcare is an issue, bring baby along in a carrier or stroller.

Soak Up Some Rays. Light therapy can also be effective for treating depression. Try getting outside for 10 minutes first thing every morning—and skip the sunglasses, contacts, or glasses for greater effect.

Try Acupuncture. Anecdotal evidence suggests that weekly acupuncture can help to keep feelings of sadness at bay.

Take a Break. A friend, family member, or even a paid helper can make it possible for you to slip away for an hour or so every day; this can be especially helpful if you've got a colicky baby.

Seek Out a Counselor. Being able to talk through your feelings about life with a newborn is extremely important. Find a trained practitioner who can help you make emotional connections, provide tools for dealing with the transition, and who can refer you to a psychiatrist, if need be.

the last word

Well, Mama, forty-ish weeks later, here we are.

It's been an honor to walk with you—albeit in a small way—during this special time. I hope your birth experience was everything you wished for and prayed for. But before you dive into caring for your newborn, I hope you take a moment to thank yourself for a job well done. Yes, you. Pat yourself on the back. Hug yourself. Grin at that beautiful face of yours in the mirror. You went the distance. You gave it your all. And now, you have one heck of a reward.

While motherhood can be daunting—and downright difficult at times—know that you are equipped for all that lies ahead. You will learn things that will astonish you—like the different colors (and meanings!) of newborn poop. Or that you really *can* carry a car seat, four bags of groceries, and talk on the phone all at the same time. There will be moments that knock you to your knees—whether you're dealing with a baby who just won't sleep or struggling through a bout with the baby blues.

You will be exhausted and delirious and crabby. You'll also be elated, ecstatic, and soooo in love. And it's all good.

Know that motherhood was never intended to be a solo act. You'll need help along the way, so don't be shy about asking for it. Build a community of other natural mamas. Trust that there's a divine plan. Lean into this miraculous season of your life, and keep your heart open for all the gifts that lie ahead.

Oh, and head over to mamanatural.com to sign up for our week-to-week emails or text series on baby's first year—all from a natural perspective, of course.

Until we meet again, blessings to you and your sweet family!

XO,
Genevieve

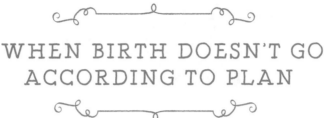

WHEN BIRTH DOESN'T GO ACCORDING TO PLAN

You read this book cover to cover. You did your exercises, went to a chiro, and took a birth class. You even ate your dates and drank your red raspberry leaf tea. And yet, your birth didn't go as you'd hoped it would.

((((Deep sigh))))

I'm so sorry, Mama.

If you're feeling bad about it—allow yourself to grieve, so that you can let go.

I know this is easier said than done. For some mamas, it can be incredibly difficult. I had a terrible time forgiving myself for getting—for *needing*—Pitocin during my son's birth. Here I was, Mama Natural, and I still couldn't pull it off without an intervention. Ugh.

The thing is, interventions save lives. According to the World Health Organization, for example, a 10 percent Cesarean rate isn't just normal, it's *healthy*. When rates fall below 10 percent, it means that mamas and babies are dying due to a lack of quality medical care. So thank God we have the interventions that we do.

The club of "natural mamas" can sometimes feel cliquey. You're either one of them, or you're not. But let me tell ya: My kids hated the baby carrier, we never practiced bedsharing, and I didn't like eating my placenta. And some people think I'm uber crunchy, so go figure. It's really a natural-living spectrum and there is *so* much more to being a natural mama than childbirth. You're just at the beginning of a lifelong journey, really.

The simple truth is that it takes strength and patience and courage and determination to bring a new life into this world. But more than anything else, it takes love. No matter your birth circumstances, you are a childbirth warrior. And you're about to embark on one of life's greatest gifts: motherhood. It'll break you open in the most marvelous way, and it will heal you.

PART FIVE

WHAT TO ASK YOUR PROSPECTIVE

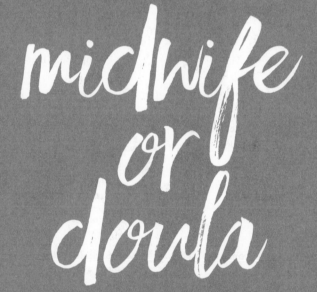

*midwife
or
doula*

plus: QUESTIONS TO ASK
WHEN TOURING
HOSPITALS AND BIRTH CENTERS

WHAT TO ASK WHEN INTERVIEWING A MIDWIFE

The midwife you're interviewing might seem amazing on paper—intense training, oodles of experience, sterling recommendations—but if your personalities don't mesh, don't hesitate to keep looking. Keep in mind that you'll likely end up asking some of these same questions when touring prospective hospitals and birth centers, too.

○ Are you licensed by the state?

○ Are you certified? From where did you receive certification?

○ Can you describe your midwifery training (school or apprenticeship program)? Do you take continuing education classes?

○ Have you completed training in neonatal resuscitation?

○ How many years have you been practicing?

○ How many babies have you delivered? How many do you deliver each year, on average?

○ Do you have experience with postpartum hemorrhage, shoulder dystocia, breech deliveries, or cord prolapse?

○ Do you offer water births?

○ Do you perform VBACs? (Vaginal Births After Cesarean—we talk more about VBACs in Week 26.)

○ At what point do your clients become too high-risk to continue working together?

○ What percentage of your patients end up having an epidural?

○ What is your C-section rate? What about forceps assistance or vacuum extraction deliveries?

○ Have you ever lost a baby or a mother during delivery?

○ Do you work with a consulting physician(s)? Do you have a collaborative agreement with a doctor in place? Which physicians are you affiliated with in the event that my pregnancy becomes high-risk? Do you have personal relationships with them?

○ Do you have hospital privileges?

○ Do you encourage mamas to work with a doula?

○ How many prenatal appointments will I have?

○ What will happen during each appointment?

○ Do you require ultrasound and/or vaginal exams?

○ Do you require the use of a Doppler? Do you have a fetoscope?

○ Can I bring a family member(s) to my appointments?

○ Will I see only you for prenatal care, or a team of midwives (if interviewing at a birth center)?

○ Will I be attended by you during my birth, or whichever midwife is on call?

○ How long after my due date can I continue to see you before my care is transferred and/or I must be induced?

○ What are my options for pain management during labor?

○ What happens if I decide that I want an epidural?

○ What does the first hour after birth look like for your patients? Do you encourage skin-to-skin contact between baby and mama? Do you allow delayed cord clamping? Delayed bathing? Do you encourage mamas to breastfeed? Do you have lactation consultants on staff?

○ What type of payment plan do you offer and what do your fees include?

○ Why should I choose you to be my midwife?

The following *additional* questions are intended for midwives attending a home-birth:

- ○ Do you recommend that I see a physician at some point during my pregnancy? Do you work with a consulting physician for this purpose?

- ○ Do you support VBACs and breech births at home? When is a home birth not recommended?

- ○ Do you carry malpractice insurance?

- ○ What sort of equipment will you bring with you on the day of the birth? (Midwives attending home births should be equipped with gloves, gauze, drop cloths, oxygen, a fetoscope, items to suture a tear, emergency medications, instruments to start an IV, and infant resuscitation equipment, at minimum.)

- ○ What kinds of supplies will I have to provide?

- ○ What preparations, if any, will I have to make to my home?

- ○ In what circumstances might you arrange an in-labor transfer?

- ○ In the event of a non-emergency transfer, how will I get to the hospital? What if there's an emergency?

WHAT TO ASK WHEN INTERVIEWING A DOULA

Just like when interviewing prospective midwives, you'll want to find a doula with whom you have professional chemistry, too. Think about other times in your life when you were stressed, overwhelmed, or confused—what brought you back to yourself? A gentle hand, a sharp fist (figuratively speaking, of course), or somewhere in between? The following questions can help you zero in on someone with the right training and skills, but at the end of the day, many mamas chose their doulas based on gut instinct.

- ○ Are you certified? Where did you receive your certification?

- ○ How many births have you attended? Do you have experience with birth complications?

- ○ Have you attended a birth that ended in Cesarean?

- ○ Have you attended a home birth?

- ○ How would you describe your "style" or bedside manner?

- ○ What kinds of pain relief/pain management techniques can you offer?

- ○ What's your philosophy when it comes to working alongside a husband/partner?

- ○ Describe how you work alongside a midwife/doctor. What happens if we have to deviate from my birth plan?

- ○ Do you offer pre-birth visits? How many?

- ○ May I call or email you with questions throughout my pregnancy?

- ○ At what point during my labor should I call you? What if I go into labor in the middle of the night?

- ○ Will you come to my home, or will you meet me at the hospital/birth center?

- ○ Do you have a back up doula? When and how often is she used? Can I meet her?

- ○ Do you have experience/training in lactation consulting?

- ○ Do you offer postpartum/follow-up care? Is that included in your fee?

- ○ What are you fees? Do you offer a payment plan?

WHAT TO ASK WHEN TOURING A BIRTH CENTER

Whether you're touring freestanding or hospital-affiliated birth centers, or both, you'll want to ask lots of questions about the care you can expect to receive. Demand direct answers—numbers, stats, percentages; if the person giving the tour doesn't know or can't tell you, consider that a sign to go elsewhere.

○ Are you licensed by the state? (Licensure and regulation of birth center varies *widely* from state to state. In states that don't grant licenses, birth centers could theoretically be owned and operated by, well, just about anybody, with little to no oversight. Unlicensed facilities should be approached with caution—are they accredited? Are they insured? Are the midwives licensed? Now's not the time to be shy—ask!)

○ Are you accredited by the Commission for the Accreditation of Birth Centers?

○ Does the birth center have its own staff (meaning, will you be required to see one of the center's affiliated practitioners for your prenatal care)?

○ Do you have physicians (ob-gyns, perinatologists) with whom you regularly consult?

○ Do you have a transfer agreement in place with a local hospital? Which hospital? (Note how far away that hospital is from the center itself.)

○ When and why might I be transferred to a hospital?

○ How long can I be in labor before transfer to a hospital becomes necessary? (Some birth centers will not let women labor indefinitely, due to an increased risk of complications and infection, especially after your water breaks. Freestanding centers will typically let you go longer before mandatory drug intervention, such as Pitocin, becomes necessary.)

○ Do the midwives have hospital privileges?

○ When and how often does the birth center rely on hospital staff vs. midwifery care (if hospital-affiliated)?

○ What is your transfer rate? (Hint: it shouldn't be higher than 10 to 15 percent. If it is, ask why.)

○ What is your Cesarean rate? (Hint: it shouldn't be higher than 10 to 15 percent.)

○ Can I bring a doula?

○ Can I bring a videographer and/or does the birth center allow photography?

○ Is there a limit on how many people, such as friends and extended family, can be in the delivery room? Is there an age-limit on who may visit (meaning, can children be present during the birth)? Can my visitors stay with me during recovery?

○ Do I have to be hooked up to an electronic fetal monitor or an IV during labor?

○ How long is the typical postpartum stay? (Being able to go home the day-of *could* be a plus. At the same time, you don't want to be shooed out the door if you'd prefer to rest for a night or two.)

○ What kind of postpartum care do you provide? Do you offer home visits?

○ Do you offer breastfeeding assistance, or have lactation consultants on staff?

WHAT TO ASK WHEN TOURING A HOSPITAL

Heads up, Mama: the following questions are geared specifically toward standard hospital (not birth center) deliveries.

○ Is this hospital baby-friendly? (Use those *exact* words. "Baby-friendly" is a real designation awarded to hospitals and birth centers that prioritize mama/baby bonding and breastfeeding.)

○ Can I be attended by a midwife?

○ What is your Cesarean rate? (The ideal Cesarean rate, according to the World Health Organization, is between 10 and 15 percent of all births; 33 percent of American women, however, will wind up having a C-section. Anything above 30–35 percent should raise some *serious* red flags. The lower the C-section rate, the better.)

○ What's your epidural rate? (Some hospitals have epidural rates as high as 90 percent—it may be harder for you to decline interventions in these settings.)

○ Do you have an anesthesiologist on-call 24/7? If not, what happens if I want an epidural? (Some smaller hospitals only offer epidurals during "office hours.")

○ Do you have a NICU? (There are four distinct levels of neonatal care, ranging from a Level I unit, which is a basic nursery for healthy, full-term newborns, to a Level IV facility, which can treat the most serious, acute conditions, including complex congenital defects.)

○ Can I eat and/or drink during labor?

○ Can I walk around and/or move freely during labor?

○ Is continuous electronic fetal monitoring part of hospital policy? What about IV fluids?

○ Can I choose what position I'd like to give birth in?

○ Is there a "time limit" to give birth? (Be advised that some hospitals will mandate the use of Pitocin or other labor-inducing drugs if your labor stalls or doesn't progress "quickly enough," according to their standards.)

○ Can I bring a doula? (Doulas can be amazing advocates in all cases, but they can be especially helpful at hospital births. See more about doulas in Week 16.)

○ Do you have natural birthing equipment, like birthing balls or birthing stools?

○ Are recording devices allowed? Can I bring a photographer and/or videographer?

○ Do you offer LDRs and/or LDRPs? Can I stay in the same room the entire time?

○ Can my baby "room in" with me (meaning, spend the night)?

○ Can papa (or a friend or family member) stay overnight after the baby is born?

○ What are the hospital's visiting hours?

○ Are there restrictions on who is allowed in the labor and/or delivery room? Is there an age limit or restriction for younger kids?

○ How long is the typical postpartum stay?

○ Does the hospital support breastfeeding? Is there an International Board Certified Lactation Consultant (IBCLC) on staff?

pregnancy loss

MISCARRIAGE AND STILLBIRTH

WHEN THE UNTHINKABLE HAPPENS:
COPING WITH MISCARRIAGE AND STILLBIRTH

To have seen your unborn child via ultrasound or heard his heartbeat, to have imagined kissing and holding your newborn, to have begun planning for baby's future only to have those dreams taken from you is among the most devastating tragedies a person can endure. The sad truth is that pregnancies sometimes end prematurely, and though heartbreaking, loss of pregnancy is actually more common than you may think. Somewhere between 10 percent and 25 percent of all known pregnancies end in miscarriage. The one bright spot is that loss of pregnancy is almost always a one-time occurrence, and the majority of women who experience a miscarriage or stillbirth go on to deliver perfectly healthy children.

You are not alone, even though at times it may feel that way. Loss of pregnancy is not often discussed openly; many women don't announce that they're expecting until the second trimester, and so many never disclose a loss to people other than very close friends and family. Some women may choose not to share the news at all.

This section will explain the various types of miscarriage and stillbirth, what happens after a loss of pregnancy, and ways to help you cope with your grief.

EARLY MISCARRIAGE

A miscarriage occurs when a pregnancy ends naturally, before a baby is able to survive outside the womb. *Early* miscarriages occur in the first trimester. The vast majority of early miscarriages—anywhere from 50 percent to 75 percent—occur shortly after implantation. In these cases, a chromosomal abnormality prevents the egg from implanting properly, and it's passed from the uterus, resembling a regular period. Many women, therefore, may not even realize they have conceived. These are known as *chemical pregnancies*. Beyond that, miscarriage may be classified in a number of different ways:

Complete Miscarriage: A complete miscarriage occurs when the budding life spontaneously passes from the uterus on its own, without assistance. Complete miscarriages typically involve a fair amount of bleeding and cramping, and may be confirmed via ultrasound.

Missed Miscarriage: A missed miscarriage occurs when the baby dies in utero, but doesn't pass from the womb. Some women may not realize they've miscarried until a routine ultrasound reveals the absence of a heartbeat. Others may no longer "feel" pregnant, and may experience a lessening of pregnancy signs and symptoms, including morning sickness. The miscarriage may continue naturally within days or weeks, or may require surgical removal (more on that in a moment).

Recurrent Miscarriage: The majority of women who experience a miscarriage will not go on

---

SIGNS OF EARLY MISCARRIAGE

Spotting or bleeding

Pink mucus-y discharge

Cramping or lower back pain

Passing tissue and clots from the vagina

Reduction in signs of pregnancy

to have another. Roughly 1 percent of couples attempting to conceive, however, will experience recurrent miscarriage, which is defined as two or more pregnancy losses.

Anembryonic Pregnancy: Also called a blighted ovum, an anembryonic pregnancy occurs when a fertilized egg implants into the uterine wall, but fetal development doesn't begin. A woman might notice signs of pregnancy, but an ultrasound will reveal that the gestational sac is empty, or that there is no heartbeat. The miscarriage may continue naturally, or may require surgical removal.

Ectopic Pregnancy: An ectopic pregnancy occurs when a fertilized egg implants somewhere other than inside the uterus (typically the fallopian tube). Treatment is necessary to stop development of the egg in order to avoid health complications for the mother.

Molar Pregnancy: A molar pregnancy is caused by a genetic mix-up during fertilization—the placenta *overgrows*, turning into a jumbled mass of cells (called a hydatidiform mole); the embryo, meanwhile, doesn't develop at all. Treatment is necessary to remove the tissue from the womb in order to avoid health complications for the mother.

LATE MISCARRIAGE AND STILLBIRTH

Most people know that a baby who dies during labor or childbirth is said to be stillborn, but stillbirths are actually defined as a fetal death that occurs any time after week 20. Fetal death that occurs during the *first* part of the second trimester (between weeks 14 and 20) is referred to as a *late miscarriage.*

Depending on how far along a woman is in her pregnancy, the signs of late miscarriage and stillbirth are often the same as those of early miscarriage. The most common sign, however, is an absence of movement in the womb. Late miscarriages and stillbirths can be confirmed via ultrasound.

HOW CAN I FIND OUT WHAT CAUSED MY MISCARRIAGE?

Depending on how far along you are in a pregnancy, your healthcare provider may attempt to determine the cause of the miscarriage or stillbirth via physical exam, laboratory tests, amniocentesis (to check for chromosomal abnormalities), tissue sampling, and/or autopsy. You may discuss all of these options with your midwife or doctor. Yet even a thorough examination may leave you with more questions than answers. When it comes to loss of pregnancy, sometimes we just don't know the cause.

HOW CAN I PREVENT THIS FROM HAPPENING AGAIN?

The majority of miscarriages are a random, one-time occurrence, that no one can possibly anticipate or avoid. An examination after a late miscarriage or stillbirth, however, may provide information that would be helpful in a future pregnancy. For example, mothers with cervical insufficiency may be candidates for a procedure called cerclage, in which the cervix

NATURAL MISCARRIAGE

NURSE/DOULA *maura's story*

When I found out that I was pregnant a second time, I knew instantly that I'd have another home birth—the experience of delivering at home had been so precious and empowering. But as I was nearing the end of my first trimester, I started to experience cramping and spotting, and I knew something wasn't right. An ultrasound confirmed there was no heartbeat, and that's when I became committed to letting the miscarriage unfold naturally, in the comfort and privacy of my own home.

Despite being overcome with grief, I found that allowing my body to take care of the process was empowering in its own way. I was far enough along that I was able to see my tiny baby, as well as the placenta. This gave me a sense of closure, too.

If you're faced with an impending early miscarriage, I encourage you to speak with your provider about your options, which might include natural miscarriage in addition to surgical or pharmacological techniques. You should discuss the potential risks or benefits associated with various herbal methods (I used a tincture of black cohosh to expedite the process). Natural aids, meanwhile, such as red raspberry leaf tea (to tone the uterus and help with contractions), a warm rice sock (to soothe cramping), or MegaFood Blood Builder (an iron-rich multivitamin) may ease some of the physical symptoms. No matter how early you were in the pregnancy, grief is a normal, healthy part of the healing process. Give yourself permission to experience the roller coaster of emotions that accompanies any loss. Allowing my pregnancy to end in my home, rather than a medical setting, happened to be the best, most comfortable choice for me.

is sewn shut to help prevent loss or premature birth. Chronic medical conditions such as diabetes, high blood pressure or Antiphospholipid Antibody Syndrome (an autoimmune disorder that may cause recurrent miscarriage) can be strictly managed and monitored in partnership with your healthcare team. Mothers who experience recurrent miscarriages may also request, or may be offered, genetic counseling. Taking excellent care of your health can also reduce your risk of pregnancy loss, too. A preconception visit with your midwife or doctor may help you identify and treat any issues that might threaten a future pregnancy.

AFTER A MISCARRIAGE— WHAT HAPPENS NOW?

In the event of a complete miscarriage, the body will naturally pass the tissue on its own, so the entire process will likely be over before you've ever paid a visit to your midwife or doctor. Sometimes, however, tissue may remain in the womb. This is what's known as an *incomplete miscarriage*, and it requires some form of intervention in order to lower the risk of infection and hemorrhage. Mothers experiencing a late miscarriage or stillbirth, meanwhile, may need to choose from among several different methods of delivering the baby. Your midwife or doctor will help you determine what's most appropriate for you, and your options will depend on the gestational age of the baby, your health, as well as other factors related to your particular situation.

Natural miscarriage. If an ultrasound confirms the absence of a heartbeat but the process of miscarriage has not yet begun, you may have the option of waiting for nature to take its course; this is also known as "expectant management." The majority of first trimester miscarriages will progress on their own, but this may take anywhere from a few days to a few weeks. Others may prefer to expedite the process, in part to move forward with grieving and healing. Note that after 10 weeks' gestation, the risks of having an incomplete miscarriage begin to rise, in which case you may require medication or surgery.

Medication. Instead of waiting for a miscarriage to complete on its own, some women may choose to expedite the miscarriage via medication. Among the most common medications is misoprostol (brand name: Cytotec), which may be prescribed orally or as a vaginal suppository. The drug brings on cramping and contractions in the uterus.

Surgical removal (D&C). Dilation and curettage (D&C) is a surgical procedure during which

your doctor will use instruments (perhaps in addition to medication) to dilate the cervix, and then to scrape the uterine lining. The procedure itself lasts only 10 to 15 minutes, but requires some form of anesthesia (either local or general). Side effects are rare, though there is a small risk of infection.

Surgical removal (D&E). Dilation and evacuation (D&E) is a similar procedure to a D&C, although it's typically reserved for second-trimester miscarriages or stillbirths, and often incorporates the use of suction. The procedure usually takes close to 30 minutes.

Induction of labor. Mothers in the second or third trimester—in particular, those who are nearing their due date—may have the option of waiting for labor to begin spontaneously, or may choose to induce labor (in some cases, induction of labor may be the safest option). The process of delivering the baby will not differ much from any other vaginal birth. Some women may prefer this option, as it may provide a natural sense of closure. Hospital staff will ask if you'd like to see, touch, or hold your baby upon delivery. There is no right answer. Some families may choose to take pictures of the baby and decide whether or not they'd like to look later on.

Cesarean. Mothers nearing their due date may need to deliver via Cesarean if the baby is positioned in such a way that makes vaginal delivery difficult (for example, a transverse presentation). An elective Cesarean may be an option, too.

GRIEVING THE LOSS OF YOUR PREGNANCY

No matter when a loss of pregnancy occurs, you have the right to grieve as much and for as long as is right for you. Know that while

you may anticipate feelings of sadness, other emotions may arise that surprise you. It's not uncommon to feel shame or guilt or anger that your body somehow "failed" you, for example, or to feel jealous of friends who are pregnant or already parenting little ones. Even those closest to you may be unsure of how best to give you the support you need. Well-meaning comments like "Don't be sad, you'll have a successful pregnancy next time" may be cold comfort.

Loss of pregnancy is a deeply personal experience; everyone will process it differently. There is no "right" way to handle it, nor is it possible to feel too much—or too little—pain. The following information, however, may prove helpful on your journey to healing.

Take all the time that you need. If possible, take some time off from work or let friends watch your older children if you need some alone time. Also, let your partner know if you need some alone time as a couple. Avoid events that you're not yet ready for, such as baby showers or first-birthday parties. This isn't an act of selfishness; it's self-preservation. It's okay now to take care of *you*.

Find ways to honor your baby. If you haven't already, consider naming the baby—even if you didn't know the baby's sex. You can reach out to the nonprofit organization Now I Lay Me Down to Sleep, which offers remembrance photography. You might also consider whether a memorial service or private ceremony would help you observe the loss.

Seek out a support system. Talk about what's happened with your partner, with family, with friends, or with a therapist, counselor, or spiritual advisor. Many hospitals and community centers offer grief counseling in group settings, or it may be helpful to talk with others who understand exactly what you're going through. Online support groups can provide comfort, too.

Watch out for physical symptoms. Grief can manifest itself physically. If you begin to experience sleeplessness, fatigue, headaches, loss of appetite, aches, pains, or other stress-related symptoms, don't hesitate to speak with your healthcare provider.

Feel what you're feeling. Even if your emotions surprise you, or if they're not what you think you "should" be feeling, know that they are exactly right for you. A sense of peace will come from having gone through the process of grieving.

AFTER THE STORM

The majority of mamas who experience miscarriage or stillbirth will go on to deliver perfectly healthy children. In fact, the experience is so common that there's a name for children born *after* a miscarriage, stillbirth, or infant loss—they're called rainbow babies, since they bring about a sense of hope and solace after the storm. If you choose to become pregnant again, know that you may still experience waves of grief, fear, guilt, or even anger. Connecting with other moms of rainbow babies can be hugely helpful during this time. Check out the nonprofit organization Pregnancy After Loss Support (PALS). Or connect with Hope Mommies or M.E.N.D. (Mommies Experiencing Neonatal Death), which are Christian organizations with local chapters for in-person support.

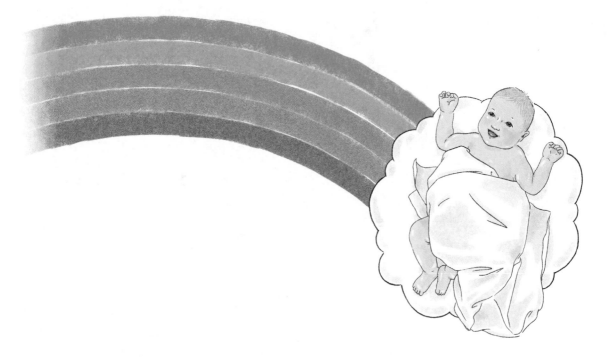

acknowledgments

Writing a book is similar to giving birth.

In the first stage there's excitement and anticipation, along with a tinge of fear: *Honey, we get to do this book! It's gonna be so much fun! (But will anyone want it?)*

In the active stage of book labor, things get more serious: *Whoa. This is a lot harder than I thought. Can we really pull this off?*

The transition stage saw me in total meltdown mode: *I really can't do this. Can we have someone else take over? I'm going to go take a nap; let me know when this is over!*

Finally, the pushing stage near the book's deadline: *Each edit brings me that much closer to the finish line. I can't wait to see my baby! (But I gotta be honest: this hurts!)*

And now, at long last, the book is here. And, like any new mom, I've got a *ton* of people to thank, as I did not do this alone!

First and most important, to Michael, my beloved partner in life. We walked hand in hand throughout the creation of this book, and I could never have given birth to this baby without you. Thank you for bringing your A game to this project and being the strategic architect. You also managed the visual and design elements of this book with excellence. You are the best husband, friend, father, and person I know. I love you!

To the Mama Natural Community: It is an honor to walk alongside you. You continually inspire, amaze, and challenge me by your commitment to natural living. Thank you for your love and support throughout the years—it means the world to me!

Courtney Hargrave: Thank you for understanding the mission and making this book infinitely better because of your skilled hands. I love your humor, smarts, and style—and how you shine under pressure. (In other words, thanks for the all-nighters!) You helped us navigate this new world of publishing, and we are incredibly grateful for you!

To Michele Martin at North Star Way: You truly were the "north star" of this project. From the very first meeting, you caught the vision and were our biggest supporter. Your kindness was such a bright spot for us and made the whole process a joy.

To my editor, Diana Ventimiglia: Thank you for your patience and steady hand throughout this process. I am so blessed to be with a team and publishing house that honors, supports, and encourages their writers so much.

To contributors Cynthia Mason and Maura Winkler: Thank you for your careful review of the manuscript and sharing your important insights. This book so needed your perspectives, and I admire the work you do in this world. I'm honored to call you friends. Thank you!

To illustrator Alice Rutherford: wow, wow, wow. You are so incredibly talented and creative, and you perfectly captured the crunchy vibe we were looking for in this book. Thank you for making this text come alive with your three-hundred-plus illustrations and for our cover art, too! You were ever the professional, meeting all deadlines with ease and excellence.

To our designer, Karla Baker: Your joyful, upbeat, and creative presence is felt on every page. I know this was a beastly manuscript to wrangle into a design format but you nailed it. Thank you for sharing your gifts!

To Kristy Rybarski, creative director and friend: You played a pivotal role in our final cover and nudging us toward the illustration style that was perfect for this book. Thank you!

To agent Steve Troha: Thank you for starting us off on this journey and getting the project proposal into the right hands at the right time. We are so thankful!

To Vani Hari (a.k.a. Food Babe): You saw the vision before we did! Thank you for your persistence in connecting us with Steve.

To Maggie Greenwood-Robinson: Thank you for helping us put together a stellar book proposal. You hit it out of the park!

To Rachel Menoher: Thank you for testing many of the book's recipes and keeping sanity in our home.

To my friends and colleagues Cathy Grennan (God mama), Carol Godart (brainstorming buddy), Julia Pryce (soul sistah), Ali Niederkorn (inspired fusion), Suzanne Bowen, Katie Wells, Heather and Daniel Dessinger, Katie and Kris Kimball, Emily and Antony Bartlett, Stephanie and Ryan Langford, Seth Spears, Erin and Will Odom, Carrie Vitt, Sara McFall, Becky Webb, Lauren Catanese, and Kate Doubler: Thank you for being my pals and pushing me to be the very best I can be in business and life. God bless you!

To all the midwives, doulas, lactation consultants, and holistically minded ob-gyns in the trenches who empower women and support babies with their fantastic care: So grateful for the work that you do!

To nonprofits that support maternal and neonatal care in the most vulnerable communities around the world: You make such a difference!

To my amazing aunts (blessed Mary Margaret and the five fabulous O'Hanley sisters), my endless cousins, sweet mother-in-law Sandy Sparks, and other wonderful in-laws: How did I get so lucky? Thank you for believing in our crazy dreams and always being there. I love you!

To my oldest friends—Beth, Julie, Susie, Jill, Carrie, Alexis, Kelli, Tiffany, and the Ladies' Night crew: You are my roots and the source of much love and laughter.

To my mom, dad, and brother: Through thick and thin, you love me unconditionally and always have my back. You've taught me how to love, to share, and to be a better human being. I love you!

To my precious children, Griffin and Paloma, who have given me my most cherished role in life. I still can't believe I get the honor of guiding you through life. None of this would have been possible without you, my eternal inspiration. I love you always!

And finally, to my Heavenly Father, Son, and Holy Spirit. Your joyful love and ever-present grace make my life heaven on earth.

about the author

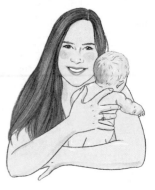

Genevieve Howland is the woman behind the number one blog and YouTube channel for natural pregnancy and childbirth, *Mama Natural*. Her work has been featured on *The Dr. Oz Show, ABC News, The Daily Mail, Newsweek*, and more. This is her first book. The author is donating 10 percent of her net income from this book to charities that support maternal and children's health.

REFERENCES

Find links to all the research, studies, and historical data referred to in this book at
www.mamanatural.com/book/references/

index

Page numbers in *italics* refer to illustrations.

breastfeeding (*cont.*)
   and kangaroo care, 450
   mothers' body preparing
      for, 311
   noting on birth plan, 273, 275
   and nursing bras, 319
   positions for, 456–57
   rooms for, 110
   second-night tips, 454
   stages of breast milk, 452
   toddler and newborn, 456–57
   see also lactation
      consultants
Breastfeeding Inc., 337
Breastfeeding USA, 337
Breast Milkshare, 339
breast pumps, 341
breathing, 351
breech presentations, 320–33,
      326, 331, 367
   natural techniques to flip,
      323–28, 327
   options for, 402–3
   reasons for, 322–23
Brewer, Thomas, 32
Brewer Diet, 32, 215
bris, 448
*British Journal of Obstetrics and
   Gynaecology,* 165
bronchioles, 259
Bumbleride Indie stroller,
      182–83
bumGenius, 187
burp cloths, 188–89
buybuy Baby, 180

Caesar, Julius, 260
caffeine, 33–34
calcium, 18, 20, 171
California, University of:
   at Berkeley, School of Public
      Health of, 14
   at Davis, Davis Medical
      Center of, 334
   at San Francisco, 50

cameras, 387
Canadian Mother and Child, The,
      40
cancer, 335
CAPPA, *see* Childbirth and
      Postpartum Professional
      Association
carbohydrates:
   to avoid, 26
   healthy, 26, *26*
cardio exercise, 45
carpal tunnel syndrome, 105
carriers, 191
car seats, 183–84, 191, 355
Cascade of Intervention, xvii
Case Western Reserve
      University. Frances Payne
      Bolton School of Nursing,
      xxii
castor oil, 418, 419
catecholamine, 377
catheters, xviii
CBC test (complete blood
      count), 148–49
CBI, *see* Childbirth
      International
CCHD, *see* critical congenital
      heart disease
CDC, *see* Centers for Disease
      Control
cell-free DNA screening,
      90–91
cell phones, 96–98, 101
Centers for Disease Control
      (CDC), 12
   on bacterial infection, 78
   on consumption of raw
      milk, 37
   on flu shots for pregnant
      women, 88
   guidelines for GBS, 358–59,
      360, 363
   on Hepatitis B vaccine,
      442–43
   Tdap shot, 125

on women persisting with
      breastfeeding, 335
   on the Zika virus, 174
cephalopelvic disproportion,
      94
certified midwives (CM), 63
certified nurse-midwives
      (CNM), 62, 63, 64
certified professional
      midwives (CPM), 63
cervical exams, 370
Cervidil, 205
Cesarean birth (C-section),
      298–99
   and cord cutting, 434
   delivery, 260
   disadvantages of, xvi, xix
   effect upon breastfeeding
      and kangaroo care, 453–55
   frequency of, xv, 49, 392, 469
   and gestational diabetes,
      149
   mandatory for transverse
      position, 325
   photographing, 308
   recovering from, 465
   standard vs. gentle, 395–97
   for stillbirths, 481
   and weight of baby, 282
cfmidwifery.org, 66
changing tables, 251–52
chargers for electronic
      devices, 387
checkups and screenings:
   declining or delaying,
      273–74
   during first trimester, 80–91
   during second trimester,
      142–51
   during third trimester,
      280–87
   laws regarding, 444
   website for, 447
   see also specific tests
chemical pregnancies, 478

vitamins:
  prenatal, 19–21, 61, 123, 134,
    171, 226
  to treat morning sickness,
    74–75
  see also specific vitamins
VKDB, *see* vitamin K
    deficiency bleeding
volatile organic compounds
  (VOCs), 180, 181, 249, 251

walking, 43–44
Wall Street Journal, 284
washcloths, 190
Washington, University of, 75
Washington Post, 12
water, for soaking grains and
  beans, 29
  see also hydration
water birth, 57–59
watermelon water, 137
waters, breaking of, 373–76
Water Wipes, 188
websites, *see specific websites*
Webster technique, 179,
  323–27
weight gain, 381
West Nile virus, 15

Weston A. Price Foundation,
  28, 339
white-noise machine, 186, 198
WHO, *see* World Health
  Organization
Whole Foods, 77
Wi-Fi, 96, 97–98
Wilkes University, 207
Williams, Robin, 212
Winfrey, Oprah, 127
Winkler, Maura, xxi, xxiii, 35,
  164, 167, 208, 217, 272, 274,
  309, 315, 454, 480
wipes, 188
World Health Organization
  (WHO), 96
  on dangers of VOC
    exposure, 249
  on delaying baby's first
    bath, 269, 442
  on EMF exposure, 95
  flu shot recommendations,
    88
  on ideal Cesarean rate, xv,
    469, 475
  on late cord clamping, 434
  recommendations for
    breastfeeding, 334

on spacing pregnancies,
  312
on x-rays as known
  carcinogen, 94
wraps, 191

x-rays, 94

yawning, 179
Year After Childbirth, The
  (Kitzinger), 177
yeast (food), 35, 206
  see also recipes; weekly
    meal plans
yeast infections:
  differentiating from UTIs,
    208
  natural remedies for, 204
Yelp, 54
yoga, 44
Young v. United Parcel Service,
  106–7
YouTube, xii, 269, 315
  see also videos

Zika virus, 15, 174
zinc, 18
zygote, 5–6, 5, 23